Rare Diseases

Edited by Zhan He Wu

Published in London, United Kingdom

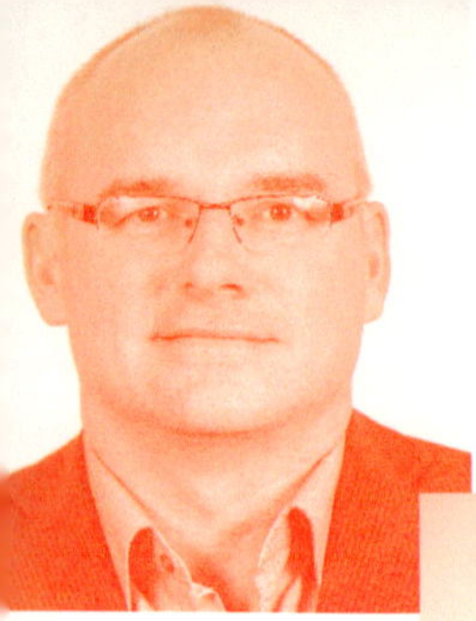
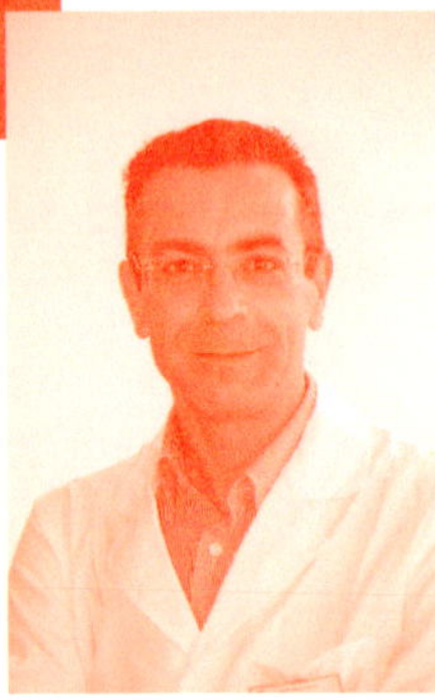
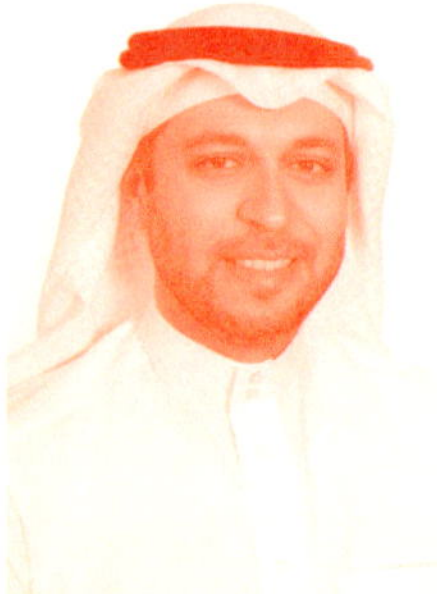
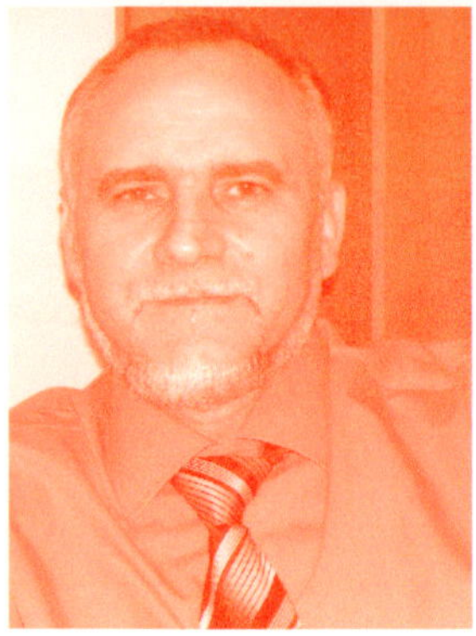
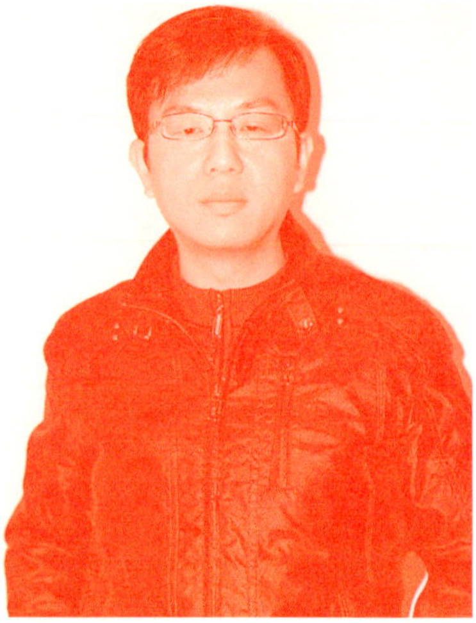
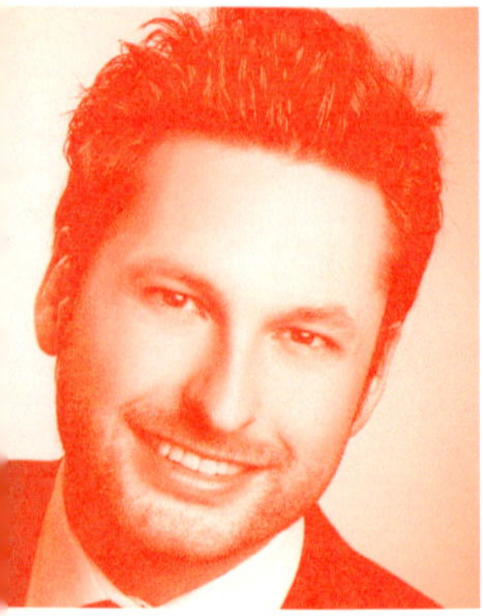
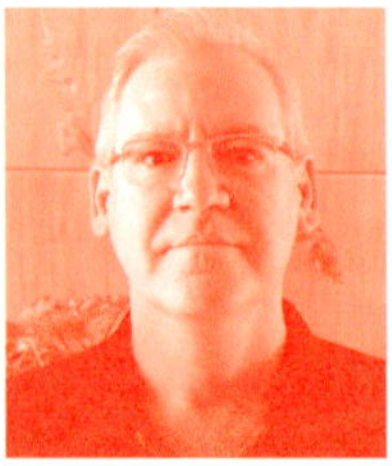

IntechOpen

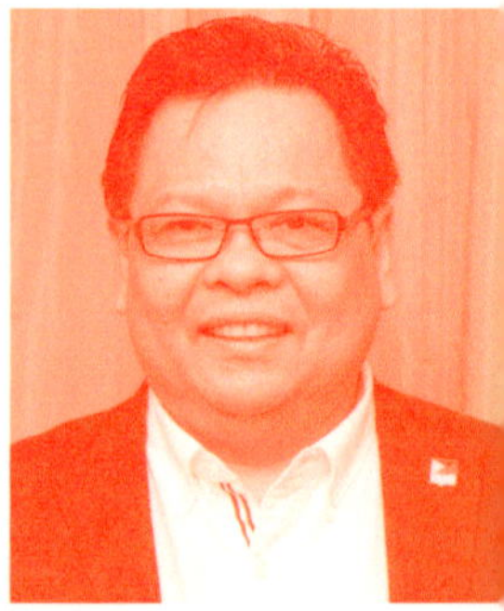
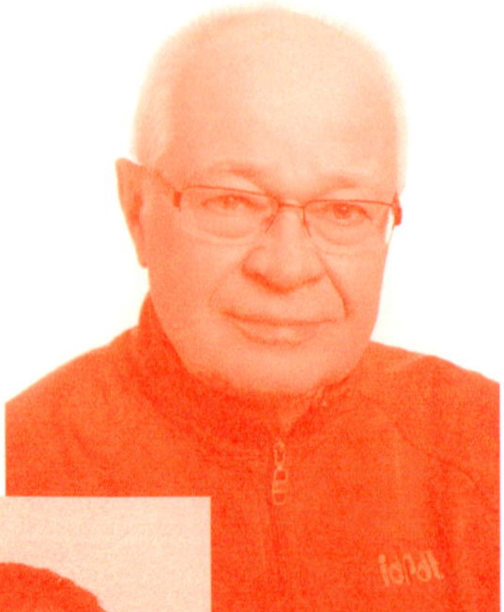
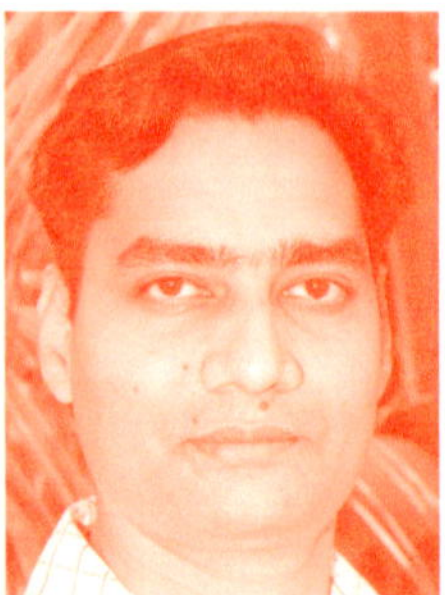
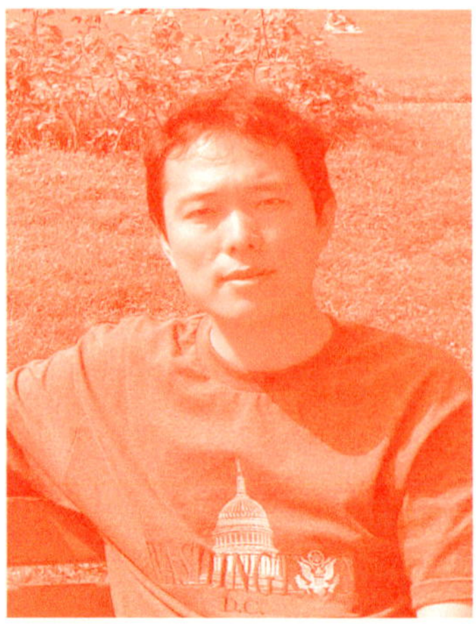
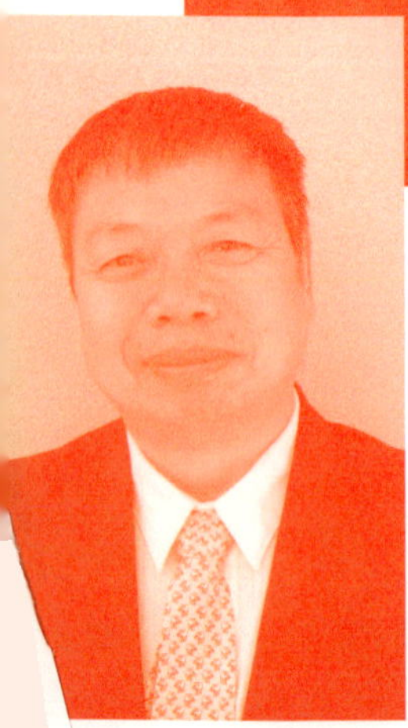
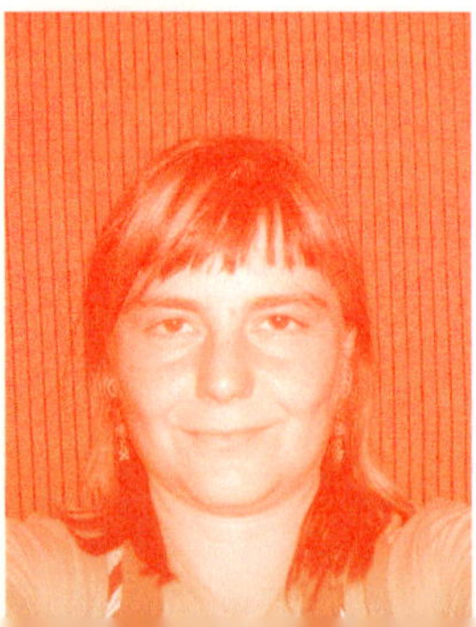

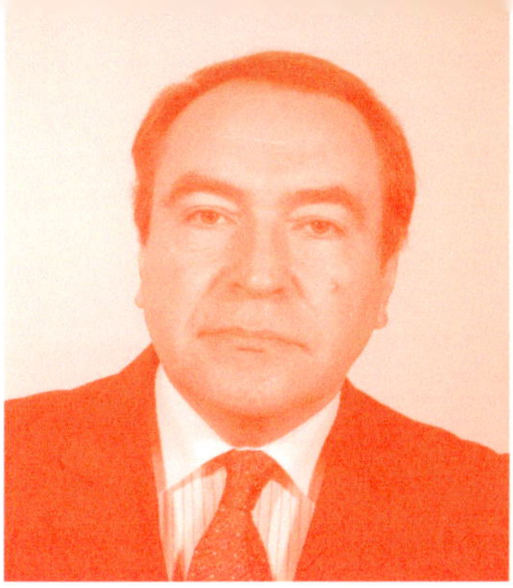
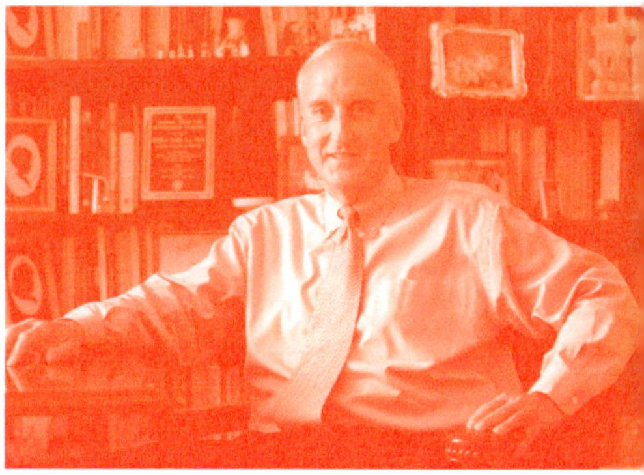
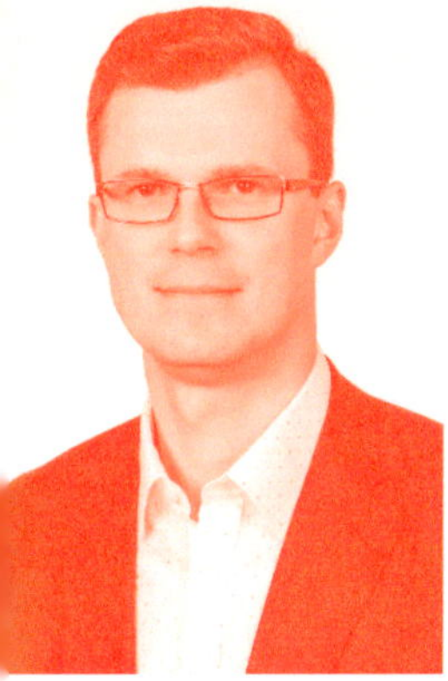
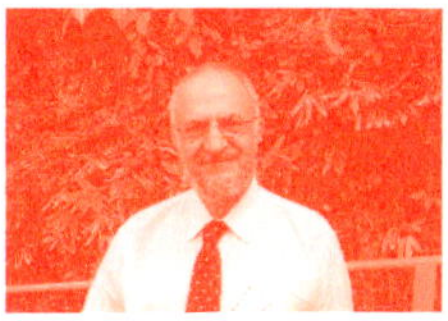
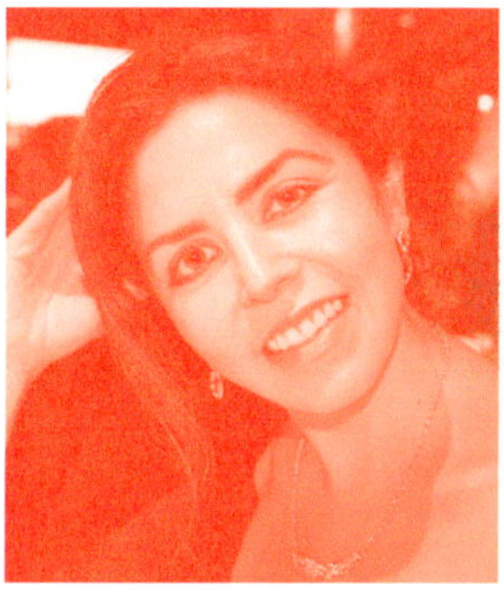

Supporting open minds since 2005

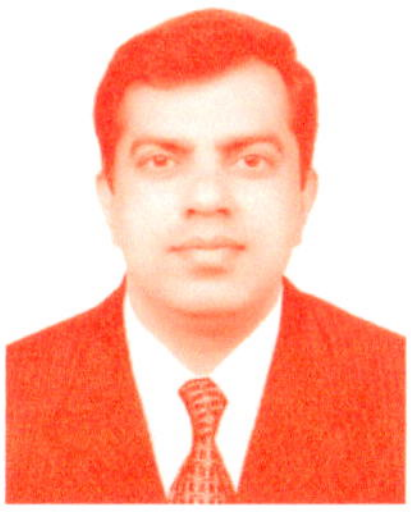
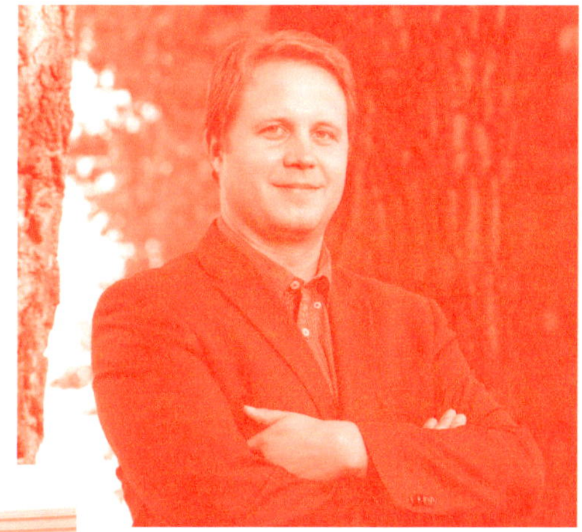
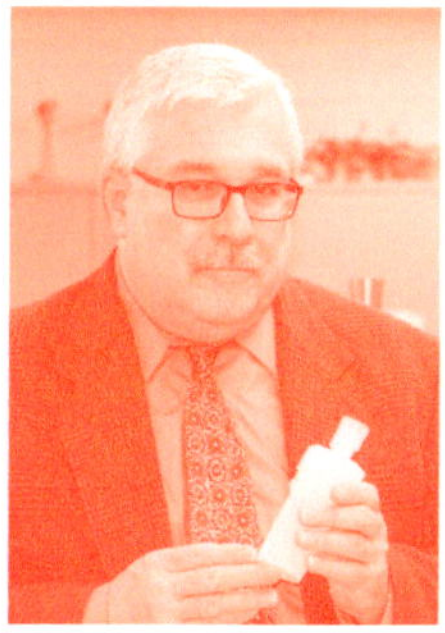
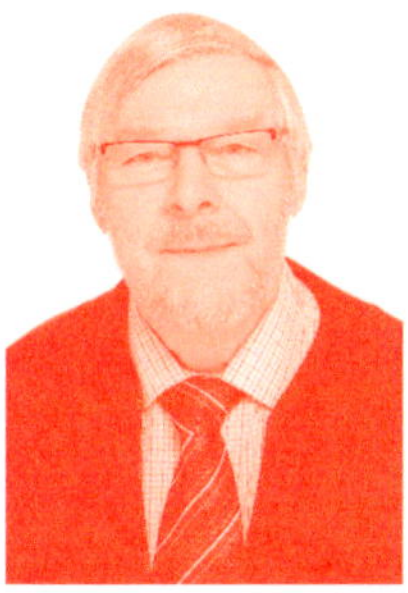
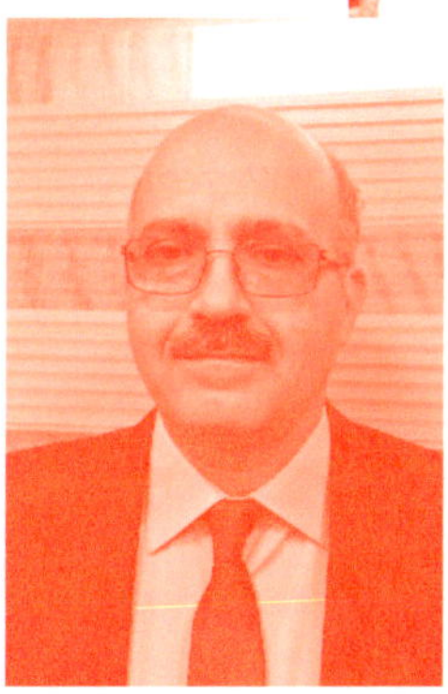
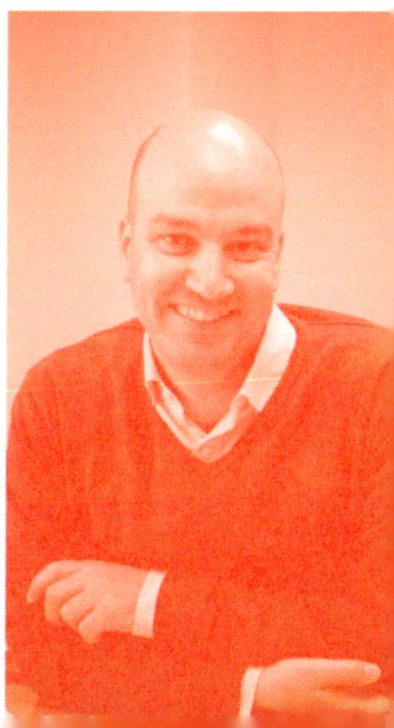
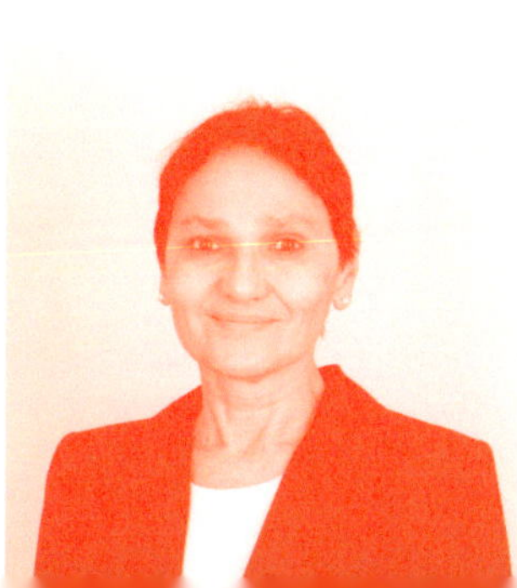

Rare Diseases
http://dx.doi.org/10.5772/intechopen.83131
Edited by Zhan He Wu

Contributors
Eva Hanusovska, Sabina Sufliarska, Hana Cechova, Lucie Pavlatova, Monika Leontovycova, Milena Vrana, Joan-Lluis Vives Corrons, Wenxiu Liu, Xinhua Yin, Zhan He Wu, Bigyan Raj Gyawali, Yanfei Qi, Long Hoa Chung, Carmine Ungaro, Teresa Sprovieri, Letícia Antunes Muniz Ferreira, Qurratulain Hasan, Yashodhara Bhattacharya, Gayatri Iyer, Aruna Priya K, Subhadra Poornima, Keerthi K J, Renfen Chen, Nahla Mousa, Ahmed Osman, Ahmed Abdellatif, Nagia Fahmy, Hassan El Fawal, Suher Kamal Zada, Branislava Medic, Bojan Stopić, Katarina Savic Vujovic, Nevena Divac, Sonja Vuckovic, Radan Stojanovic, Dragana Srebro, Milos Basailovic, Milica Prostran, Adrian Thorogood

First published in London, United Kingdom, 2020 by IntechOpen
IntechOpen is the global imprint of INTECHOPEN LIMITED, registered in England and Wales, registration number: 11086078, 7th floor, 10 Lower Thames Street, London, EC3R 6AF, United Kingdom
Printed in Croatia

British Library Cataloguing-in-Publication Data
A catalogue record for this book is available from the British Library

Additional hard and PDF copies can be obtained from orders@intechopen.com

Rare Diseases
Edited by Zhan He Wu
p. cm.
Print ISBN 978-1-83880-023-9
Online ISBN 978-1-83880-024-6
eBook (PDF) ISBN 978-1-83880-459-6

For EU product safety concerns:
IN TECH d.o.o., Prolaz Marije Krucifikse Kozulić 3, 51000 Rijeka, Croatia, info@intechopen.com or visit our website at intechopen.com.

Meet the editor

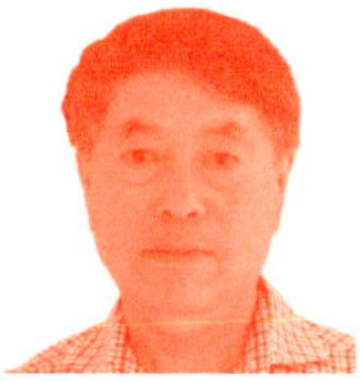

Dr. Zhan He Wu graduated from Harbin Medical University, China, and received his Master's degree in 1985 from the same university. He received his PhD degree in 1993 from the University of New South Wales, Australia. Since 1996, he has been working in the field of human genetics disease studies in the Sydney Genome Diagnostics, Western Sydney Genetics Program, The Children's Westmead, affiliated to the University of Sydney, mainly on hematological malignancies such as leukemia and lymphoma, and inherited bone marrow failure syndromes, including Fanconi anemia (called the prone cancer syndrome and is a paradigm for cancer and aging research). Dr. Zhan He Wu has published more than 60 original articles, more than 60 scientific conference presentations, and five chapters in books. He was granted Founding Fellow of the Royal College of Pathologists for Australasia in 2011. He has been invited to organize a number of national scientific conferences. He has been involved in medical journal reviewing and editing and has been invited by nine international journals as a reviewer, associate editor, guest editor, editor, column chair, and so on. He has also edited two professional medical books in English by IntechOpen: Germline Mutations Associated Leukemia and Rare Diseases.

Contents

Preface

Rare diseases, also referred to as orphan diseases, are diseases affecting a low percentage of the population compared with common diseases. However, more people suffer from rare diseases than cancer and AIDS combined. About 350 million people worldwide are suffering from rare diseases. It is estimated that there are about 7000–8000 different types of rare diseases/disorders. These diseases are rare in some populations but may be common in others, such as Fanconi anemia, which is more prevalent in some regions due to founder mutations in Ashkenazi Jews, the Roma population of Spain, and black South Africans. Evidence and facts from the accumulated data indicate that rare diseases are quite common.

Genetics-causing diseases are classified as chromosomal abnormalities, single gene defects, multifactorial problems, teratogenic problems, and mitochondrial disorders by their etiology.

Most rare diseases are genetics based. Any abnormality of one of the above four categories could result in rare diseases being phenotypic, including some types of malignancies.

Studies of rare diseases offer exciting opportunities and challenges. Knowledge and experience obtained from these studies not only increase our understanding of the correlations between phenotype and genotype, but also have enlightened other areas, particularly in personalized medicine when translating into therapies.

The aim of this book is to increase awareness and exchange experiences and knowledge from experts in field to reduce the challenges and increase an understanding of the nature of rare diseases. As a result, diagnosis/management and care of those suffering from these diseases will hopefully improve.

This book contains 15 chapters covering epidemiology, pathogenesis, clinical characteristics, classification, diagnosis, and disease monitoring using modern technologies, therapies, prevention techniques, data management, and analysis.

To meet the special needs, nine comprehensive literature review chapters were edited focusing on specific types of rare diseases analyzing the past and present and predicting the future of these types of diseases systemically.

We hope this edition will be a helpful and useful book for those studying rare diseases. Most importantly it will benefit patients and improve their quality of life, as well as help families and society reduce social burdens.

Therefore, we would like to express our special thanks to these experienced authors for their valuable contributions to this work.

We would also like to thank the Author Service Manager Ms. Marijana Francetic for her skillful organizational ability and great effort.

Dr. Zhan He Wu, MD, PhD, FFSc (RCPA)
Western Sydney Genome Diagnostics,
Western Sydney Genetics Program,
The Children's Hospital at Westmead,
Affiliated to the University of Sydney,
Sydney, NSW, Australia

Section 1

Introduction

Chapter 1

Introductory Chapter: Advances in the Diagnosis and Management of Rare Diseases

Zhan He Wu

1. Introduction

Rare diseases, also known as orphan diseases, are a group of disorders that affects a small percentage of the population which it commonly presented in early life, but it can also be seen in adulthood with chronic phase. These diseases are frequently progressive, disabling and life threatening. Approximately 30% of children suffering will die at 5 years of age [1–4].

Rare diseases not only have a severe impact on patients and families psychologically and financially but also create a huge burden to communities/societies and counties.

It is estimated that there are approximately 7000–8000 distinct rare diseases in existence. The majority of rare diseases are genetic based on their aetiology and pathology with huge variations of clinical phenotypes [5–8].

According to the estimation from the Global Genes Project, there are approximately 300 million people worldwide who have been affected by rare diseases, some types of rare solid cancers and haematological malignancies (liquid cancers), for example, myelodysplasia syndrome (MDS) and myeloproliferative neoplasms (MPN) including polycythemia vera, essential thrombocythemia, primary myelofibrosis, and chronic myeloid leukaemia [9, 10].

Although there are some definitions relating to rare diseases based on the number of people living with a disease, including several factors such as the existence of adequate treatments or the severity of the disease, unfortunately, there is no single, widely accepted definition for rare diseases [11]. Actually, the most accepted definition is no disease is rare when it affects someone you love.

Nowadays the treatment of infectious and nutritional disorders has been well established. In contrast, paediatric onset genetic disorders and cancer in children constitute a substantial load in paediatric clinics, and rare diseases are the major clinical load.

2. Advances in the diagnosis and management of rare diseases

In the past, diagnosis of rare diseases was very difficult due to the lack of diagnostic technologies. The detection rate for rare diseases was very low before the genomic era. Therefore, delayed or wrong diagnosis was not uncommon which resulted in stress, frustration and worry for patients and families.

Studies showed that only 36% of rare patients/individuals can be diagnosed earlier; about 25% of these got a different diagnosis, 15% sought a second opinion and 5% had unnecessary management and care [3].

In the last two decades, the study on rare diseases is the hallmark of genetic era in medicine from clinical symptomatic to pathological aetiology phase with the development of new technologies. With the advances of genomic technologies, the detection rate on genetic-based rare diseases dramatically increased.

The applications of next-generation sequencing technology have been bringing benefits to patients with rare diseases first. Excitingly, the concept and practice on rare diseases have been changing dramatically in the last decades.

In approximately 50% of the estimated 7000 rare diseases, responsible genes have been identified for the determination of their molecular aetiology, and it is predicted that the remaining 50% genes will be identified by 2020. This will be speeded up by the next-generation sequencing technology [12].

In order to guide the care for rare diseases and accelerate progress of rare disease research through international cooperation and collaboration, the International Rare Diseases Research Consortium (IRDiRC) was formed in 2011, and policies and guidelines were documented in 2013 [13].

Much effort has been made in the last 10 years to increase knowledge of the epidemiology of rare diseases, including recognition of the specificity of rare diseases; develop information for patients; increase the health professionals and the general public concerning their diseases; train health professionals to better identify rare diseases; organise screening and access diagnostic tests; improve access to treatment and the quality of patient care; continue efforts in favour of orphan drugs; respond to the specific accompanying needs of people suffering from rare diseases; promote research on rare diseases; and develop national and international partnerships [14, 15].

National Coordinated and Collaborative Approach, Data Collection and Use, Coordinated Care, Equitable Access to Services, Equitable Access to Diagnostics and Treatments, Nationally Coordinated Research both in malignant and non-malignant phenotypes have been established [16, 17].

Huge steps have been made for the caring and therapies of rare diseases internationally. The last day of February each year is recognised as the Rare Disease Day. In 2015 and 2016, the Food and Drug Administration (FDA) approved 47% of the novel drugs for the therapies of rare diseases. It is aimed to develop 200 new therapies for rare diseases in 2020 [15].

3. Advances in rare disease research

In the past, rare diseases were under-researched in many aspects and were also impeded due to the lack of population-based epidemiology, aetiology study of disease-related mechanisms, clinical treatment trials, diagnostic tools, research on health service and familial/communities and social researches.

In the recent years, the studies on the disease cause of genetic and environment and their interactions on rare diseases have become the key area in medical research. It is believed such studies hold the key for conquering human diseases. Studies on rare disease became the main stream from the branch stream in the paediatric research field.

High-throughput sequencing approaches (whole genome sequencing and whole exome sequencing) have revolutionised research and translated into accurate and specific diagnosis and effective treatment.

The discoveries on disease-causing genes, identification of inherited mutations and detection of genetic variations provided huge benefits to patients and families with rare diseases.

Knowledge and experience obtained from the studies on rare diseases not only increased our understanding of the correlations between phenotype and genotype, but also such studies have been enlightening the other medical areas, particularly in personalized medicine. Such research findings have been translating into the development in therapies.

Studies on rare diseases provided exciting opportunities in the identification of human disease-causing genes, understanding of common disease and the translation of genetic findings into clinical bedside.

Fanconi anaemia (FA) is the most classical, representative rare disease and the best example with the most successful achievements. FA is an inherited rare disease which is characterised with developmental abnormalities, progressive bone marrow failure and cancer predisposition commonly in acute myeloid leukaemia [18, 19] and first reported and named as a disease which was in 1927 by the Swiss paediatrician—Guido Fanconi [20].

FA has several synonyms such as Fanconi pancytopenia, inherited aplastic anaemia, inherited pancytopenia, constitutional aplastic anaemia, inherited bone marrow failure syndrome, premalignant disorder, chromosome breakup syndrome and DNA repair disorder [21]. The incidence is 1 in 160,000 in the general population, but it is 1 in 20,000 in some ethnic groups [22].

So far, 23 responsible genes were identified [23], and interestingly, several of them are genes also found to be associated with other types of cancers, including breast cancer genes BRCA 1 and BRCA2 [24–26].

It was the first successful example in cord blood stem cell transplantation in 1988 [27]. So the study on Fanconi anaemia is named as a paradigm for the understanding of cancer and aging [28].

4. Conclusion

The achievements in the last two decades in the diagnosis, management and research on rare diseases have been unprecedented. The advancing studies of rare diseases toward genetic causes and effective therapies have been progressing rapidly.

Policies and guidelines concerning rare diseases have been issued in different regions and countries. Life quality of patients with rare diseases has been improving with such advances internationally.

Increases in research funding support have been providing more and more coordination in different disciplines/areas of management to provide the forming of best practice.

Awareness of rare disease has been raising quality of life, and the ensuing impact on patients has been improving, although we are still facing challenges in medical and nonmedical issues.

Challenges from medical and nonmedical issues have been reducing with more knowledge and awareness of rare diseases in the community/society in the healthcare strategies and established in vitro diagnostic and bioinformatics systems.

Further and deep studies on rare diseases across different levels and aspects, including the cell types, tissues and organs, are associated with rare diseases and the interactions between different cell types to explore mysteries.

Rare disease is named historically with the limitation of technologies in the symptomatic era under the condition from clinical data to distinguish from the common diseases, such as nutritional and infectious diseases which were relatively and predominantly higher.

However, it is believed that more rare diseases will be identified and reclassified in the future in the genomic era since we know that "rare disease" is probably not a proper terminology to be used currently to classify such a disease genetic base affecting such a large population worldwide.

Author details

Zhan He Wu
Western Sydney Genome Diagnostics, Western Sydney Genetics Program, The Children's Hospital at Westmead, Sydney, NSW, Australia

*Address all correspondence to: zhan.wu@health.nsw.gov.au

References

[1] Carter CO. Monogenic disorders. Journal of Medical Genetics. 1977;**14**:316-320

[2] Baird PA, Anderson TW, Newcombe HB, et al. Genetic disorders in children and young adults: A population study. American Journal of Human Genetics. 1988;**42**:677-693

[3] Jaffe A, Zurynski Y, Beville L, et al. Call for a national plan for rare diseases. Journal of Paediatrics and Child Health. 2010;**46**(1-2):2-4

[4] Anderson M, Elizabeth J, Elliott EJ, et al. Australian families living with rare disease: Experiences of diagnosis, health services use and needs for psychosocial support. Orphanet Journal of Rare Diseases. 2013;**8**:22, 1-9

[5] Zurynski Y, Firth K, Leonard H, et al. Rare childhood diseases: How should we respond? Archives of Disease in Childhood. 2008;**93**:1071-1074

[6] Samuels ME. Saturation of the human phenome. Current Genomics. 2010;**11**:482-499

[7] Knight AW, Senior TP. The common problem of rare disease in general practice. The Medical Journal of Australia. 2006;**185**:82-83

[8] Rath A, Valérie Salamon V, Peixoto S, et al. A systematic literature review of evidence-based clinical practice for rare diseases: What are the perceived and real barriers for improving the evidence and how can they be overcome? Trials. 2017;**18**:556, 1-11

[9] Swerdlow SH, Campo E, Harris NL, et al. World Health Organisation (WHO) Classification of Tumours of Haematopoietic and Lymphoid Tissues. Lyon, France: IARC; 2008. pp. 75-104

[10] Arber DA, Orazi A, Hasserjian R, et al. The 2016 revision to the World Health Organization classification of myeloid neoplasms and acute leukemia. Blood. 2016;**127**(20):2391-2405

[11] Richter T, Nestler-Parr S, Babela R, et al. Rare disease terminology and definitions—A systematic global review: Report of the ISPOR rare disease special interest group. Value in Health. 2015;**18**(6):906-914

[12] Boycott KM, Vanstone MR, Bulman DE, et al. Rare-disease genetics in the era of next-generation sequencing: Discovery to translation. Nature Reviews Genetics. 2013;**14**:618-691

[13] Hennekam RC. Care for patients with ultra-rare disorders. European Journal of Medical Genetics. 2011;**54**(3):220-224

[14] Groft SC. Rare diseases research: Expanding collaborative translational research opportunities. Chest. 2013;**144**:16-23

[15] Abbott A. Rare-disease project has global ambitions. Nature. 2011;**472**:17

[16] Lochmller H, Farnell TJ, Cam YL, et al. The International Rare Diseases Research Consortium: Policies and guidelines to maximize impact. European Journal of Human Genetics. 2017;**25**:1293-1302

[17] Dharssi S, Wong-Rieger D, Harold M, et al. Review of 11 national policies for rare disease. Orphanet Journal of Rare Diseases. 2017;**12**:63, 1-13

[18] Alter BP. Cancer in Fanconi anemia, 1927-2001. Cancer. 2003;**97**:425-440

[19] Tischkowitz MD, Hodgson SV. Fanconi anaemia. Journal of Medical Genetics. 2003;**40**:1-10

[20] Fanconi G. Familiäre infantile perniziosaartige Anämie (pernizioses Blutbild und Konstitution). Jahrbuch fur Kinderheilkunde. 1927;**117**:257-280

[21] Wu Z-H. The concept and practice of Fanconi anemia: From the clinical bedside to the laboratory bench. Translational Pediatrics. 2013;**2**(3):112-119

[22] Tipping AJ, Pearson T, Morgan NV, et al. Molecular and genealogical evidence for a founder effect in Fanconi anemia families of the Afrikaner population of South Africa. Proceedings of the National Academy of Sciences of the United States of America. 2001;**98**:5734-5739

[23] Fanconi Anemia Mutation Database. Available online: www.rockefeller.edu/fanconi

[24] Wu ZH. Inherited bone marrow failure and chromosome instability syndromes and their cancer predisposition. In: Zakaria M, Hassan T, editors. Contemporary Pediatric Hematology and Oncology. IntechOpen; 2019. pp. 25-44

[25] D'Andrea AD. BRCA1: A missing link in the Fanconi anemia/BRCA pathway. Cancer Discovery. 2013;**3**(4):376-378

[26] Meyer S, Marc Tischkowitz M, Kate Chandler K, et al. Fanconi anaemia, BRCA2 mutations and childhood cancer: A developmental perspective from clinical and epidemiological observations with implications for genetic counselling. Journal of Medical Genetics. 2014;**51**:71-75

[27] Gluckman E, Broxmeyer HA, Auerbach AD, et al. Hematopoietic reconstitution in a patient with Fanconi's anemia by means of umbilical-cord blood from an HLA identical sibling. NEJM. 1989;**321**:1174-1178

[28] Schindler D, Hoehn H. Fanconi Anemia. A Paradigmatic Disease for the Understanding of Cancer and Aging. Switzerland: Karger; 2007

Section 2

Clasical Genetic Based Rare Diseases

Chapter 2

Duchenne Muscular Dystrophy (DMD) Diagnosis: Past and Present Perspectives

Nahla O. Mousa, Ahmed Osman, Nagia Fahmy, Ahmed Abdellatif, Suher Zada and Hassan El-Fawal

Abstract

Duchenne muscular dystrophy (DMD) is a fatal X-linked disorder, characterized by progressive skeletal muscle wasting. The disease is caused by various types of mutations in the dystrophin gene (DMD). The disease occurs at a frequency of about 1 in 5000 male births, making it the most common severe neuro-muscular disease. In addition to clinical examinations of muscle strength and function, diagnosis of DMD usually involves a combination of immunological assays using muscle biopsies, typically immunohistochemistry and western blotting, and molecular techniques such as DMD gene sequencing or Multiplex Ligation Dependent Probe Amplification (MLPA) using blood samples. In fact, precise molecular diagnosis is a prerequisite for determining the appropriate personalized therapeutic approach such as exon-skipping, gene therapy or stem cell-based therapies in conjunction with gene editing techniques like CRISPR-Cas9. However, the quest for reliable biomarkers with high sensitivity and specificity for DMD from liquid biopsy is still a hotspot of research, as such non-invasive biomarker(s) would not only facilitate disease diagnosis but would also help in carrier detection, which will eventually result in better disease management. In this chapter, we will illustrate the detailed current and prospect strategies for disease.

Keywords: DMD, diagnosis, biomarkers

1. Introduction

Dystrophin protein is present in myocytes in skeletal, cardiac, and smooth muscles, acting to connect the actin microfilaments, via N-terminus of the protein, to the extracellular matrix by binding membrane—bound (sarcolemma) glycoprotein complex (dystrophin associated glycoprotein complex; DGC) to the C-terminal end of the protein, and thus, plays an important role in normal muscle function [1]. Inactivating mutations occurring in DMD gene causes immature termination of protein translation, giving rise to C-terminally truncated protein product that fails to transmit muscle impulses, which causes increasing intracellular Ca^{2+} influx and thus, activating apoptotic machineries and eventually causes cell death and muscle atrophy/necrosis [2]. Death usually occurs in the third decade of life as a result of respiratory or heart failure [3].

IntechOpen

2. Methods for DMD diagnosis

2.1 Clinical picture

Affected DMD boys are usually normal at birth but in early childhood they suffer from inability to get up from floor or climb stairs or run and they fell very often. Also, enlarged calf muscles (pseudo hypertrophy) are always noticed [4]. From the age of 7–12, the cases become more deteriorated, and the patients start to suffer from scoliosis [5], and joint contracture [6]. Also, patients will have an apparent reduction in bone-mineral density and will have hypocalciuria and osteoporosis [7].

Because the disease affects proximal as well as distal muscles, thus, in early teenage, DMD boys usually get respiratory infections and sleep apnea [8], and later, the patient will develop cardiomyopathy and eventually heart failure [9].

2.2 Circulating blood biomarkers

2.2.1 CK levels and other proteins/enzymes

One of the dystrophin protein main functions is to stabilize the muscle tissue, since it exists and binds to sarcolemma. The absence of dystrophin will eventually lead to the increased permeability of the muscular tissue and consequently the release of the muscle proteins [10], of which the creatine kinase (CK) enzyme that is responsible for the production of phosphocreatine and ADP from creatine and ATP as part of energy homeostasis. In normal condition, normal myocytes turnover, serum levels of CK ranges from 20 to 200 U/L, however, it can be slightly increased in some neurological disorders. On the other hand, in case of DMD boys, due to the accelerated muscular destruction, it may reach higher levels reaching several thousands of units/L, and in severe muscle damage it can reach 200,000 U/L [11–13]. However, CK levels sometimes can be misleading because in advanced stages of DMD, CK levels may come within normal range due to progressive muscular atrophy [14].

CK is considered one of the most used serum biomarkers in DMD diagnosis, however, many studies were performed to detect alterations in other muscle related proteins using immunoassay and MS-based detection to screen for other potential diagnostic biomarkers (**Table 1**).

2.2.2 MicroRNA

MicroRNAs (miRNAs) are a tissue—specific class of small, non-coding RNA molecules that function as gene regulators/silencers and consequently they are considered sensitive indicators for different cellular contexts. MiRNAs act through binding to a specific region in the 3′-UTR in the target mRNA molecules, thus, inducing mRNA degradation and inhibiting the translation process [42]. The circulating levels of miRNAs in serum reflect the intracellular status and hence, they are excellent biomarkers for many pathological conditions as they can be detected from liquid biopsies and/or tissue specimens [43]. Many studies attempted to study the modulation in the levels of different miRNAs (**Table 2**).

2.2.3 Lipids, metabolites, amino acid, and organic acid

In addition to the previously mentioned biomarkers, lipid profile and metabolites in the blood or urine are also very important parameters that reflect the status

Tested marker	Levels (high or low) in DMD patients and/or other MDs	Location (serum/muscle)	Detection method	Ref.
Alkaline phosphatase (AP)-A	Elevated in Grade 1 and Grade 2 patients	Serum	Measuring enzyme activities	[15]
AP-B	No change			
Gly-AP	Elevated in Grade 1 and Grade 2			
Ala-AP	Elevated in Grade 1			
Ser-AP	Elevated in Grade 1,2,3			
Leu-AP	Elevated in Grade 1			
Met-AP	No Change			
Phe-AP	Elevated in Grade 1,2,3			
Trp-AP	Elevated h in Grade 1,2,3			
Gly-pro-AP	Elevated in Grade1 Reduced in Grade 3			
Gly-Pro-Leu-AP	Reduced in Grade1 and Grade 2			
Trypsin	Reduced in Grade 1			
Cathepsin C	Reduced in Grade 1 and Grade 2			
Sulphatase	No change			
Phosphatase	No change			
Acetyl-choline esterase	Reduced in Grade 2			
Esterase	Elevated in Grade 1,2,3			
RNase	Reduced in Grade 1 and Grade 2			
Angiotensin Converting enzyme	Reduced in Grade 3			
Myostatin (Growth and differentiation factor 8; GDF8)	Elevated in DMD patients	Serum	ELISA	[16]
Interleukin 17	Elevated in Emery-Dreifuss MD and Limb-Girdle MD 1B	Serum	ELISA	[17, 18]
TGF-β2	Elevated in Emery-Dreifuss MD and Limb-Girdle MD 1B			
IL6	Variable			
Skeletal troponin I (sTnI),	Elevated in DMD, BMD, LGMD2B	Serum	ELISA	
Myosin light chain 3 (Myl3),	Elevated in DMD, BMD, LGMD2B			
Fatty acid binding protein 3 (FABP3)	Elevated in DMD, BMD, LGMD2B			
Muscle-type creatine kinase (CKM)	Elevated in DMD, BMD, LGMD2B			

Tested marker	Levels (high or low) in DMD patients and/or other MDs	Location (serum/muscle)	Detection method	Ref.
N-terminal α Dystroglycan (αDG-N)	Reduced in DMD patients	Serum	ELISA	[19]
Fibronectin	Elevated in DMD Normal in BMD	Serum	ELISA	[20]
Basic fibroblast growth factor	Elevated in DMD patients	Serum	ELISA	[21]
cardiac myosin light chain I	Elevated in DMD patients (correlated with CK levels)	Serum	Immunoradiometric assay	[22]
Troponin I, fast skeletal muscle	Elevated in DMD	Serum	SOMAscan assay "Aptamer-based proteomic technology"	[23]
Carbonic anhydrase 3	Elevated in DMD			
Fatty acid-binding protein, heart	Elevated in DMD			
Troponin I, cardiac muscle	Elevated in DMD			
Creatine kinase M-type	Elevated in DMD			
Mitogen-activated protein kinase 12	Elevated in DMD			
Alanine aminotransferase 1	Elevated in DMD			
Myoglobin	Elevated in DMD			
Fibrinogen	Elevated in DMD			
Phospholipase A2, membrane associated	Elevated in DMD			
Acidic leucine-rich nuclear phosphoprotein 32 family member B	Elevated in DMD			
Hepatoma-derived growth factor-related protein 2	Elevated in DMD			
40S Glucose-6-phosphate isomerase ribosomal protein S7	Elevated in DMD			
Heparin cofactor 2	Elevated in DMD			
Persephin	Elevated in DMD			
Calcium/calmodulin-dependent protein kinase II α	Elevated in DMD			
Malate dehydrogenase, cytoplasmic	Elevated in DMD			
l-lactate dehydrogenase B chain	Elevated in DMD			
Aminoacylase-1	Elevated in DMD			
Proteosome subunit α type-2	Elevated in DMD			

Tested marker	Levels (high or low) in DMD patients and/or other MDs	Location (serum/muscle)	Detection method	Ref.
C-X-C motif chemokine 10	Elevated in DMD			
cAMP-dependent protein kinase catalytic subunit α	Elevated in DMD			
Heat-shock 70 kDa protein 1A/1B	Elevated in DMD			
Proto-oncogene tyrosine-protein kinase receptor Ret	Reduced in DMD			
Growth/differentiation factor 11	Reduced in DMD			
Complement decay-accelerating factor	Reduced in DMD			
Cadherin-5	Reduced in DMD			
Tumor necrosis factor receptor superfamily member 19 L	Reduced in DMD			
Gelsolin	Reduced in DMD			
Wnt inhibitory factor 1	Reduced in DMD			
Contactin-5	Reduced in DMD			
Prolyl endopeptidase FAP	Reduced in DMD			
Jagged-1	Reduced in DMD			
Netrin receptor UNC5C	Reduced in DMD			
Kunitz-type protease inhibitor 1	Reduced in DMD			
Protein SET	Reduced in DMD			
Disintegrin metalloproteinase domain-containing protein 9	Reduced in DMD			
Cell adhesion molecule L1-like	Reduced in DMD			
Osteomodulin	Reduced in DMD			
WAP, Kazal, Ig, Kunitz and NTR domain-containing protein 1	Reduced in DMD			
Bone sialoprotein 2	Reduced in DMD			
Interleukin-34	Reduced in DMD			
Neurogenic locus notch homolog protein 3	Reduced in DMD			
Cytoplasmic aspartate aminotransferase	Elevated in DMD	Serum	Measuring enzyme activity	[24]
mitochondrial aspartate aminotransferase	Elevated in DMD			

Tested marker	Levels (high or low) in DMD patients and/or other MDs	Location (serum/muscle)	Detection method	Ref.
Alanine transaminase (ALT)	Elevated in DMD	Serum	ELISA	[25]
Aspartate transaminase (AST)	Elevated in DMD			
Muscle-specific enolase (MSE, beta beta and alpha beta enolases)	Elevated in DMD and another progressive muscular dystrophies	Serum	Enzyme immunoassay	[26]
Serum carbonic anhydrase III (CA-III)	Elevated in DMD, limb-girdle dystrophy, facioscapulohumeral dystrophy and congenital dystrophy	Serum	Enzyme immunoassay	[27]
Creatine kinase (CK) isoenzymes (MM, MB, and BB)	Elevated in DMD	Serum	Sensitive enzyme immunoassay	[28]
Matrix metalloproteinase-9 (MMP-9)	Elevated in DMD	Serum	ELISA	[29]
Tissue inhibitors of metalloproteinase-1 (TIMP-1)	Elevated in DMD			
Osteopontin (OPN)	Normal			
MT-1-MMP	Elevated in autosomal dominant EDMD	Serum	ELISA and zymography	[30]
MMP2	Elevated in autosomal dominant EDMD and in X-linked EDMD			
MMP9	Non-significant elevation			
TIMP-1	Normal in AD-EDMD Elevated in X-linked EDMD	Serum	ELISA sandwich immunoassay	[31]
TIMP-2	Non-significant decrease AD-EDMD/X-EDMD cases			
TIMP-3	Reduced in AD-EDMD/X-EDMD			
Carbonic anhydrase III (CA-III, EC 4.2.1.1)	Elevated in DMD, congenital (Fukuyama-type), limb-girdle, also elevated in: polymyositis myotonic dystrophy amyotrophic lateral sclerosis spinal progressive muscular atrophy or Kugelberg-Welander disease and in carriers of DMD	Serum	Radioimmunoassay	[32]
Vitamin D binding protein (GC)	Reduced in DMD	Serum	2D-HPLC off-line coupled to LC-MALDI-TOF-MS verified with ELISA	[33]
Fibulin-1 (FBLN1)	Elevated in DMD			

Tested marker	Levels (high or low) in DMD patients and/or other MDs	Location (serum/muscle)	Detection method	Ref.
Gelsolin (GSN)	Reduced in DMD			
Carbonic anhydrase 1 (CA1)	Elevated in DMD			
Apolipoprotein B100	Reduced in DMD			
ALT, AST, LDH, and ALP	Elevated in DMD	Serum	Enzymatic assay	[34]
ALT, AST, and LDH	Elevated in BMD and LGMD			
FSHD and EDMD	lack of abnormal serum enzyme levels			
ALP	Highly elevated in LGMD2B Elevated in non-LGMD2B			
Vascular endothelial growth factor	Highly elevated in BMD Elevated in Bedridden DMD, spinal muscular atrophy, myotonic dystrophy	Serum	ELISA	[35]
Creatine kinase MB fraction	Elevated in DMD	Serum	Multiplex, microsphere-based immune-fluorescent assay	[36]
Tissue-type plasminogen activator PLAT	Slightly elevated in DMD			
Myoglobin	Slightly elevated in DMD			
Epidermal growth factor	Slightly elevated in DMD			
Chemokine (C-C motif) ligand 2	Slightly elevated in DMD			
CD 40 ligand	Slightly elevated in DMD			
Vitronectin	Slightly elevated in DMD			
Carboxyterminal propeptide of type I procollagen	No significant alteration	Serum	Radioimmunoassay	[37]
Aminoterminal propeptide of type III procollagen	No significant alteration			
Laminin P1	No significant alteration			
Creatine kinase	Elevated in DMD and BMD	Serum	Measuring enzyme activity	[38]
Pyruvate kinase	Elevated in DMD and BMD			
Myosin light chain—3	Elevated in DMD	Serum	affinity proteomics-based screening approach using an antibody suspension bead array	[39]
Carbonic anhydrase III	Elevated in DMD			
Electron transfer flavoprotein A	Elevated in DMD			

Tested marker	Levels (high or low) in DMD patients and/or other MDs	Location (serum/muscle)	Detection method	Ref.
Mitochondrial malate dehydrogenase 2	Elevated in DMD			
Electron transfer flavoprotein B	Reduced in DMD			
Fast skeletal muscle troponin T	Elevated in DMD			
Matrix metalloproteinase 9	Elevated in DMD	Serum	Immunoassay	[40]
Matrix metalloproteinase 2	Reduced in BMD			
Myostatin (GDF-8)	Reduced in DMD			
Follistatin (FSTN)	Elevated in DMD and BMD			
N-terminal fragment of titin	Elevated in DMD patients	Urine	ELISA	[41]

Table 1.
List of potential protein biomarkers that could be utilized in the diagnosis of Duchenne muscular dystrophy.

of the muscles and thus, they could be measured to indicate the extent of muscular dystrophy and can serve as good candidates for diagnostic purposes (**Table 3**).

2.3 Muscle imaging

Magnetic resonance imaging (MRI) is now used to visualize the composition of skeletal muscles and detect structural abnormalities in the of DMD patients [61]. The produced images can reveal the presence of fat infiltration of muscle tissue, a characteristic consequence of DMD, and thus, can be used for monitoring disease progression and response to treatment [62].

2.4 Genetic diagnosis

2.4.1 RFLP

Detecting the mutation, especially non-sense point mutations, in the 2.4 Mb gene represents a challenging task. In this context, restriction fragment length polymorphism (RFLP) analysis could be used by digesting the genomic DNA using specific restriction endonucleases followed by Southern blotting using DMD-specific DNA probes (genomic or cDNA probes). At 1985, Bamkan et al. developed 11 RELP markers that are present in the X chromosome and can be used for diagnosis. However, RFLP can detect only small percentage of the mutation and hence it cannot be used as gold standard technique in the diagnosis process [63–65].

2.4.2 Multiplex PCR

Multiplex PCR is one of the modified PCR protocols that allows the co-amplification of multiple products using different primer pairs that specially bind complementary regions in the target segment. This method showed a great potential

microRNA	Status	Disease	Location	Ref.
miR-133a	Upregulated	DMD, BMD, LGMD, FSHD	Serum and skeletal muscles	[44–47]
miR-206	Upregulated	DMD, BMD, LGMD, FSHD	Serum and skeletal muscles	
miR-1	Upregulated	DMD, BMD, LGMD, FSHD	Serum and skeletal muscles	
miR-499	Upregulated	DMD	Serum	[45]
miR-208a	Upregulated	DMD	Serum	
miR-208b	Upregulated	DMD	Serum	
miR-95	Upregulated	DMD	Serum	[48]
miR-539	Downregulated	DMD	Serum	
miR-30c	Upregulated	DMD	Serum	[49]
miR-181a	Upregulated	DMD	Serum	
miR-21	Downregulated	DMD	Urine	[50]
miR-29	Downregulated	DMD	Urine	
miR-23	Downregulated	DMD	Urine	
miR-181a	Upregulated	DMD	Serum	[51]
miR-4538	Upregulated	DMD	Serum	
miR-4539	Upregulated	DMD	Serum	
miR-606	Upregulated	DMD	Serum	
miR-454	Downregulated	DMD	Serum	
miR-483	Upregulated	DMD	Serum	[52]
hsa_miR_146b, hsa_miR_368, hsa_miR_381, hsa_miR_487b, hsa_miR_495, hsa_miR_376a, hsa_miR_299_5p, hsa_miR_155, hsa_miR_382, hsa_miR_199a, hsa_miR_379, hsa_miR_335, ambi_miR_5021, hsa_miR_432, hsa_miR_199b, hsa_miR_369_5p, hsa_miR_21, hsa_miR_34a, hsa_miR_199a*, hsa_miR_154, hsa_miR_221, hsa_miR_214, hsa_miR_518a_2*, hsa_miR_409_3p, hsa_miR_452, ambi_miR_2537, hsa_miR_127, hsa_miR_493_3p, hsa_miR_130a, ambi_miR_4983, ambi_miR_13145, hsa_miR_148a, hsa_miR_210, hsa_miR_485_5p, hsa_miR_299_3p, hsa_miR_134, hsa_miR_222, hsa_miR_181d, ambi_miR_13258	Upregulated	DMD	Serum	[53]
hsa_miR_423, hsa_miR_361, hsa_miR_197, hsa_miR_92, hsa_miR_26a, ambi_miR_7075, hsa_miR_30b, hsa_miR_30e_5p, hsa_miR_29a, ambi_miR_13156, hsa_miR_30a_5p, hsa_miR_193b, hsa_miR_331, hsa_miR_486, hsa_miR_30d, hsa_miR_29b, hsa_miR_101, hsa_miR_30c, hsa_miR_22	Downregulated			

Table 2.
List of different microRNAs that could be used as potential biomarkers in the diagnosis of DMD.

Tested marker	Levels (high or low)	Location (serum/ muscle)	Ref.
24,25(OH)2D3	Reduced in DMD	Serum	[54]
1,25(OH)2D3	No change		
25(OH)D3	No change		
Creatinine	Reduced in DMD, BMD, LGMD2A and LGMD2B	Serum	[55]
Imidazole acetic acid	Reduced in DMD and LGMD2B		
5α Dihydrotestosterone glucuronide // androsterone glucuronide // Etiocholan-3alpha-ol-17-one 3-glucuronide	Reduced in DMD		
DL-p-Hydroxyphenyllactic acid // Isohomovanillic acid	Reduced in DMD		
Creatine	Elevated in DMD, DM1, LGMD2Aand LGMD2B		
Guanidinoacetic acid	Reduced in DMD, BMD, DM1 and LGMD2A		
p-Coumaric acid	Reduced in DMD		
Citrulline	Reduced in DMD		
5-Methoxyindoleacetate // Indoleacetic acid	Reduced in DMD		
L-Aspartic acid	Reduced in DMD		
Ornithine	Reduced in DMD		
2-Hydroxycaproic acid	Reduced in DMD		
L-Serine	Reduced in DMD		
Dehydroisoandrosterone 3-sulfate	Reduced in DMD		
Erythrose	Reduced in DMD, BMD, FSHD		
Glutamine	Reduced in DMD, BMD, LGMD-2B, FSHD and elevated in DM-1	Serum	[56]
Acetate	Elevated in DMD, BMD, FSHD, LGMD-2B and DM-1		
Tyrosine	Elevated in BMD		
Lysine	Reduced in FSHD, LGMD-2B and DM-1		
Citrate	Reduced in FSHD Elevated in LGMD-2B		
Lactate	Reduced in LGMD-2B		
Histidine	Reduced in FSHD		
Serum creatinine	Elevated in BMD Decreased in DMD	Serum	[57]
3-Methylhistidine	Deduced in DMD and LGMD	Urine	[58]
N epsilon,N epsilon-dimethyllysine	No alteration		
N epsilon, N epsilon, N epsilon-trimethyllysine	No alteration		
NG,NG-dimethylarginine	Elevated in DMD and LGMD		
NG,N'G-dimethylarginine	No alteration		

Tested marker	Levels (high or low)	Location (serum/muscle)	Ref.
Tetranor PGDM (PGD2 metabolite)	Elevated in DMD	Urine	[59]
Nitric oxide	Reduced in DMD	Serum	[60]

Table 3.
List of metabolites that can be used as potential biomarkers in DMD diagnosis.

to diagnose DMD since the multiple primers covered commonly mutated locations across the entire DMD gene, hotspot regions [66–68]. This technique was first developed by Chamberlain et al. [69] through utilization of 6 primer sets that were modified to 9 sets and later to 10 by Beggs et al. [70] (to amplify exons 45, 48, 19, 17, 51, 8, 12, 44, 4). If no amplification take place, this will confirm deletion of this exon. The developed primer sets were successfully able to detect deletion mutations in the hot spot regions. One of the limitations of such technique was its inability to diagnose all cases with other deletion mutation in other regions, or patients with SNPs or deep intronic mutation.

2.4.3 Multiplex ligation dependent probe amplification (MLPA)

In order to simultaneously investigate the status of the 79 exons of the DMD gene, a PCR-based technique was developed to diagnose DMD in a multiplex PCR reaction. The assay uses multiple probes to target different exons in the DMD gene. Each probe consists of two oligonucleotides; one consists of a 5′-adapter and a 3′-exon-specific region, and vice versa for the second oligonucleotide, where the 3′-end of the first primer and the 5′-end of the second hybridize to two adjacent nucleotides in the target exon. Hybridized probes are subjected to ligation reaction, thus, only hybridized probes get ligated, amplified by PCR using adapter-specific primers and separated by capillary electrophoresis. Positive PCR product indicates the presence of the target exon, while deleted exon(s) will not produce corresponding product(s). In this assay, it is also possible to detect exon duplication, which will be detected as larger peak [71, 72]. However, this assay cannot detect non-sense nor in/del point mutations.

2.4.4 Microarray

High-throughput methods such as DNA microarrays were adopted using specific oligonucleotide probes that cover the entire 2.4 mbp DMD gene (targeted high density comparative genomic hybridization (CGH) microarray). Such method could effectively be used to detect known as well as novel intronic mutations [73–75].

2.4.5 Next generation sequencing (NGS)

The development of NGS and the massively parallel sequencing allowed the sequencing of 100 s of millions of independent short reads (100–300 bp) at the same time. Such approaches generate huge amount of data that uses bioinformatic analysis for annotations and alignments of the generated sequences to produce sequence information for large genes such as DMD and titin and delineate the exact locations of mutations [76]. One major advantage of resorting to NGS for DMD diagnosis is that it could be used for the analysis of MLPA-negative samples that could have small deletions/duplications or single nucleotides variants [77].

Also, RNA sequencing by NGS (RNA-seq) is very useful in detecting the splicing pattern that occur in the DMD transcripts in the muscles through different developmental stages, muscle breakdown or muscle regeneration [78–80].

2.4.6 Muscle biopsy

In some cases, muscle biopsy is required to fully characterize the phenotypic effect of the mutation. The muscle tissue is used in immunoassays, using different antibodies targeting different regions of dystrophin protein (C-terminal, Rod and N-terminal domains), such as western blotting [81–83] or immunohistochemistry [83]. Uchino et al. [83] developed a multiplex western blotting assay to analyze the expression of other muscle proteins like dysferlin, merosin, different forms of sarcoglycan (alpha, beta, gamma, delta), and calpain in addition to dystrophin protein, due to the frequent epigenetic changes incited in these proteins as a consequence to the alteration in dystrophin expression.

3. Conclusion

In this chapter, we have presented a comprehensive review for the methods that have been used in the diagnosis of DMD. Because of the nature of the disease, an X-linked disorder, DMD symptoms of the first affected male births of asymptomatic carrier mothers are usually go unnoticed until the age of 5, where the progressive muscle weakness becomes obvious and fibrotic fatty tissue infiltration is prominent. However, it is well known that early diagnosis and treatment results in better disease management and improve the clinical outcomes. In fact, some studies have pointed out to the fact that initiating corticosteroids therapy early enough has delayed the loss of ambulation in most cases by about 2 years [84]. In addition, with the fast-paced progress in molecular/personalized therapies such as exon-skipping and gene-editing based approaches, precise diagnosis and mutation detection becomes a necessity. Moreover, the genetic testing has been extensively used in prenatal diagnosis and has assisted in decreasing disease burden by aborting affected male pregnancies. In a retrospective study conducted in the Netherland, the authors reported 145 abortions of male fetuses over 26 years that had been found to carry inactivating mutations of the DMD gene [85]. Furthermore, identifying female carriers, is gaining momentum to decrease the possibility of giving birth to affected males and consequently contributes to the overall disease management.

Author details

Nahla O. Mousa[1,2], Ahmed Osman[3,4]*, Nagia Fahmy[5], Ahmed Abdellatif[1], Suher Zada[1] and Hassan El-Fawal[1]

1 Biology Department, and Biotechnology Program, School of Sciences and Engineering, The American University in Cairo, Cairo, Egypt

2 Biotechnology Program, Chemistry Department, Faculty of Science, Cairo University, Giza, Egypt

3 Biotechnology Department, Basic and Applied Sciences Institute, Egypt-Japan University of Science and Technology, Borg Al Arab, Alexandria, Egypt

4 Biochemistry Department, Faculty of Science, Ain Shams University, Cairo, Egypt

5 Neuromuscular Unit, Neuropsychiatry Department, Faculty of Medicine, Ain Shams University, Cairo, Egypt

*Address all correspondence to: ahmed.osman@ejust.edu.eg

References

[1] Pasternak C, Wong S, Elson EL. Mechanical function of dystrophin in muscle cells. The Journal of Cell Biology. 1995;**128**(3):355-361

[2] Vila MC, Rayavarapu S, Hogarth MW, Van der Meulen JH, Horn A, Defour A, et al. Mitochondria mediate cell membrane repair and contribute to Duchenne muscular dystrophy. Cell Death and Differentiation. 2017;**24**(2):330-342

[3] Gao QQ, McNally EM. The Dystrophin complex: Structure, function, and implications for therapy. Comprehensive Physiology. 2015;**5**(3): 1223-1239

[4] Bushby K, Finkel R, Birnkrant DJ, Case LE, Clemens PR, Cripe L, et al. Diagnosis and management of Duchenne muscular dystrophy, part 1: Diagnosis, and pharmacological and psychosocial management. Lancet Neurology. 2010;**9**(1):77-93

[5] Archer JE, Gardner AC, Roper HP, Chikermane AA, Tatman AJ. Duchenne muscular dystrophy: The management of scoliosis. Journal of Spine Surgery. 2016;**2**(3):185-194

[6] Choi YA, Chun SM, Kim Y, Shin HI. Lower extremity joint contracture according to ambulatory status in children with Duchenne muscular dystrophy. BMC Musculoskeletal Disorders. 2018; **19**(1):287

[7] Kervin T, Thangarajh M. The relationship between bone mineral density and cardiovascular function in Duchenne muscular dystrophy: A retrospective cohort study. PLOS Currents. 2018;**10**:pii: ecurrents.md. ee7ac0ec8c19a47b114737f9c2714779. DOI: 10.1371/currents.md.ee7ac0ec8c 19a47b114737f9c2714779

[8] Sawnani H. Sleep disordered breathing in Duchenne muscular dystrophy. Paediatric Respiratory Reviews. 2019;**30**:2-8

[9] Kamdar F, Garry DJ. Dystrophin-deficient cardiomyopathy. Journal of the American College of Cardiology. 2016; **67**(21):2533-2546

[10] Gumerson JD, Michele DE. The dystrophin-glycoprotein complex in the prevention of muscle damage. Journal of Biomedicine & Biotechnology. 2011; **2011**:210797

[11] Okinaka S, Kumagai H, Ebashi S, Sugita H, Momoi H, Toyokura Y, et al. Serum creatine phosphokinase. Activity in progressive muscular dystrophy and neuromuscular diseases. Archives of Neurology. 1961;**4**:520-525

[12] Birnkrant DJ, Bushby K, Bann CM, Apkon SD, Blackwell A, Brumbaugh D, et al. Diagnosis and management of Duchenne muscular dystrophy, part 1: Diagnosis, and neuromuscular, rehabilitation, endocrine, and gastrointestinal and nutritional management. Lancet Neurology. 2018; **17**(3):251-267

[13] Efstratiadis G, Voulgaridou A, Nikiforou D, Kyventidis A, Kourkouni E, Vergoulas G. Rhabdomyolysis updated. Hippokratia. 2007;**11**(3):129-137

[14] Rosalki SB. Serum enzymes in disease of skeletal muscle. Clinics in Laboratory Medicine. 1989;**9**(4):767-781

[15] Aoyagi T, Wada T, Kojima F, Nagai M, Miyoshino S, Umezawa H. Two different modes of enzymatic changes in serum with progression of Duchenne muscular dystrophy. Clinica Chimica Acta. 1983;**129**(2):165-173

[16] Awano H, Takeshima Y, Okizuka Y, Saiki K, Yagi M, Matsuo M. Wide ranges of serum myostatin concentrations in

Duchenne muscular dystrophy patients. Clinica Chimica Acta. 2008;**391**(1–2): 115-117

[17] Bernasconi P, Carboni N, Ricci G, Siciliano G, Politano L, Maggi L, et al. Elevated TGF beta2 serum levels in Emery-Dreifuss muscular dystrophy: Implications for myocyte and tenocyte differentiation and fibrogenic processes. Nucleus. 2018;**9**(1):292-304

[18] Burch PM, Pogoryelova O, Goldstein R, Bennett D, Guglieri M, Straub V, et al. Muscle-derived proteins as serum biomarkers for monitoring disease progression in three forms of muscular dystrophy. Journal of Neuromuscular Diseases. 2015;**2**(3): 241-255

[19] Crowe KE, Shao G, Flanigan KM, Martin PT. N-terminal alpha Dystroglycan (alphaDG-N): A potential serum biomarker for Duchenne muscular dystrophy. Journal of Neuromuscular Diseases. 2016;**3**(2): 247-260

[20] Cynthia Martin F, Hiller M, Spitali P, Oonk S, Dalebout H, Palmblad M, et al. Fibronectin is a serum biomarker for Duchenne muscular dystrophy. Proteomics. Clinical Applications. 2014;**8**(3–4): 269-278

[21] D'Amore PA, Brown RH Jr, Ku PT, Hoffman EP, Watanabe H, Arahata K, et al. Elevated basic fibroblast growth factor in the serum of patients with Duchenne muscular dystrophy. Annals of Neurology. 1994;**35**(3):362-365

[22] Fukunaga H, Higuchi I, Usuki F, Moritoyo T, Okubo R. Clinical significance of serum cardiac myosin light chain I in patients with Duchenne muscular dystrophy. Nō to Shinkei. 1992;**44**(2):131-135

[23] Hathout Y, Brody E, Clemens PR, Cripe L, DeLisle RK, Furlong P, et al. Large-scale serum protein biomarker discovery in Duchenne muscular dystrophy. Proceedings of the National Academy of Sciences of the United States of America. 2015;**112**(23): 7153-7158

[24] Janik P, Nowak I, Niebroj-Dobosz I. Serum cytoplasmic and mitochondrial aspartate aminotransferase in Duchenne's progressive muscular dystrophy. Materia Medica Polona. 1994;**26**(3):101-104

[25] McMillan HJ, Gregas M, Darras BT, Kang PB. Serum transaminase levels in boys with Duchenne and Becker muscular dystrophy. Pediatrics. 2011; **127**(1):e132-e136

[26] Mokuno K, Riku S, Matsuoka Y, Sobue I, Kato K. Serum muscle-specific enolase in progressive muscular dystrophy and other neuromuscular diseases. Journal of the Neurological Sciences. 1984;**63**(3):345-352

[27] Mokuno K, Riku S, Matsuoka Y, Sobue I, Kato K. Serum carbonic anhydrase III in progressive muscular dystrophy. Journal of the Neurological Sciences. 1985;**67**(2):223-228

[28] Mokuno K, Riku S, Sugimura K, Takahashi A, Kato K, Osugi S. Serum creatine kinase isoenzymes in Duchenne muscular dystrophy determined by sensitive enzyme immunoassay methods. Muscle & Nerve. 1987;**10**(5): 459-463

[29] Nadarajah VD, van Putten M, Chaouch A, Garrood P, Straub V, Lochmuller H, et al. Serum matrix metalloproteinase-9 (MMP-9) as a biomarker for monitoring disease progression in Duchenne muscular dystrophy (DMD). Neuromuscular Disorders. 2011;**21**(8):569-578

[30] Niebroj-Dobosz I, Madej-Pilarczyk A, Marchel M, Sokolowska B, Hausmanowa-Petrusewicz I. Matrix

metalloproteinases in serum of Emery-Dreifuss muscular dystrophy patients. Acta Biochimica Polonica. 2009;**56**(4): 717-722

[31] Niebroj-Dobosz IM, Sokolowska B, Madej-Pilarczyk A, Marchel M, Hausmanowa-Petrusewicz I. Tissue inhibitors of matrix metalloproteinases in serum are cardiac biomarkers in Emery-Dreifuss muscular dystrophy. Kardiologia Polska. 2015;**73**(5):360-365

[32] Ohta M, Itagaki Y, Itoh N, Hayashi K, Nishitani H, Ohta K. Carbonic anhydrase III in serum in muscular dystrophy and other neurological disorders: Relationship with creatine kinase. Clinical Chemistry. 1991;**37**(1):36-39

[33] Oonk S, Spitali P, Hiller M, Switzar L, Dalebout H, Calissano M, et al. Comparative mass spectrometric and immunoassay-based proteome analysis in serum of Duchenne muscular dystrophy patients. Proteomics Clinical Applications. 2016; **10**(3):290-299

[34] Zhu Y, Zhang H, Sun Y, Li Y, Deng L, Wen X, et al. Serum enzyme profiles differentiate five types of muscular dystrophy. Disease Markers. 2015;**2015**:543282

[35] Saito T, Yamamoto Y, Matsumura T, Fujimura H, Shinno S. Serum levels of vascular endothelial growth factor elevated in patients with muscular dystrophy. Brain & Development. 2009;**31**(8):612-617

[36] Statland J, Donlin-Smith CM, Tapscott SJ, van der Maarel S, Tawil R. Multiplex screen of serum biomarkers in facioscapulohumeral muscular dystrophy. Journal of Neuromuscular Diseases. 2014;**1**(2):181-190

[37] von Moers A, Danne T, Moller P, Scheffner D. Serum levels of carboxyterminal propeptide of type I procollagen, aminoterminal propeptide of type III procollagen and laminin P1 in Duchenne muscular dystrophy. Acta Paediatrica. 1997;**86**(4):377-380

[38] Zatz M, Rapaport D, Vainzof M, Passos-Bueno MR, Bortolini ER, Pavanello Rde C, et al. Serum creatine-kinase (CK) and pyruvate-kinase (PK) activities in Duchenne (DMD) as compared with Becker (BMD) muscular dystrophy. Journal of the Neurological Sciences. 1991;**102**(2):190-196

[39] Ayoglu B, Chaouch A, Lochmuller H, Politano L, Bertini E, Spitali P, et al. Affinity proteomics within rare diseases: A BIO-NMD study for blood biomarkers of muscular dystrophies. EMBO Molecular Medicine. 2014;**6**(7):918-936

[40] Anaya-Segura MA, Garcia-Martinez FA, Montes-Almanza LA, Diaz BG, Avila-Ramirez G, Alvarez-Maya I, et al. Non-invasive biomarkers for Duchenne muscular dystrophy and carrier detection. Molecules. 2015;**20**(6): 11154-11172

[41] Awano H, Matsumoto M, Nagai M, Shirakawa T, Maruyama N, Iijima K, et al. Diagnostic and clinical significance of the titin fragment in urine of Duchenne muscular dystrophy patients. Clinica Chimica Acta. 2018;**476**:111-116

[42] O'Brien J, Hayder H, Zayed Y, Peng C. Overview of microRNA biogenesis, mechanisms of actions, and circulation. Frontiers in Endocrinology. 2018;**9**:402

[43] Finotti A, Fabbri E, Lampronti I, Gasparello J, Borgatti M, Gambari R. MicroRNAs and long non-coding RNAs in genetic diseases. Molecular Diagnosis & Therapy. 2019;**23**(2):155-171

[44] Zaharieva IT, Calissano M, Scoto M, Preston M, Cirak S, Feng L, et al. Dystromirs as serum biomarkers for

monitoring the disease severity in Duchenne muscular dystrophy. PLoS One. 2013;**8**(11):e80263

[45] Li X, Li Y, Zhao L, Zhang D, Yao X, Zhang H, et al. Circulating muscle-specific miRNAs in Duchenne muscular dystrophy patients. Molecular Therapy–Nucleic Acids. 2014;**3**:e177

[46] Hu J, Kong M, Ye Y, Hong S, Cheng L, Jiang L. Serum miR-206 and other muscle-specific microRNAs as non-invasive biomarkers for Duchenne muscular dystrophy. Journal of Neurochemistry. 2014;**129**(5):877-883

[47] Matsuzaka Y, Kishi S, Aoki Y, Komaki H, Oya Y, Takeda S, et al. Three novel serum biomarkers, miR-1, miR-133a, and miR-206 for limb-girdle muscular dystrophy, facioscapulohumeral muscular dystrophy, and Becker muscular dystrophy. Environmental Health and Preventive Medicine. 2014;**19**(6):452-458

[48] Jeanson-Leh L, Lameth J, Krimi S, Buisset J, Amor F, Le Guiner C, et al. Serum profiling identifies novel muscle miRNA and cardiomyopathy-related miRNA biomarkers in Golden retriever muscular dystrophy dogs and Duchenne muscular dystrophy patients. The American Journal of Pathology. 2014;**184**(11):2885-2898

[49] Llano-Diez M, Ortez CI, Gay JA, Alvarez-Cabado L, Jou C, Medina J, et al. Digital PCR quantification of miR-30c and miR-181a as serum biomarkers for Duchenne muscular dystrophy. Neuromuscular Disorders. 2017;**27**(1):15-23

[50] Catapano F, Domingos J, Perry M, Ricotti V, Phillips L, Servais L, et al. Downregulation of miRNA-29, -23 and -21 in urine of Duchenne muscular dystrophy patients. Epigenomics. 2018;**10**(7):875-889

[51] Liu DZ, Stamova B, Hu S, Ander BP, Jickling GC, Zhan X, et al. MicroRNA and mRNA expression changes in steroid naive and steroid treated DMD patients. Journal of Neuromuscular Diseases. 2015;**2**(4):387-396

[52] Coenen-Stass AML, Sork H, Gatto S, Godfrey C, Bhomra A, Krjutskov K, et al. Comprehensive RNA-sequencing analysis in serum and muscle reveals novel small RNA signatures with biomarker potential for DMD. Molecular Therapy–Nucleic Acids. 2018;**13**:1-15

[53] Eisenberg I, Eran A, Nishino I, Moggio M, Lamperti C, Amato AA, et al. Distinctive patterns of microRNA expression in primary muscular disorders. Proceedings of the National Academy of Sciences of the United States of America. 2007;**104**(43):17016-17021

[54] Shapira YA, Patz D, Menczel J, Schwartz L, Meyer S, Frutkoff IW, et al. Low serum 24,25 dihydroxyvitamin D in Duchenne muscular dystrophy. Neurology. 1984;**34**(9):1192-1196

[55] Spitali P, Hettne K, Tsonaka R, Sabir E, Seyer A, Hemerik JBA, et al. Cross-sectional serum metabolomic study of multiple forms of muscular dystrophy. Journal of Cellular and Molecular Medicine. 2018;**22**(4):2442-2448

[56] Srivastava NK, Annarao S, Sinha N. Metabolic status of patients with muscular dystrophy in early phase of the disease: In vitro, high resolution NMR spectroscopy based metabolomics analysis of serum. Life Sciences. 2016;**151**:122-129

[57] Wang L, Chen M, He R, Sun Y, Yang J, Xiao L, et al. Serum creatinine distinguishes Duchenne muscular dystrophy from Becker muscular dystrophy in patients aged ≦3 years: A

retrospective study. Frontiers in Neurology. 2017;**8**:196

[58] Inoue R, Miyake M, Kanazawa A, Sato M, Kakimoto Y. Decrease of 3-methylhistidine and increase of NG,NG-dimethylarginine in the urine of patients with muscular dystrophy. Metabolism. 1979;**28**(8):801-804

[59] Nakagawa T, Takeuchi A, Kakiuchi R, Lee T, Yagi M, Awano H, et al. A prostaglandin D2 metabolite is elevated in the urine of Duchenne muscular dystrophy patients and increases further from 8 years old. Clinica Chimica Acta. 2013;**423**: 10-14

[60] Gucuyener K, Ergenekon E, Erbas D, Pinarli G, Serdaroglu A. The serum nitric oxide levels in patients with Duchenne muscular dystrophy. Brain & Development. 2000;**22**(3):181-183

[61] Schreiber A, Smith WL, Ionasescu V, Zellweger H, Franken EA, Dunn V, et al. Magnetic resonance imaging of children with Duchenne muscular dystrophy. Pediatric Radiology. 1987;**17**(6):495-497

[62] Gaur L, Hanna A, Bandettini WP, Fischbeck KH, Arai AE, Mankodi A. Upper arm and cardiac magnetic resonance imaging in Duchenne muscular dystrophy. Annals of Clinical Translational Neurology. 2016;**3**(12): 948-955

[63] Hofker MH, van Ommen GJ, Bakker E, Burmeister M, Pearson PL. Development of additional RFLP probes near the locus for Duchenne muscular dystrophy by cosmid cloning of the DXS84 (754) locus. Human Genetics. 1986;**74**(3):270-274

[64] Laing NG, Siddique T, Bartlett RJ, Yamaoka LH, Chen JC, Walker AP, et al. RFLP for Duchenne muscular dystrophy cDNA clone 44-1. Nucleic Acids Research. 1988;**16**(14B):7209

[65] Walker AP, Bartlett RJ, Laing NG, Siddique T, Yamaoka LH, Chen JC, et al. RFLP for Duchenne muscular dystrophy cDNA clone 30-2. Nucleic Acids Research. 1988;**16**(18):9072

[66] Kawamura J. Detection of mutation in dystrophin gene in Duchenne muscular dystrophy–multiplex PCR and southern blot analysis. Nihon Rinsho. 1997;**55**(12):3126-3130

[67] Ma S. Rapid screening of the Duchenne muscular dystrophy gene deletion by two multiplex PCR. Zhongguo Yi Xue Ke Xue Yuan Xue Bao. 1993;**15**(1):74-78

[68] Singh R, Vijjaya, Kabra M. Multiplex PCR for rapid detection of exonal deletions in patients of duchenne muscular dystrophy. Indian Journal of Clinical Biochemistry. 2006;**21**(1): 147-151

[69] Chamberlain JS, Chamberlain JR, Fenwick RG, Ward PA, Caskey CT, Dimnik LS, et al. Diagnosis of Duchenne and Becker muscular dystrophies by polymerase chain reaction. A multicenter study. Journal of the American Medical Association. 1992; **267**(19):2609-2615

[70] Beggs AH, Koenig M, Boyce FM, Kunkel LM. Detection of 98% of DMD/ BMD gene deletions by polymerase chain reaction. Human Genetics. 1990; **86**(1):45-48

[71] Janssen B, Hartmann C, Scholz V, Jauch A, Zschocke J. MLPA analysis for the detection of deletions, duplications and complex rearrangements in the dystrophin gene: Potential and pitfalls. Neurogenetics. 2005;**6**(1):29-35

[72] Schwartz M, Duno M. Improved molecular diagnosis of dystrophin gene mutations using the multiplex ligation-dependent probe amplification method. Genetic Testing. 2004;**8**(4): 361-367

[73] Hegde MR, Chin EL, Mulle JG, Okou DT, Warren ST, Zwick ME. Microarray-based mutation detection in the dystrophin gene. Human Mutation. 2008;**29**(9):1091-1099

[74] Ishmukhametova A, Khau Van Kien P, Mechin D, Thorel D, Vincent MC, Rivier F, et al. Comprehensive oligonucleotide array-comparative genomic hybridization analysis: New insights into the molecular pathology of the DMD gene. European Journal of Human Genetics. 2012;**20**(10):1096-1100

[75] del Gaudio D, Yang Y, Boggs BA, Schmitt ES, Lee JA, Sahoo T, et al. Molecular diagnosis of Duchenne/Becker muscular dystrophy: Enhanced detection of dystrophin gene rearrangements by oligonucleotide array-comparative genomic hybridization. Human Mutation. 2008;**29**(9):1100-1107

[76] Ng SB, Buckingham KJ, Lee C, Bigham AW, Tabor HK, Dent KM, et al. Exome sequencing identifies the cause of a mendelian disorder. Nature Genetics. 2010;**42**(1):30-35

[77] Singh B, Mandal K, Lallar M, Narayanan DL, Mishra S, Gambhir PS, et al. Next generation sequencing in diagnosis of MLPA negative cases presenting as Duchenne/Becker muscular dystrophies. Indian Journal of Pediatrics. 2018;**85**(4):309-310

[78] Bouge AL, Murauer E, Beyne E, Miro J, Varilh J, Taulan M, et al. Erratum: Targeted RNA-Seq profiling of splicing pattern in the DMD gene: Exons are mostly constitutively spliced in human skeletal muscle. Scientific Reports. 2017;**7**:45414

[79] Bouge AL, Murauer E, Beyne E, Miro J, Varilh J, Taulan M, et al. Targeted RNA-Seq profiling of splicing pattern in the DMD gene: Exons are mostly constitutively spliced in human skeletal muscle. Scientific Reports. 2017;**7**:39094

[80] Gonorazky H, Liang M, Cummings B, Lek M, Micallef J, Hawkins C, et al. RNAseq analysis for the diagnosis of muscular dystrophy. Annals of Clinical Translational Neurology. 2016;**3**(1):55-60

[81] Nicholson LV, Davison K, Falkous G, Harwood C, O'Donnell E, Slater CR, et al. Dystrophin in skeletal muscle. I. Western blot analysis using a monoclonal antibody. Journal of the Neurological Sciences. 1989;**94**(1–3):125-136

[82] Beekman C, Janson AA, Baghat A, van Deutekom JC, Datson NA. Use of capillary Western immunoassay (Wes) for quantification of dystrophin levels in skeletal muscle of healthy controls and individuals with Becker and Duchenne muscular dystrophy. PLoS One. 2018;**13**(4):e0195850

[83] Uchino M, Tokunaga M, Mita S, Uyama E, Ando Y, Teramoto H, et al. PCR and immunocytochemical analyses of dystrophin-positive fibers in Duchenne muscular dystrophy. Journal of the Neurological Sciences. 1995;**129**(1):44-50

[84] Koeks Z, Bladen CL, Salgado D, van Zwet E, Pogoryelova O, McMacken G, et al. Clinical outcomes in Duchenne muscular dystrophy: A study of 5345 patients from the TREAT-NMD DMD global database. Journal of Neuromuscular Diseases. 2017;**4**(4):293-306

[85] Helderman-van den Enden AT, Madan K, Breuning MH, van der Hout AH, Bakker E, de Die-Smulders CE, et al. An urgent need for a change in policy revealed by a study on prenatal testing for Duchenne muscular dystrophy. European Journal of Human Genetics. 2013;**21**(1):21-26

Chapter 3

Lipodystrophy - A Rare Condition with Serious Metabolic Abnormalities

Long Hoa Chung and Yanfei Qi

Abstract

Lipodystrophy is a rare lipid storage disorder that is characterized by a loss of adipose tissue. It can be inherited due to monogenic mutation or acquired by medication and autoimmune illness. Two primary forms of inherited lipodystrophy are congenital generalized lipodystrophy manifested as a near-complete loss of fat tissue since birth and familial partial lipodystrophy with progressive, partial loss of fat tissue during late childhood and puberty. Lipodystrophy results in severe metabolic conditions, including insulin resistance, type 2 diabetes, hepatosteatosis, polycystic ovary syndrome, acanthosis nigricans, and hypertension. This chapter summarizes the symptoms, causes, and treatments of inherited and acquired lipodystrophy.

Keywords: adipose tissue, adipogenesis, metabolic syndrome, lipid disorders, ectopic lipid

1. Introduction

In order to survive and adapt to challenging environment, living organisms have equipped themselves with different mechanisms of energy storage that can be accessed when there is a shortage of food supply. In mammals, fat is mainly stored in adipose tissues [1]. There are two types of adipose tissues: white adipose tissue that stores the majority of the body fat and also functions as an endocrine organ and brown adipose tissue that generates the body heat [2]. In adipocytes, fat is stored in lipid droplets (LDs) in the form of neutral lipids, e.g., triacylglycerol (TAG) and cholesteryl ester (CE). White adipocytes contain unilocular LDs that occupy up to 90% of the cytoplasmic space, while brown adipocytes contain multilocular LDs. Obesity is characterized by both increase in the size and number of white adipocytes [3]. Fat storage in white adipose tissue is essential for proper metabolic homeostasis [4]. In contrast, when fat storage in white adipose tissue is compromised or overwhelmed, the ectopic fat accumulation in non-adipose tissues will result in severe metabolic disorders [5].

Lipodystrophy is an extreme fat storage condition, in which white adipose tissue is selectively lost [6]. Partial or generalized loss of fat in this condition causes an array of complications including insulin resistance, type 2 diabetes and acanthosis nigricans, hypertriglyceridemia, hepatic steatosis, hypertension, polycystic ovarian syndrome, and proteinuric kidney disease [7, 8]. The severity of lipodystrophy depends on the level of adipocyte depletion in the body. Fat loss can occur in nearly the entire body known as congenital generalized lipodystrophy (CGL) or partial loss in small and discrete areas known as familial partial lipodystrophy (FPLD). While CGL is manifested early in life at birth or soon after, partial fat loss in FPLD occurs during late childhood and puberty. CGL can be determined by measurements of skinfold thickness with calipers or by whole-body magnetic resonance imaging (MRI) scan [9]. Since lipodystrophy is a monogenetic disorder, it can also be diagnosed and confirmed by genotyping.

Lipodystrophy is a very rare genetic disease (1 in 10 million for CGL). Currently, there have been around 300–500 CGL cases and 1000 FPLD cases reported; however, the number of undiagnosed patients is suspected to be three times more [10]. Nearly 20 loci for different subtypes of lipodystrophy have been identified. These genes are implicated in the regulation of either the development of white adipose tissue or the expansion of LDs in white adipocytes. In this chapter, we will outline these lipodystrophy-causative gene loci as well as describe in brief the acquired condition of lipodystrophy.

2. Genetics of congenital generalized lipodystrophy

There are four different genetic subtypes of CGL that result from different mutations.

2.1 Type 1 CGL (CGL1) and AGPAT2

Mutations that are responsible for CGL1 (Online Mendelian Inheritance in Man [OMIM] #608594) occur in the region of 1-acylglycerol-3-phosphate O-acyltransferase 2 (*AGPAT2*) on chromosome 9q34. Only 4% of compound heterozygotes with a null and a missense mutation still maintain some residual enzymatic activity [7]. Also, homozygous missense mutations have been reported to be 2% of CGL1 patients. Interestingly, there is no strong correlation between the type of mutation and lipodystrophy phenotype (the level of adipocyte malfunction) [7, 11]. On the contrary, a founder mutation variant might exist in a particular population [11]. In fact, almost all patients that have African origin have the founder mutation in intron 4, c589-2A>G of one or both alleles [7, 12]. In the past 5 years, several novel variants of *AGPAT2* have been identified in CGL patients: c.144C>A, c.667_705delinsCTGCG, c.268delC, and c.316+1G>T; c.134C>A and c.216C>G [13]; c.514G>A [14]; c.685G>T, and c.514G>A [15]. In addition, a very rare case of dual mutations (c.493-1G>C and c.299G>A) in *AGPAT2* was identified in two Chilean sisters [16].

AGPAT2 is a member of lysophosphatidic acid acyltransferases (LPAATs) including AGPAT family (AGPAT1–AGPAT11) and others such as CGI-58 and endophilin [17]. In fact, AGPAT2 was identified with AGPAT1 by searching an EST database for human homologs of yeast LPAAT in 1997 [18]. There are 11 isoforms of AGPATs that are involved in the de novo synthesis of phospholipids (PLs) and triacylglycerol from glycerol-3-phosphate (G3P). *AGPAT2* is predominantly expressed in adipose tissue, and its mRNA level increases by 30-fold during the differentiation of adipocytes [19]. Patients with CGL1 normally suffer extreme loss of all metabolically active adipose tissue in most subcutaneous areas, intra-abdominal areas, intrathoracic regions, and bone marrow; however, it is postulated that the redundancy of other AGPAT isoforms or the enhanced expression of other *AGPAT* genes helps preserve mechanical fat depots located in the palms, soles, under the scalp, retro-orbital, periarticular regions, perineum, vulva, and pericalyceal regions of the kidneys [7, 20].

In adipose tissue, the synthesis of PLs and TAG begins with the acylation of G3P with FA-CoA by glycerol phosphate acyltransferase (GPAT) at the S_N1 position to form 1-acylglycerol-3-phosphate or lysophosphatidic acid (LPA). Then AGPAT2 catalyzes the conversion of LPA into phosphatidic acid (PA) via an acylation reaction at the S_N2 position. PA is a pivotal intracellular signaling lipid for it sits at the branching point of de novo PL and TAG synthesis pathway and acts as a precursor for the lipin-mediated production of diacylglycerol (DAG), followed by phosphatidylcholine (PC), phosphatidylethanolamine (PE), and TAG, and as the substrate for the cytidine diphosphate synthase (CDS)-mediated generation of cytidine diphosphate diacylglycerol (CDP-DAG), followed by phosphatidylinositol (PI), phosphatidylglycerol (PG), and cardiolipin [21]. PA is a cone-shaped lipid that has the capacity to alter the curvature of the membranes, and it has been shown to mediate membrane fusion in both soluble N-ethylmaleimide-sensitive factor attachment protein (NSF)-receptor (SNARE)-dependent and SNARE-independent fashions [22, 23]. It has been implicated in the fusion of multiple LDs to form a gigantic LD [24]. In addition, PA is believed to be an endogenous antagonist of peroxisome proliferator-activated receptor gamma (PPARγ) that is the master transcription factor in adipocyte differentiation [25]. The malfunctioned *AGPAT2* in CGL1 is assumed to cause dysregulated PL and TAG synthesis, leading to defective adipose tissue development [11, 19]. However, the exact mechanism of how AGPAT2 deficiency causes lipodystrophy remains unraveled. Intriguingly, the same effect cannot be achieved by knocking out other key enzymes in the TAG synthesis including glycerol-3-phosphate acyltransferase 1 (GPAT1), GPAT4, lipin, and diacylglycerol acyltransferase 1 (DGAT1) and DGAT2 [26–30].

Ablation of *Agpat2* induces severe lipodystrophy in mice with the loss of both WAT and BAT during the first week of postnatal period, due to inflammatory infiltration to adipose tissue and massive adipocyte cell death [31]. In addition, both male and female mice have extreme insulin resistance, type 2 diabetes, hepatic steatosis, as well as organomegaly including hepatosplenomegaly, nephromegaly, and elongated small intestines as seen in human CGL [32]. Since almost all adipose tissues have disappeared, *Agpat2*$^{-/-}$ mice are not an ideal model to study the development of lipodystrophy; however, this type of animals can be particularly useful for the investigation of lipodystrophy-induced metabolic disorders in non-adipose tissues such as severe hepatic insulin resistance and steatosis in CGL [20]. Up to 90% of the total AGPAT activity is compromised in the liver tissue of *Agpat2*$^{-/-}$ mice and that can be restored by adenoviral delivery of *Agpat1* or *Agpat2*. However, overexpression of *Agpat1* or Agpat2 in *Agpat2*$^{-/-}$ liver failed to alleviate hepatic steatosis, indicating that the ectopic hepatic lipid accumulation was derived from insulin resistance and loss of body fat [33]. While reduced AGPAT activity is supposed to result in a reduction in PA synthesis, the PA level was seen to increase in the liver of male *Agpat2*$^{-/-}$ mice, which suggests an alternative pathway for PA synthesis with a compensatory activation of DAG kinase or phospholipase D [32, 34]. A high level of PA predisposes *Agpat2*$^{-/-}$ liver to elevated hepatic glucose production, which is attributed to insulin resistance [34]. PA accumulation was also found in differentiated *Agpat2*$^{-/-}$ murine embryonic fibroblast (MEF) adipocytes [31]. At day 6 of the differentiation, ultrastructural alterations in mitochondria, plasma membrane, and autophagosomes were found in *Apgat2*$^{-/-}$ MEF adipocytes, suggesting that in the absence of AGPAT2, cells can initiate adipogenesis, but a variety of cellular abnormalities eventually block the terminal phase of adipogenesis [31]. Enforcing adipocyte differentiation by overexpression of PPARγ, the master regulator of adipogenesis can also promote adipogenesis of *Agpat2*$^{-/-}$ MEFs; nevertheless, massive cell death occurred before they reached full differentiation [31]. In agreement with this finding, preadipocytes from *Agpat2*$^{-/-}$ interscapular BAT underwent progressive cell death during the adipogenic induction with no activation of caspase 3 [35].

In addition, these BAT-derived preadipocytes exhibit an increased expression of autophagy-related proteins but a decreased autophagic flux [35]. In isolated muscle-derived multipotent cells (MDMCs) from CGL1 patients and 3T3-L1 preadipocyte cells with the knockdown of AGPAT2, cell death also proceeds during adipogenesis, which might be associated with defective Akt activation as a result of altered PI composition [36, 37]. The constitutively active Akt and PPARγ agonist pioglitazone partially rescued the adipogenic defect in the *Agpat2*$^{-/-}$ cells [37]. In addition, regarded as a therapy for CGL patients, leptin treatment normalizes the levels of plasma TAG, insulin, and glucose as well as improves hepatic steatosis in *Agpat2*$^{-/-}$ mice, which is independent of hepatic leptin receptor [38]. The role of AGPAT2 in LD biology has been rarely reported. In contrast to WT adipose tissue that manifests large unilocular LDs, *Apgat2*$^{-/-}$ adipocytes are featured by smaller multilocular LDs. Although LDs in *Apgat2*$^{-/-}$ MEFs are smaller than *Apgat2*$^{+/+}$ cells, they are still normally coated with perilipin 1 (Plin1) [31].

2.2 Type 2 CGL (CGL2) and SEIPIN

In CGL2 (OMIM #269700), mutations happen in the *BSCL2* gene located on chromosome 11q13. The *BSCL2* gene encodes Seipin. Null mutations found in CGL2 patients occupy approximately 75% of all mutations in the *BSCL2* gene, and the rest are missense mutations [39]. Phenotypically, there are no significant differences between patients with null and missense mutations. However, mutagenic truncated forms of Seipin fail to bind lipin-1, while missense mutants still preserve this type of interaction. Although CGL2 affects a diverse range of people from Europe, Mediterranean and Middle Eastern Arabs, and Japanese, patients that have Lebanese origin share a common homozygous *BSCL2* mutation of c.315_319delGTATC (p. Tyr106Cysfs*6) [20, 40].

Unlike patients with CGL1, patients with CGL2 suffer a near-total loss of both metabolically active and mechanical adipose tissues [41]. In addition, these patients have significantly low median serum levels of leptin (0.01 ng/ml) and adiponectin (3.3 μg/ml) as compared to normal healthy individuals who had median serum levels of 4.6 ng/ml and 7.8 μg/ml for leptin and adiponectin, respectively [42]. Also, they suffer cardiomyopathy and mild mental retardation in a more prevalent way [7, 8, 43]. One single patient with CGL2 has been reported to have teratozoospermia, a condition characterized by sperm defects including abnormalities in sperm morphology and bundled sperm with two or more sperms joined together by large ectopic LDs [44]. Additionally, three patients in a family from Pakistan with *BSCL2* mutations have been reported to suffer spastic gait, a movement-related complication due to upper motor neuron [45]. While null mutations in *BSCL2* can also result in early-onset, fatal neurodegenerative syndrome as reported in four patients, gain-of-function heterozygous *BSCL2* mutations located in the N-glycosylation motif causes distal hereditary motor neuropathy [46].

SEIPIN is a 398 amino acid transmembrane protein in the endoplasmic reticulum (ER), which regulates the transport of macromolecules including proteins and lipids between the ER and the LD [47]. Therefore, it plays a role as a docking protein to regulate LD biogenesis and adipogenesis [48, 49]. Seipin, an integral ER membrane, participates in lipid homeostasis via various complex mechanisms. One of them is to assist LD assembly and fusion as well as adipocyte differentiation [50]. In fact, SEIPIN deficiency in mammals or its yeast ortholog Fld1p/Sei1p can lead to changes in LD morphology, manifested as clustering of multiple small LDs or supersized LDs [5]. Recently, SEIPIN/Fld1p has been found to be stabilized to

ER-LD contacts to assist the protein and lipid trafficking into growing LDs. SEIPIN strengthens the contact site between ER and LD to regulate the growth of immature LDs [51]. The protein might also be involved in PL and TAG synthesis by its binding and interaction with phosphatidic acid phosphatase lipin-1 and AGPAT2 [52, 53].

Bscl2$^{-/-}$ mice manifest complete loss of WAT and have most metabolic complications including hyperinsulinemia, insulin resistance, and hepatic steatosis [54–56]. These animals have low plasma levels of glucose and TAG compared to their wild-type (WT) counterparts but have postprandial hypertriglyceridemia [54, 57]. Insulin signaling in the liver of *Bscl2*$^{-/-}$ mice was diminished after 4 h of fasting but improved after 16 h [57]. Knocking out *Bscl2* specifically in adipose tissue causes the mice to have an adipocyte hypertrophy with enlarged LDs, reduced lipolysis, adipose tissue inflammation, progressive loss of both WAT and BAT, insulin resistance, and hepatic steatosis [40].

Bscl2$^{-/-}$ MEFs and stromal vascular cells failed to differentiate due to uncontrolled lipolysis activated by cyclic AMP (cAMP)-dependent protein kinase A (PKA) [55, 58]. It causes loss of LDs and subsequently impaired adipogenesis by silencing the expression of adipose-specific transcription factors. This loss of function can be rescued by inhibitors of lipolysis but not by a PPARγ agonist. Thiazolidinediones, antidiabetic drugs, are able to restore adipogenesis but unable to intervene the unbridled lipolysis happening in *Bscl2*$^{-/-}$ MEFs [56]. Interestingly, LDs in lymphoblastoid cell lines have been reported to have an increase in numbers but shrinkage in size from 12 patients with CGL2 with null *BSCL2* mutations [59]. In addition, it has been observed that there is a shift in the proportion of monounsaturated fatty acids to saturated fatty acids in hepatic triglycerides and phosphatidylethanolamine, implicating a defect in acyl-CoA desaturase activity in these cell lines [59].

2.3 Type 3 CGL (CGL3) and CAV1

CGL3 (OMIM #612526) is induced by mutations in the *CAV1* gene located on chromosome 7q31. The *CAV1* gene encodes caveolin-1. Kim et al. first described a CGL3 patient from Brazil who has a homozygous "loss of function" mutation at p.E38X in the *CAV1* gene [60]. This patient possesses generalized lipodystrophy with near-total loss of metabolically active adipose tissue but preserves mechanical adipose tissue and fat in the bone marrow. She also manifests acanthosis nigricans, severe hypertriglyceridemia, hepatic steatosis and splenomegaly, short stature, functional megaesophagus, hypocalcaemia, primary amenorrhea, and chronic diarrhea. She also developed diabetes mellitus at age 13 [60]. Almost at the same time, Cao et al. reported a case of a typical partial lipodystrophy caused by heterozygous frame-shift mutation in *CAV1*, designated I134 fsdelA-X137 and −88deltaC [61]. This female patient has subcutaneous fat loss in the upper part of her body and face but spared her legs, gluteal region, and visceral fat stores [61]. Since 2015, two novel variants of *CAV1* have been identified: de novo heterozygous null mutations, c.424C>T (p.Q142X) and c.479_480delTT (p.F160X) in a 7-year-old male and a 3-year-old female of European origin, respectively [62]. Both of the patients have generalized fat loss, thin mottled skin, and progeroid features at birth [62]. The male patient has cataracts requiring extraction at 30 months of age, and the female patient has pulmonary arterial hypertension [62–64].

Caveolin-1 is the scaffolding protein primarily constituting specialized vesicular invaginations of 50–100 nm called caveolae [1, 36]. It was discovered by Anderson Lab in 1992 [65, 66]. Its potential function in vesicle transport was reported by Glenney using cDNA encoding caveolin-1 from lungs [67]. There are three caveolin isoforms: CAV1, CAV2, and CAV3. While CAV3 is muscle specific, CAV1 and CAV2 are predominantly expressed in adipose tissue, endothelial cells, and fibroblasts [68, 69]. As the main component of caveolae, caveolin-1 plays an essential role in the caveolae assembly alongside with other caveolar proteins, such as cavinl–cavin4, Pacsin2, and EH domain-containing 2 (EHD2) [70]. In addition to its essential role in caveolae formation, caveolin-1 is also a key determinant of normal lipid homeostasis, vesicular trafficking, and signaling transduction [71]. Caveolae plays a regulatory role in maintaining the integrity and function of the LDs as well as binding and transporting fatty acids and cholesterol by budding off the plasma membrane [70]. Moreover, they serve as a platform for augmenting insulin and PKA signaling [72]. In adipocyte cells, the expression of caveolin-1 is increased 10-fold during adipogenesis [73, 74]. The abundance level of caveolin-1 determines the PL and surface protein composition in LDs and the LD growth. In fact, the expression of *Cav1* in adipose cell lines and mice leads to an increase in the density of caveolae and enhances adipocytes' capacity to have larger LDs and promote cell growth through increased glucose utilization [75].

Similar to caveolin-1 deficiency, lacking another caveolar protein cavin-1 in humans also causes another type of congenital generalized lipodystrophy (type 4 CGL) [76–78]. Interestingly, subcutaneous injection of caveolin-1 overexpressed preadipocytes could form fat pads and larger adipocytes [75]. Both caveolin-1 and cavin-1 are the strong indicators of adipogenic differentiation in human tumors and liposarcoma [79]. Taken together, these data indicate the critical role of adipocyte caveolae in adipose tissue development.

Cav1$^{-/-}$ mice show complete loss of morphologically identifiable caveolae in endothelial and adipose tissue [74]. Likewise, primary cells derived from *Cav1*$^{-/-}$ MEFs fall short of functional caveolae [74]. *Cav1*$^{-/-}$ mice have dramatically smaller fat pads, reduced adipocyte size, and poorly differentiated white adipose parenchyma than their WT littermates [80]. While the animals are hyperphagic, they are resistant to dietinduced obesity [20, 81]. Their BAT undergoes hypertrophy [80, 82].

2.4 Type 4 CGL (CGL4) and PTRF

CGL4 (OMIM #613327) is an autosomal recessive condition caused by mutations in the *PTRF* gene that is located on chromosome 17q21. *PTRF* gene encodes cavin-1 protein. The coincidence of generalized lipodystrophy and muscular dystrophy was found in some Omani patients as early as 2002 [83, 84]; however, the genetic basis underlies this new subtype of generalized lipodystrophy was not identified until 2009 [85]. CGL4 patients normally do not have severe lipodystrophy at birth but gradually develop progressive fat loss from infancy or early childhood [85]. Similar to CGL3, CGL4 subjects lose metabolically active adipose tissue but preserve mechanical adipose tissue and fat in bone marrow [83]. In contrast to the "classic" lipodystrophies, CGL4 is comprising congenital myopathy with high circulating creatine kinase, smooth and skeletal muscle hypertrophy, cardiac arrhythmias, osteopenia, distal metaphyseal deformation with joint stiffness, pyloric stenosis, atlantoaxial instability, as well as percussion-induced muscle mounding and local protracted muscle contractions [78, 83, 86, 87]. Since 2013, a few homozygous *PTRF* mutations identified in CGL4 patients have been reported: c.259C>T (p.Gln87*) and c.481–c.482insGTGA (p.Lys161Serfs*41) in two female Turkish teenagers [43, 88]; c.176A>T (p.Asp59Val) and c.471G>C (p.Gln157Hisfs*52) in patients from Switzerland and Egypt, respectively [89]; c.550G>T (p.Glu184*) in a Saudi family [90]; c.947delA in child of Moroccan origin [76]; and c.696_697insC in a Japanese boy [91].

As mentioned before, cavin-1 interacts with caveolin proteins to form caveolae and to mediate cellular trafficking and lipid turnover [70, 85]. Cavin-1 can stabilize caveolae and caveolin proteins probably via its interactions with cytoskeleton [20]. In agreement with this finding, *Ptrf*$^{-/-}$ mice do not possess morphologically detectable caveolae and exhibit dramatically impaired expression of all three caveolin isoforms [92]. Specifically, cavin-1 colocalizes with caveolin-1 in adipocytes [93]. Paradoxically, it is believed that PTRF deficiency, as seen with loss of *CAV1*, causes generalized lipodystrophy due to the defects in caveolar formation [1, 20]. Recently, Liu and Pilch have demonstrated that the insulin-induced phosphorylation of cavin-1 results in its translocation to the nucleus where it regulates ribosomal transcription [94]. Primary and cultured cavin-1-deficient adipocytes have much lower levels of ribosomal RNA and proteins, resulting in ribosomal stress, which in turn leads to fat loss over time. This caveolae-independent cavin-1 function provides a novel explanation to CGL4 phenotype [95]. *PTRF* also serves as a terminator transcription factor via its interactions with both the thyroid transcription factor 1 (TFF-1) and RNA polymerase 1. cDNA cloning and functional characterization were initially reported by Jansa et al. in 1998 [94].

Ptrf$^{-/-}$ mice are viable with no overt change in body weight; nonetheless, they exhibit considerably reduced adipose tissue mass, high circulating triglyceride levels, glucose intolerance, and hyperinsulinemia, phenocopying lipodystrophy as seen in humans [92]. Notably, there is no morphologically detectable caveolae in *Ptrf*$^{-/-}$ mice, due to the absence of cavin-1 protein [85, 92]. Epididymal white adipocytes from *Ptrf*$^{-/-}$ mice were smaller as the result of reduced triglyceride accumulation due to decreased fatty acid uptake and incorporation [92]. In addition, they are insensitive to insulin; as a result, lacked insulin-stimulated glucose transport [96]. Both *Cav1*$^{-/-}$ and *Ptrf*$^{-/-}$ white adipocytes are resistant to lipolytic stimulation due to impaired perilipin phosphorylation [72, 96]. Much as *Ptrf*$^{-/-}$ mice are resistant to diet-induced obesity as seen in cav1$^{-/-}$ mice, BAT and liver exhibited abnormal lipid metabolism [96].

3. Familial partial dystrophy

3.1 Type 1 FPLD (FPLD1)

Type 1 FPLD (OMIM #608600), also known as Köbberling-type lipodystrophy, was first reported by Köbberling et al. in 1971 [97]. The syndrome manifests loss of subcutaneous fat in the extremities and gluteus, with normal or increased fat deposition in the face, neck, and trunk [97]. The ratio of skin thickness from the abdomen to the thigh is significantly higher in these subjects, which can be used as a diagnostic method [98]. Diabetes and other metabolic complications including hypertension, insulin resistance, and severe hypertriglyceridemia develop during adulthood, with higher severity in women than men [98, 99]. Similar to other types of lipodystrophy, FPLD1 is an extremely rare genetic condition whose chance of occurrence is 1 in 15 million [6, 36]. Unfortunately, the causative loci for FPLD1 have not been identified to unravel the underlying genetic mechanism of the syndrome.

3.2 Type 2 FPLD (FPLD2) and LMNA

FPLD2 (OMIM #151660) is an autosomal dominant condition that is caused by heterozygous mutations in the *LMNA* gene located on chromosome 1q21–1q22. In contrast to FPLD1 patients who preserve trunk fat, FPLD2 subjects suffer variable and progressive fat loss from the anterior abdomen and chest that occurs after the gradual loss of subcutaneous fat in extremities [6]. Accompanying the loss of subcutaneous fat is the accumulation of intramuscular (in limbs) and intra-abdominal fat [100]. Despite the similar pattern of fat loss in men and women, women are more prone to develop diabetes, dyslipidemia, and cardiovascular diseases [99].

Most cases of FPLD2 are caused by mutations in the lamin A/lamin C (*LMNA*) gene at the codon position 482 in exon 8 with a variety of mutations, such as p.R482W, p.R482Q, and p.R482L [101, 102]. Subsequently, many more missense mutations in *LMNA* have been reported including p.D230N, p.R399C, p.R439C, p.G465D, p.R471G, p.P485R, p.K486 N, and p.H506D [6, 103, 104]. In the past 3 years, several novel variants of LMNA have been identified such as c.1634G>A (p.R545H) [105], c.1001_1003delGCC (p.S334del) [106], c.175C>CG (p.L59 V) [107], c.683A>T (p.E228V) [108], c.139G>A (p. D47N) [109], and c.1543A>G (p.K515E) [110]. Notably, mandibuloacral dysplasia type A (MADA), an autosomal recessive disorder, is also caused by homozygous mutations of the *LMNA* gene. Although MADA is a form of lipodystrophy, it is distinctive from FPLD2 [101].

The *LMNA* gene encodes proteins lamin A and lamin C in the nuclear lamina [102]. The lamin proteins have been shown to be able to interact with and affect other regulatory proteins such as chromatin and transcription factors [101]. Therefore, any defects in this structural protein might disrupt the formation and integrity of the nuclear envelope, leading to premature cell death in many tissues, including adipocytes [6, 12]. Recently, lamin A and lamin C have been shown to interact with sterol response element-binding protein 1 (SREBP1), a transcription factor for genes involved in lipid metabolism and adipocyte differentiation [111]. Interestingly, the overexpression of the R482W mutation in primary human preadipocytes and endogenous expression of A-type lamins R482W in fibroblasts of FPLD2 patient fibroblasts impaired the interaction with SREBP1 and thus upregulate many SREBP1target genes [112]. This implies overexpression of SREBP1might lead to the inhibition of adipogenic in FPLD2, which opens a window of SREBP1-targeting therapies against FPLD2 [112].

Lmna$^{-/-}$ mice have been employed to study dilated cardiomyopathy and muscular dystrophy [113]. In both WAT and BAT of *Lmna*$^{-/-}$ mice, rapamycin inhibits mTORC1 but not mTORC2, leading to the suppression of lipolysis and the restoration of thermogenic uncoupling protein 1 (UCP1) levels, respectively. It indicates that altered mTOR signaling in *Lmna*$^{-/-}$ mice contributes to lipodystrophic phenotype that can be rescued with rapamycin [113].

Lamin A is maturated from pre-lamin A via multiple-step posttranslational modifications [114]. This process involves a cleavage reaction carried out by an endoplasmic reticulum membrane protease full name ZMPSTE24 located on chromosome 1p34 [115]. Mutations in ZMPSTE24 have been shown to cause mandibuloacral dysplasia type B and autosomal-dominant FPLD2, due to the lack of functional lamin A [116]. Nonetheless, the question as to whether there is an accumulation of pre-lamin A remains controversial. On the one hand, using lamin A/lamin C antibodies and pre-lamin A-specific monoclonal antibodies, one recent study has shown that fibroblasts carrying lipodystrophy-related LMNA mutations (R482W, I299V, C591F, T528 M) do not exhibit an accumulation of pre-lamin A as compared with their WT counterpart [117]. On the other hand, one prior study has demonstrated that the pre-lamin A level is upregulated in *zmpste24*$^{-/-}$ mice [117].

3.3 Type 3 FPLD (FPLD3) and PPRAG

FPLD3 (OMIM #151660) is caused by mutations in the *PPRAG* gene on chromosome 3p25. The *PPRAG* gene encodes PPARγ, a nuclear hormone receptor involved in glucose metabolism, adipocyte differentiation, inflammation, and carcinogenesis [118–126]. Importantly, PPARγ is the master transcription factor that governs 60% of genes involved in adipogenesis [127]. Differential RNA splicing along with alternative

PPARγ gives rise to different isoforms of PPARγ. While PPARγ 1 and PPARγ3 are ubiquitously expressed in most differentiated cells, PPARγ 2 and PPARγ 4 are strictly found in adipose tissue [126]. PPARγ has three functional domains: a ligand-binding domain (LBD), a DNA-binding domain (DBD), and an A/B domain [126]. Mutations in the PPARγ gene that lead to FLPD have been reported since 1999, mainly in the LBD and DBD [121, 126]. These mutations cause either haploinsufficiency or dysfunction in the normal receptor protein. It has been found that four out of seven mutations in the LBD result in reduced PPARγ activity [118]. For the mutations in the DBD, three out of six cause dysfunction in the wild-type protein [122]. In some cases, loss of function mutations in one of the alleles is also able to induce FLPD3 [126]. A D424N mutation found in two FPLD3 patients in the LBD leads to the downregulation of PPARγ-related transcriptional activity [124]. This loss-of-function effect can be rescued and corrected by the PPARγ agonist rosiglitazone [122]. In fact, treatment with 1 μmol/l or 10 μmol/l of rosiglitazone is able to normalize transcriptional activity of D424N PPARγ [126].

FPLD3 patients with PPARγ-induced FPLD suffer metabolic disorders including hypertriglyceridemia, insulin resistance with raised serum triglyceride and cholesterol levels and raised aminotransferase, and γ-glutamyltranspeptidase activities as well as manifest the symptoms of FPLD including subcutaneous fat loss from the arms, muscular hypertrophy in the legs, and arterial hypertension while having the subcutaneous fat buildup in the face, chin, trunk, and abdomen [128].

3.4 Type 4 FPLD (FPLD4) and PLIN1

It has been reported that null mutations in the *PLIN1* gene causes FPLD4 (OMIM #613877). *PLIN1* encodes perilipin 1 which is found in adipocytes as a LD surface protein [129]. Dysfunction of this protein is likely to cause FPLD4 via in the regulation of LDs and reduced fat mass [130]. However, a latest study using targeted next-generation sequencing of the *PLIN1* gene from 2208 individuals has revealed that haploinsufficiency in *PLIN1* does not result in FPLD [107].

3.5 Type 5 FPLD (FPLD5) and CIDEC

The rare FPLD5 (OMIM #615238) is caused by a homozygous nonsense mutation in the LD protein cell death-inducing Dffa-like effector C (*CIDEC*). The FPLD5 condition is manifested in a 19-year-old Ecuadorian girl with muscular lower limbs and prominent acanthosis nigricans [131]. The mutation induces a premature truncation of the CIDEC protein, and thus it restricts the LD expansion [132]. In fact, *Cidec*$^{-/-}$ mice have a reduced fat mass and impaired white adipocyte differentiation with multilocular LDs [133]. They are resistant to diet-induced obesity and insulin resistance as seen in the patient [133]. It is deduced from the observations in this study that CIDEC plays an indispensable role in the LD fusion, particularly for the development of unilocular LDs [108].

3.6 Type 6 FPLD (FPLD6) and LIPE

Exome sequencing has revealed another novel case of FPLD6 (OMIM #615980) that is caused by a homozygous nonsense mutation in the *LIPE* gene on chromosome 19. *LIPE* gene encodes hormone-sensitive lipase (HSL). HSL plays a vital role in lipolysis in which TAG and DAG are hydrolyzed to fatty acids in time of energy need [109]. Patients with FPLD6 have reduced lipolysis, small adipocytes, insulin resistance, and inflammation [134]. In addition, these patients exhibit downregulation of the PPARγ-induced genes in their adipose tissue, which suggests an inhibitory effect on the regulation of adipogenesis. Two FPLD6 patients from Italy have been reported to have mild muscular dystrophy with an increased serum creatine kinase level as well as other metabolic features such as dyslipidemia and diabetes [135]. In rodents, HSL also plays an important role in reproduction, specifically in male testes where it participates in steroid hormone synthesis from cholesterol [136]. In fact, *Lipe*$^{-/-}$ mice manifest impaired spermatogenesis, azoospermia, and male infertility [136].

3.7 Type 7 FPLD (FPLD7) and CAV1

FPLD7 (OMIM #606721) is also caused by the mutation in the *CAV1* gene on chromosome 7q31. Different from the CGL3 that is caused by homozygous mutation in *CAV1*, FPLD7 results from a heterozygous mutation in the gene. *CAV1* gene encodes caveolin-1 [60]. Very few cases of FPLD7 have been reported in humans. These FPLD7 patients share common symptoms and complications of FPLD including deficiency in subcutaneous fat, poor weight gain, development of congenital cataracts, insulin resistance, hyperlipidemia, and muscle weakness [62].

4. Acquired partial lipodystrophy (APL)

4.1 Barraquer-Simons syndrome

Barraquer-Simons syndrome (OMIM #608709) is named after Barraquer and Simons who first described the disease in the 1900s. Unlike other lipodystrophies, Barraquer-Simons syndrome occurs not due to inherited genetic mutations but normally derives from an acute viral transfection, such as measles [60]. Barraquer-Simons syndrome is extremely rare, with approximately 250 cases that have been reported in the literature with a male-to-female ratio of 1:4 [137]. The syndrome results in loss of subcutaneous fat mainly in the upper part of the body (face, neck, arms, and thorax) and upper abdomen; however, some adipose tissues are preserved in the gluteal regions and lower extremities [138]. Fortunately, Barraquer-Simons syndrome does not normally induce other metabolic complications such as insulin resistance, diabetes, and hypertriglyceridemia [137].

4.2 Highly active antiretroviral therapy (HAART)-induced lipodystrophy (LD-HIV)

LD-HIV can develop in some HIV-infected individuals who are undergoing antiretroviral therapy of more than 2 years [139]. Several cases have been reported since 1998 [140]. The toxicity of the treatment might result from HIV-1 protease inhibitors and nucleoside reverse-transcriptase inhibitors [141]. The latter ones have been shown to disrupt lipid metabolism and mitochondrial functions [141]. In patients with LD-HIV, subcutaneous fat loss occurs in the arms, legs, and face throughout the treatment course and does not cease after the therapy is discontinued [139]. Fortunately, this type of APL does not result in diabetes and insulin resistance, but some individuals might experience some conditions such as hypertriglyceridemia and coronary heart disease [139].

5. Management

Patients with lipodystrophy normally seek medical treatments toward the specific symptoms that they encounter. Since the disease affects its patients in multiple aspects, care and management require a multidisciplinary team involving pediatricians, surgeons, cardiologists, endocrinologists, nutritionists, and psychiatrists [20]. Mental health supports should also be made to patients who suffer depressions from the diagnosis and anxieties about their appearance [142]. In addition, special education might be necessary for those who have an intellectual disability [142]. Furthermore, such cosmetic surgery as reconstructive facial surgery and bilateral gluteus maximus muscle flap advance might benefit the patients in improving their appearance and quality of life [20].

Dietary restriction is of paramount importance in the disease management. Particularly, those with CGL should follow a high-carb and low-fat diet, since it can raise very-low-density lipoprotein (VLDL) TAG levels while alleviating chylomicronemia [143]. Sufficient energy supply along with regular exercise is highly important in children with CGL to ensure their normal growth [20]. However, strenuous exercise is not recommended for CGL4 patients who can be treated with β-adrenergic blockers along with other antiarrhythmic medications to prevent catecholaminergic polymorphic ventricular tachycardia [144]. Also, in this case, an implantable pacemaker or defibrillator can be quite beneficial [144]. It remains unclear whether patients with CGL2 and cardiomyopathy should restrict exercise [145].

The first-line therapy for diabetes mellitus, such as metformin and sulphonylureas, can be prescribed to patients with CGL [146]. The lack of subcutaneous fat in the abdomen and thighs might pose a potential barrier for insulin injection, and the patients might necessitate higher doses of insulin [147]. Furthermore, kidney damage such as diabetic nephropathy and end-stage renal disease might occur in patients with long-standing diabetes as the result high blood glucose exposure. Treatments for such condition might involve hemodialysis and kidney transplantation [20].

Metreleptin can be a promising therapeutic drug in the near future as recent studies have shown its potency in improving metabolic complications involving diabetes mellitus, hypertriglyceridemia, and hepatic steatosis in CGL [146, 148–151]. In fact, 63% reduction in circulating levels of TAG along with 30% increase in insulin sensitivity, and 20% reduction in liver volume are observed in seven patients treated with metreleptin over the period of 4 months [20]. Three patients with CGL2 and two patients with CGL treated with recombinant leptin therapy in Japan during the treatment course of 36 months have shown ameliorated fasting glucose and TAG levels as well as increased insulin sensitivity [152]. Metreleptin therapy can also reduce symptoms of other conditions such as macroalbuminuria, microalbuminuria, and hyperfiltration as well as improve the balance in sex hormone profile [151, 152]. Patients treated with metreleptin might suffer such adverse effects as hypoglycemia, headache, nausea, decreased weight, and abdominal pain [153, 154]. In addition, there is a rare possibility that antileptin antibodies might develop severe infections [154]. Metreleptin therapy can reduce appetite signaled from the hypothalamus, as *Agpat2*$^{-/-}$ mice with selective deletion of leptin receptor do not respond to the treatment [153]. The use of metreleptin in combination with dietary management has been approved by the Food and Drug Administration in the treatment for patients with CGL and APL in 2014, and Japan has approved it to be an anti-lipodystrophic drug in 2013 [20].

6. Conclusions

Lipodystrophy is a rare genetic disease characterized by near-total loss or partial loss of body fat. The syndrome can result in an array of metabolic complications such as insulin resistance, type 2 diabetes, hypertriglyceridemia, and hepatic steatosis. The disease is managed with dietary restriction and exercise programs in line with the leptin therapy.

Author details

Long Hoa Chung and Yanfei Qi*
Centenary Institute, The University of Sydney, Sydney, Australia

*Address all correspondence to: j.qi@centenary.org.au

References

[1] Robbins AL, Savage DB. The genetics of lipid storage and human lipodystrophies. Trends in Molecular Medicine. 2015;**21**(7):433-438

[2] Coelho M, Oliveira T, Fernandes R. Biochemistry of adipose tissue: An endocrine organ. Archives of Medical Science: AMS. 2013;**9**(2):191-200

[3] Jo J et al. Hypertrophy and/or hyperplasia: Dynamics of adipose tissue growth. PLoS Computational Biology. 2009;**5**(3):e1000324-e1000324

[4] Cohen P, Spiegelman BM. Cell biology of fat storage. Molecular Biology of the Cell. 2016;**27**(16):2523-2527

[5] Qi Y, Sun L, Yang H. Lipid droplet growth and adipocyte development: Mechanistically distinct processes connected by phospholipids. Biochimica et Biophysica Acta (BBA)—Molecular and Cell Biology of Lipids. 2017;**1862**(10, Part B):1273-1283

[6] Garg A. Acquired and inherited lipodystrophies. New England Journal of Medicine. 2004;**350**(12):1220-1234

[7] Agarwal AK et al. Phenotypic and genetic heterogeneity in congenital generalized lipodystrophy. The Journal of Clinical Endocrinology and Metabolism. 2003;**88**(10):4840-4847

[8] Van Maldergem L et al. Genotype-phenotype relationships in Berardinelli-Seip congenital lipodystrophy. Journal of Medical Genetics. 2002;**39**(10):722-733

[9] Garg A. Lipodystrophies: Genetic and acquired body fat disorders. The Journal of Clinical Endocrinology & Metabolism. 2011;**96**(11):3313-3325

[10] Brown WV et al. JCL roundtable: Diagnosis and clinical management of lipodystrophy. Journal of Clinical Lipidology. 2016;**10**(4):728-736

[11] Agarwal AK et al. AGPAT2 is mutated in congenital generalized lipodystrophy linked to chromosome 9q34. Nature Genetics. 2002;**31**(1):21-23

[12] Garg A. Clinical review#: Lipodystrophies: Genetic and acquired body fat disorders. The Journal of Clinical Endocrinology and Metabolism. 2011;**96**(11):3313-3325

[13] Haghighi A et al. Congenital generalized lipodystrophy: Identification of novel variants and expansion of clinical spectrum. Clinical Genetics. 2016;**89**(4):434-441

[14] Rostami P et al. AGPAT2 gene mutation in a child with Berardinelli-Seip congenital lipodystrophy syndrome. Annales d'endocrinologie. 2013;**74**(1):59-61

[15] Haghighi A et al. Identification of a novel nonsense mutation and a missense substitution in the AGPAT2 gene causing congenital generalized lipodystrophy type 1. European Journal of Medical Genetics. 2012;**55**(11):620-624

[16] Cortes VA et al. Divergent metabolic phenotype between two sisters with congenital generalized lipodystrophy due to double AGPAT2 homozygous mutations. A clinical, genetic and in silico study. PLoS One. 2014;**9**(1):e87173

[17] Nagle CA, Klett EL, Coleman RA. Hepatic triacylglycerol accumulation and insulin resistance. Journal of Lipid Research. 2009;**50**(Suppl):S74-S79

[18] West J et al. Cloning and expression of two human lysophosphatidic acid acyltransferase cDNAs that enhance cytokine-induced signaling responses in cells. DNA and Cell Biology. 1997;**16**(6):691-701

[19] Gale SE et al. A regulatory role for 1-acylglycerol-3-phosphate-

O-acyltransferase 2 in adipocyte differentiation. The Journal of Biological Chemistry. 2006;**281**(16):11082-11089

[20] Patni N, Garg A. Congenital generalized lipodystrophies—New insights into metabolic dysfunction. Nature Reviews. Endocrinology. 2015;**11**(9):522-534

[21] Qi Y et al. CDP-diacylglycerol synthases regulate the growth of lipid droplets and adipocyte development. Journal of Lipid Research. 2016;**57**(5):767-780

[22] Choi SY et al. A common lipid links Mfn-mediated mitochondrial fusion and SNARE-regulated exocytosis. Nature Cell Biology. 2006;**8**(11):1255-1262

[23] Vitale N et al. Phospholipase D1: A key factor for the exocytotic machinery in neuroendocrine cells. The EMBO Journal. 2001;**20**(10):2424-2434

[24] Paar M et al. Remodeling of lipid droplets during lipolysis and growth in adipocytes. The Journal of Biological Chemistry. 2012;**287**(14):11164-11173

[25] Moseti D, Regassa A, Kim W-K. Molecular regulation of adipogenesis and potential anti-adipogenic bioactive molecules. International Journal of Molecular Sciences. 2016;**17**(1):124

[26] Beigneux AP et al. Agpat6—A novel lipid biosynthetic gene required for triacylglycerol production in mammary epithelium. Journal of Lipid Research. 2006;**47**(4):734-744

[27] Buhman KK et al. DGAT1 is not essential for intestinal triacylglycerol absorption or chylomicron synthesis. The Journal of Biological Chemistry. 2002;**277**(28):25474-25479

[28] Hammond LE et al. Mitochondrial glycerol-3-phosphate acyltransferase-deficient mice have reduced weight and liver triacylglycerol content and altered glycerolipid fatty acid composition. Molecular and Cellular Biology. 2002;**22**(23):8204-8214

[29] Stone SJ et al. Lipopenia and skin barrier abnormalities in DGAT2-deficient mice. The Journal of Biological Chemistry. 2004;**279**(12):11767-11776

[30] Vergnes L et al. Agpat6 deficiency causes subdermal lipodystrophy and resistance to obesity. The Journal of Lipid Research. 2006;**47**(4):745-754

[31] Cautivo KM et al. AGPAT2 is essential for postnatal development and maintenance of white and brown adipose tissue. Molecular Metabolism. 2016;**5**(7):491-505

[32] Cortes VA et al. Molecular mechanisms of hepatic steatosis and insulin resistance in the AGPAT2-deficient mouse model of congenital generalized lipodystrophy. Cell Metabolism. 2009;**9**(2):165-176

[33] Agarwal AK et al. Human 1-acylglycerol-3-phosphate O-acyltransferase isoforms 1 and 2: Biochemical characterization and inability to rescue hepatic steatosis in Agpat2(-/-) gene lipodystrophic mice. The Journal of Biological Chemistry. 2011;**286**(43):37676-37691

[34] Sankella S et al. Hepatic gluconeogenesis is enhanced by phosphatidic acid which remains uninhibited by insulin in lipodystrophic Agpat2-/- mice. The Journal of Biological Chemistry. 2014;**289**(8):4762-4777

[35] Fernandez-Galilea M et al. AGPAT2 deficiency impairs adipogenic differentiation in primary cultured preadipocytes in a non-autophagy or apoptosis dependent mechanism. Biochemical and Biophysical Research Communications. 2015;**467**(1):39-45

[36] Nolis T. Exploring the pathophysiology behind the more common genetic and acquired lipodystrophies. Journal of Human Genetics. 2014;**59**(1):16-23

[37] Subauste AR et al. Alterations in lipid signaling underlie lipodystrophy secondary to AGPAT2 mutations. Diabetes. 2012;**61**(11):2922-2931

[38] Cortes VA et al. Leptin ameliorates insulin resistance and hepatic steatosis in Agpat2-/- lipodystrophic mice independent of hepatocyte leptin receptors. Journal of Lipid Research. 2014;**55**(2):276-288

[39] Magré J et al. Identification of the gene altered in Berardinelli-Seip congenital lipodystrophy on chromosome 11q13. Nature Genetics. 2001;**28**(4):365-370

[40] Liu L et al. Adipose-specific knockout of SEIPIN/BSCL2 results in progressive lipodystrophy. Diabetes. 2014;**63**(7):2320

[41] Simha V, Garg A. Phenotypic heterogeneity in body fat distribution in patients with congenital generalized lipodystrophy caused by mutations in the AGPAT2 or seipin genes. The Journal of Clinical Endocrinology and Metabolism. 2003;**88**(11):5433-5437

[42] Haque WA et al. Serum adiponectin and leptin levels in patients with lipodystrophies. The Journal of Clinical Endocrinology & Metabolism. 2002;**87**(5):2395-2398

[43] Akinci B et al. Natural history of congenital generalized lipodystrophy: A nationwide study from Turkey. The Journal of Clinical Endocrinology and Metabolism. 2016;**101**(7):2759-2767

[44] Lungu AO et al. Insulin resistance is a sufficient basis for hyperandrogenism in lipodystrophic women with polycystic ovarian syndrome. The Journal of Clinical Endocrinology and Metabolism. 2012;**97**(2):563-567

[45] Schuster J et al. Exome sequencing circumvents missing clinical data and identifies a BSCL2 mutation in congenital lipodystrophy. BMC Medical Genetics. 2014;**15**:71

[46] Windpassinger C et al. Heterozygous missense mutations in BSCL2 are associated with distal hereditary motor neuropathy and Silver syndrome. Nature Genetics. 2004;**36**(3):271-276

[47] Agarwal AK, Garg A. Seipin: A mysterious protein. Trends in Molecular Medicine. 2004;**10**(9):440-444

[48] Yang WL et al. BSCL2/seipin regulates adipogenesis through actin cytoskeleton remodelling. Human Molecular Genetics. 2014;**23**(2):502-513

[49] Cartwright BR et al. Seipin performs dissectible functions in promoting lipid droplet biogenesis and regulating droplet morphology. Molecular Biology of the Cell. 2015;**26**(4):726-739

[50] Szymanski KM et al. The lipodystrophy protein seipin is found at endoplasmic reticulum lipid droplet junctions and is important for droplet morphology. Proceedings of the National Academy of Sciences of the United States of America. 2007;**104**(52):20890-20895

[51] Salo VT et al. Seipin regulates ER-lipid droplet contacts and cargo delivery. The EMBO Journal. 2016;**35**(24):2699-2716

[52] Talukder MMU et al. Seipin oligomers can interact directly with AGPAT2 and lipin 1, physically scaffolding critical regulators of adipogenesis. Molecular Metabolism. 2015;**4**(3):199-209

[53] Sim MFM et al. Analysis of naturally occurring mutations in the human lipodystrophy protein

seipin reveals multiple potential pathogenic mechanisms. Diabetologia. 2013;**56**(11):2498-2506

[54] Cui X et al. Seipin ablation in mice results in severe generalized lipodystrophy. Human Molecular Genetics. 2011;**20**(15):3022-3030

[55] Chen W et al. Altered lipid metabolism in residual white adipose tissues of Bscl2 deficient mice. PLoS One. 2013;**8**(12):e82526

[56] Prieur X et al. Thiazolidinediones partially reverse the metabolic disturbances observed in Bscl2/seipin-deficient mice. Diabetologia. 2013;**56**(8):1813-1825

[57] Chen W et al. Molecular mechanisms underlying fasting modulated liver insulin sensitivity and metabolism in male lipodystrophic Bscl2/Seipin-deficient mice. Endocrinology. 2014;**155**(11):4215-4225

[58] Chen W et al. Berardinelli-seip congenital lipodystrophy 2/seipin is a cell-autonomous regulator of lipolysis essential for adipocyte differentiation. Molecular and Cellular Biology. 2012;**32**(6):1099-1111

[59] Boutet E et al. Seipin deficiency alters fatty acid Δ9 desaturation and lipid droplet formation in Berardinelli-Seip congenital lipodystrophy. Biochimie. 2009;**91**(6):796-803

[60] Kim CA et al. Association of a homozygous nonsense caveolin-1 mutation with Berardinelli-Seip congenital lipodystrophy. The Journal of Clinical Endocrinology and Metabolism. 2008;**93**(4):1129-1134

[61] Cao H et al. Heterozygous CAV1 frameshift mutations (MIM 601047) in patients with atypical partial lipodystrophy and hypertriglyceridemia. Lipids in Health and Disease. 2008;7:3

[62] Garg A et al. Whole exome sequencing identifies de novo heterozygous CAV1 mutations associated with a novel neonatal onset lipodystrophy syndrome. American Journal of Medical Genetics. Part A. 2015;**167A**(8):1796-1806

[63] Schrauwen I et al. A frame-shift mutation in CAV1 is associated with a severe neonatal progeroid and lipodystrophy syndrome. PLoS One. 2015;**10**(7):e0131797

[64] Han B et al. Characterization of a caveolin-1 mutation associated with both pulmonary arterial hypertension and congenital generalized lipodystrophy. Traffic. 2016;**17**(12):1297-1312

[65] Rothberg KG et al. Caveolin, a protein component of caveolae membrane coats. Cell. 1992;**68**(4):673-682

[66] Brown MS, Goldstein JL. Richard G.W. Anderson (1940-2011) and the birth of receptor-mediated endocytosis. The Journal of Cell Biology. 2011;**193**(4):601-603

[67] Glenney JR Jr. The sequence of human caveolin reveals identity with VIP21, a component of transport vesicles. FEBS Letters. 1992;**314**(1):45-48

[68] Williams TM, Lisanti MP. The caveolin proteins. Genome Biology. 2004;**5**(3):214-214

[69] Stan RV. Structure of caveolae. Biochimica et Biophysica Acta (BBA)—Molecular. Cell Research. 2005;**1746**(3):334-348

[70] Shvets E, Ludwig A, Nichols BJ. News from the caves: Update on the structure and function of caveolae. Current Opinion in Cell Biology. 2014;**29**:99-106

[71] Fridolfsson HN et al. Regulation of intracellular signaling and

function by caveolin. FASEB Journal. 2014;**28**(9):3823-3831

[72] Cohen AW et al. Role of caveolin-1 in the modulation of lipolysis and lipid droplet formation. Diabetes. 2004;**53**(5):1261-1270

[73] Parton RG, del Pozo MA. Caveolae as plasma membrane sensors, protectors and organizers. Nature Reviews Molecular Cell Biology. 2013;**14**(2):98-112

[74] Razani B, Lisanti MP. Caveolin-deficient mice: Insights into caveolar function human disease. The Journal of Clinical Investigation. 2001;**108**(11):1553-1561

[75] Briand N et al. Caveolin-1 expression and cavin stability regulate caveolae dynamics in adipocyte lipid store fluctuation. Diabetes. 2014;**63**(12):4032-4044

[76] Ardissone A et al. Novel PTRF mutation in a child with mild myopathy and very mild congenital lipodystrophy. BMC Medical Genetics. 2013;**14**:89

[77] Dwianingsih EK et al. A Japanese child with asymptomatic elevation of serum creatine kinase shows PTRF-CAVIN mutation matching with congenital generalized lipodystrophy type 4. Molecular Genetics and Metabolism. 2010;**101**(2-3):233-237

[78] Rajab A et al. Fatal cardiac arrhythmia and long-QT syndrome in a new form of congenital generalized lipodystrophy with muscle rippling (CGL4) due to PTRF-CAVIN mutations. PLoS Genetics. 2010;**6**(3):e1000874

[79] Codenotti S et al. Caveolin-1, Caveolin-2 and Cavin-1 are strong predictors of adipogenic differentiation in human tumors and cell lines of liposarcoma. European Journal of Cell Biology. 2016;**95**(8):252-264

[80] Zhao Y-Y et al. Persistent eNOS activation secondary to caveolin-1 deficiency induces pulmonary hypertension in mice and humans through PKG nitration. The Journal of Clinical Investigation. 2009;**119**(7):2009-2018

[81] Asterholm IW et al. Altered mitochondrial function and metabolic inflexibility associated with loss of caveolin-1. Cell Metabolism. 2012;**15**(2):171-185

[82] Martin S et al. Caveolin-1 deficiency leads to increased susceptibility to cell death and fibrosis in white adipose tissue: Characterization of a lipodystrophic model. PLoS One. 2012;**7**(9):e46242

[83] Rajab A et al. Heterogeneity for congenital generalized lipodystrophy in seventeen patients from Oman. American Journal of Medical Genetics. 2002;**110**(3):219-225

[84] Heathcote K et al. Molecular analysis of Berardinelli-Seip congenital lipodystrophy in Oman: Evidence for multiple loci. Diabetes. 2002;**51**(4):1291-1293

[85] Hayashi YK et al. Human PTRF mutations cause secondary deficiency of caveolins resulting in muscular dystrophy with generalized lipodystrophy. The Journal of Clinical Investigation. 2009;**119**(9):2623-2633

[86] Simha V et al. Novel subtype of congenital generalized lipodystrophy associated with muscular weakness and cervical spine instability. American Journal of Medical Genetics. Part A. 2008;**146A**(18):2318-2326

[87] Shastry S et al. Congenital generalized lipodystrophy, type 4 (CGL4) associated with myopathy due to novel PTRF mutations. American Journal of Medical Genetics. Part A. 2010;**152A**(9):2245-2253

[88] Akinci G et al. Spectrum of clinical manifestations in two young Turkish patients with congenital generalized lipodystrophy type 4. European Journal of Medical Genetics. 2016;**59**(6-7):320-324

[89] Salle-Teyssieres L et al. Maladaptative autophagy impairs adipose function in congenital generalized ipodystrophy due to Cavin-1 Deficiency. The Journal of Clinical Endocrinology and Metabolism. 2016;**101**(7):2892-2904

[90] Jelani M et al. Novel nonsense mutation in the PTRF gene underlies congenital generalized lipodystrophy in a consanguineous Saudi family. European Journal of Medical Genetics. 2015;**58**(4):216-221

[91] Murakami N et al. Congenital generalized lipodystrophy type 4 with muscular dystrophy: Clinical and pathological manifestations in early childhood. Neuromuscular Disorders. 2013;**23**(5):441-444

[92] Liu L et al. Deletion of Cavin/PTRF causes global loss of caveolae, dyslipidemia, and glucose intolerance. Cell Metabolism. 2008;**8**(4):310-317

[93] Liu L, Pilch PF. A critical role of cavin (polymerase I and transcript release factor) in caveolae formation and organization. The Journal of Biological Chemistry. 2008;**283**(7):4314-4322

[94] Jansa P et al. Cloning and functional characterization of PTRF, a novel protein which induces dissociation of paused ternary transcription complexes. The EMBO Journal. 1998;**17**(10):2855-2864

[95] Liu L, Pilch PF. PTRF/Cavin-1 promotes efficient ribosomal RNA transcription in response to metabolic challenges. Elife. 2016;**5**:e17508

[96] Ding SY et al. Pleiotropic effects of cavin-1 deficiency on lipid metabolism. The Journal of Biological Chemistry. 2014;**289**(12):8473-8483

[97] Kobberling J, Dunnigan MG. Familial partial lipodystrophy: Two types of an X linked dominant syndrome, lethal in the hemizygous state. Journal of Medical Genetics. 1986;**23**(2):120-127

[98] Herbst KL et al. Kobberling type of familial partial lipodystrophy: An underrecognized syndrome. Diabetes Care. 2003;**26**(6):1819-1824

[99] Garg A. Gender differences in the prevalence of metabolic complications in familial partial lipodystrophy (Dunnigan variety). The Journal of Clinical Endocrinology and Metabolism. 2000;**85**(5):1776-1782

[100] Garg A, Peshock RM, Fleckenstein JL. Adipose tissue distribution pattern in patients with familial partial lipodystrophy (Dunnigan variety). The Journal of Clinical Endocrinology and Metabolism. 1999;**84**(1):170-174

[101] Shackleton S et al. LMNA, encoding lamin A/C, is mutated in partial lipodystrophy. Nature Genetics. 2000;**24**(2):153-156

[102] Cao H, Hegele RA. Nuclear lamin A/C R482Q mutation in canadian kindreds with Dunnigan-type familial partial lipodystrophy. Human Molecular Genetics. 2000;**9**(1):109-112

[103] Scharner J et al. Mapping disease-related missense mutations in the immunoglobulin-like fold domain of lamin A/C reveals novel genotype-phenotype associations for laminopathies. Proteins. 2014;**82**(6):904-915

[104] Lanktree M et al. Novel LMNA mutations seen in patients with familial partial lipodystrophy subtype 2 (FPLD2; MIM 151660). Clinical Genetics. 2007;**71**(2):183-186

[105] Chan D et al. Familial partial lipodystrophy presenting as metabolic syndrome. Journal of Clinical Lipidology. 2016;**10**(6):1488-1491

[106] Madej-Pilarczyk A et al. Limb-girdle muscular dystrophy with severe heart failure overlapping with lipodystrophy in a patient with LMNA mutation p.Ser334del. Journal of Applied Genetics. 2017;**58**(1):87-91

[107] Guo X et al. A case of novel Lamin A/C mutation manifesting as atypical progeroid syndrome and cardiomyopathy. Canadian Journal of Cardiology. 2016;**32**(9):1166, e1129-e1131

[108] Ambrosi P et al. A novel overlapping phenotype characterized by lipodystrophy, mandibular dysplasia, and dilated cardiomyopathy associated with a new mutation in the LMNA gene. International Journal of Cardiology. 2016;**209**:317-318

[109] Kutbay NO et al. A case of familial partial lipodystrophy caused by a novel lamin A/C (LMNA) mutation in exon 1 (D47N). European Journal of Internal Medicine. 2016;**29**:37-39

[110] Chirico V et al. LMNA gene mutation as a model of cardiometabolic dysfunction: From genetic analysis to treatment response. Diabetes and Metabolism. 2014;**40**(3):224-228

[111] Lloyd DJ, Trembath RC, Shackleton S. A novel interaction between lamin A and SREBP1: Implications for partial lipodystrophy and other laminopathies. Human Molecular Genetics. 2002;**11**(7):769-777

[112] Vadrot N et al. The p.R482W substitution in A-type lamins deregulates SREBP1 activity in Dunnigan-type familial partial lipodystrophy. Human Molecular Genetics. 2015;**24**(7):2096-2109

[113] Liao CY et al. Rapamycin reverses metabolic deficits in Lamin A/C-deficient mice. Cell Reports. 2016;**17**(10):2542-2552

[114] Davies BSJ et al. The posttranslational processing of prelamin A and disease. Annual Review of Genomics and Human Genetics. 2009;**10**:153-174

[115] Lucas-Herald AK et al. Proteomic evidence of biological aging in a child with a compound heterozygous ZMPSTE24 mutation. Proteomics - Clinical Applications. 2019;**13**(2):e1800135-e1800135

[116] Novelli G et al. Mandibuloacral dysplasia is caused by a mutation in LMNA-encoding lamin A/C. American Journal of Human Genetics. 2002;**71**(2):426-431

[117] Tu Y et al. LMNA missense mutations causing familial partial lipodystrophy do not lead to an accumulation of prelamin A. Nucleus. 2016;**7**(5):512-521

[118] Barroso I et al. Dominant negative mutations in human PPARγ associated with severe insulin resistance, diabetes mellitus and hypertension. Nature. 1999;**402**(6764):880-883

[119] Agarwal AK, Garg A. A novel heterozygous mutation in peroxisome proliferator-activated receptor-γ gene in a patient with familial partial lipodystrophy. The Journal of Clinical Endocrinology and Metabolism. 2002;**87**(1):408

[120] Hegele RA et al. PPARG F388L, a transactivation-deficient mutant, in familial partial lipodystrophy. Diabetes. 2002;**51**(12):3586

[121] Al-Shali K et al. A single-base mutation in the peroxisome proliferator-activated receptor γ4 promoter associated with altered in vitro expression and partial lipodystrophy. The Journal of Clinical

Endocrinology and Metabolism. 2004;**89**(11):5655-5660

[122] Agostini M et al. Non-DNA binding, dominant-negative, human PPARγ mutations cause lipodystrophic insulin resistance. Cell Metabolism. 2006;**4**(4):303-311

[123] Francis GA et al. Peroxisomal proliferator activated receptor-gamma deficiency in a Canadian kindred with familial partial lipodystrophy type 3 (FPLD3). BMC Medical Genetics. 2006;**7**:3

[124] Hegele RA et al. A frameshift mutation in peroxisome-proliferator-activated receptor-γ in familial partial lipodystrophy subtype 3 (FPLD3; MIM 604367). Clinical Genetics. 2006;**70**(4):360-362

[125] Monajemi H et al. Familial partial lipodystrophy phenotype resulting from a single-base mutation in deoxyribonucleic acid-binding domain of peroxisome proliferator-activated receptor-γ. The Journal of Clinical Endocrinology and Metabolism. 2007;**92**(5):1606-1612

[126] Lüdtke A et al. New PPARG mutation leads to lipodystrophy and loss of protein function that is partially restored by a synthetic ligand. Journal of Medical Genetics. 2007;**44**(9):e88

[127] Lefterova MI et al. PPARgamma and C/EBP factors orchestrate adipocyte biology via adjacent binding on a genome-wide scale. Genes and Development. 2008;**22**(21):2941-2952

[128] Al-Attar SA et al. Quantitative and qualitative differences in subcutaneous adipose tissue stores across lipodystrophy types shown by magnetic resonance imaging. BMC Medical Imaging. 2007;**7**:3

[129] Itabe H et al. Perilipins: A diversity of intracellular lipid droplet proteins. Lipids in Health and Disease. 2017;**16**(1):83

[130] Kozusko K et al. Clinical and molecular characterization of a novel PLIN1 frameshift mutation identified in patients with familial partial lipodystrophy. Diabetes. 2015;**64**(1):299

[131] Rubio-Cabezas O et al. Partial lipodystrophy and insulin resistant diabetes in a patient with a homozygous nonsense mutation in CIDEC. EMBO Molecular Medicine. 2009;**1**(5):280-287

[132] Keller P et al. Fat-specific protein 27 regulates storage of triacylglycerol. The Journal of Biological Chemistry. 2008;**283**(21):14355-14365

[133] Nishino N et al. FSP27 contributes to efficient energy storage in murine white adipocytes by promoting the formation of unilocular lipid droplets. The Journal of Clinical Investigation. 2008;**118**(8):2808-2821

[134] Albert JS et al. Null mutation in hormone-sensitive lipase gene and risk of type 2 diabetes. New England Journal of Medicine. 2014;**370**(24):2307-2315

[135] Zolotov S et al. Homozygous LIPE mutation in siblings with multiple symmetric lipomatosis, partial lipodystrophy, and myopathy. American Journal of Medical Genetics. Part A. 2017;**173**(1):190-194

[136] Wang F et al. Hormone-sensitive lipase deficiency alters gene expression and cholesterol content of mouse testis. Reproduction (Cambridge, England). 2016;**153**(2):175-185

[137] Oliveira J et al. Barraquer-Simons syndrome: A rare form of acquired lipodystrophy. BMC Research Notes. 2016;**9**:175

[138] Ferrarini A et al. Two new cases of Barraquer–Simons syndrome. American

Journal of Medical Genetics Part A. 2004;**126A**(4):427-429

[139] Martínez E et al. Risk of lipodystrophy in HIV-1-infected patients treated with protease inhibitors: A prospective cohort study. The Lancet. 2001;**357**(9256):592-598

[140] Martínez E, Gatell JM. Metabolic abnormalities and body fat redistribution in HIV-1 infected patients: The lipodystrophy syndrome. Current Opinion in Infectious Diseases. 1999;**12**(1):13-19

[141] Carr A et al. Pathogenesis of HIV-1-protease inhibitor-associated peripheral lipodystrophy, hyperlipidaemia, and insulin resistance. The Lancet. 1998;**351**(9119):1881-1883

[142] Okada E, Iwahira Y, Maruyama Y. Buttock deformity repair for congenital generalized lipodystrophy. Plastic and Reconstructive Surgery. 1995;**95**(4):744-746

[143] Handelsman Y et al. The clinical approach to the detection of lipodystrophy—An AACE consensus statement. Endocrine Practice. 2013;**19**(1):107-116

[144] Napolitano C, Priori SG. Diagnosis and treatment of catecholaminergic polymorphic ventricular tachycardia. Heart Rhythm. 2007;**4**(5):675-678

[145] Simha V, Garg A. Inherited lipodystrophies and hypertriglyceridemia. Current Opinion in Lipidology. 2009;**20**(4):300-308

[146] Chan JL, Oral EA. Clinical classification and treatment of congenital and acquired lipodystrophy. Endocrine Practice. 2010;**16**(2):310-323

[147] McNally M et al. Successful renal transplantation in a patient with congenital generalized lipodystrophy: A case report. American Journal of Transplantation. 2004;**4**(3):447-449

[148] Oral EA et al. Leptin-replacement therapy for lipodystrophy. New England Journal of Medicine. 2002;**346**(8):570-578

[149] Araujo-Vilar D et al. Recombinant human leptin treatment in genetic lipodystrophic syndromes: The long-term Spanish experience. Endocrine. 2015;**49**(1):139-147

[150] Chan JL et al. Clinical effects of long-term metreleptin treatment in patients with lipodystrophy. Endocrine Practice. 2011;**17**(6):922-932

[151] Safar Zadeh E et al. The liver diseases of lipodystrophy: The long-term effect of leptin treatment. Journal of Hepatology. 2013;**59**(1):131-137

[152] Ebihara K et al. Efficacy and safety of leptin-replacement therapy and possible mechanisms of leptin actions in patients with generalized lipodystrophy. The Journal of Clinical Endocrinology and Metabolism. 2007;**92**(2):532-541

[153] Cortés VA et al. Leptin ameliorates insulin resistance and hepatic steatosis in Agpat2$^{-/-}$ lipodystrophic mice independent of hepatocyte leptin receptors. Journal of Lipid Research. 2014;**55**(2):276-288

[154] Oral EA, Chan JL. Rationale for leptin-replacement therapy for severe lipodystrophy. Endocrine Practice. 2010;**16**(2):324-333

Chapter 4

Bilateral Abductor Palsy in Neonates

Bigyan Raj Gyawali

Abstract

Paediatric airway compared to the adult has a considerable anatomical and physiological difference. Airway pathologies in neonates are very challenging in terms of diagnosis and management. Bilateral abductor paralysis is one of such situations. Despite being the second most common cause of stridor in paediatric population, the disease is still rare. Having a huge range of aetiological variations on one hand and the grievousness of pathology on the other, management of the disease is very challenging at times. Here, we present a review on various aetiological factors along with management of the disease.

Keywords: paediatric, airway, vocal fold, stridor, paralysis

1. Introduction

Airway pathologies in neonates are very challenging. Considering a wide variation in the anatomy and physiology compared to the adults, clinical approach to this population is entirely different.

Bilateral abductor paralysis means the failure of vocal cords to abduct resulting from denervation of recurrent laryngeal branch of vagus nerve. Although being a second most common cause of stridor in paediatric population, it is still a rare entity. The incidence in neonates is estimated to be 0.75 cases per million births per year [1]. There is no definite sex predilection. With no single definable cause and being a common presentation of wide range of pathologies, for example, congenital, neurological, traumatic etc., this is a topic that has to be critically explored.

2. Anatomy

2.1 Laryngeal framework

Paediatric airway differs considerably from adult airway. Location of the larynx in the neonates is high up in the neck opposite to cervical third and fourth vertebra which gradually descends down with age. Thyrohyoid membrane is short compared to the adult; thus, the thyroid notch lies either posterior or just inferior to the hyoid bone. Subglottis is the narrowest part of the larynx in neonates and the abundance of soft tissue in the subglottis and supraglottis make them vulnerable to swelling during inflammation. In the glottis, arytenoids make up the 50% of antero-posterior length and the vocal cords, next 50%.

2.2 Laryngeal musculature

Larynx comprises of two groups of muscles: intrinsic and extrinsic. Intrinsic muscles are usually responsible for various movements of vocal cords. Posterior cricoarytenoid is the only muscle of the larynx that abducts the vocal cords. Lateral cricoarytenoid and interarytenoid muscles act as adductor of the vocal cord. Thyroarytenoid and cricothyroid muscles act as tensor of the vocal cords.

2.3 Nerve supply

Both sensory and motor supplies to larynx come from vagus nerve via superior and recurrent laryngeal nerve. All the muscles of the larynx are supplied by recurrent laryngeal nerve except for the cricothyroid, which is supplied by the external branch of superior laryngeal nerve. Sensory supply of the supraglottis and glottis is provided by the internal branch of superior laryngeal nerve, and the subglottis is provided by recurrent laryngeal nerve.

The abductor fibers in the recurrent laryngeal nerve are phylogenetically newer compared to the adductor fibers and occupy the periphery of the nerve. This makes them more vulnerable to injury from any organic lesion (*Semon's law*).

3. Aetiology

3.1 Congenital causes

Congenital bilateral abductor palsy may present immediately or within few days of birth. Child may present with stridor, weak cry, cyanosis, or difficulty in feeding. Aetiological factors can be broadly classified into genetic or nongenetic.

3.1.1 Genetic

Bilateral abductor palsy presenting with the genetic etiology is very rare. Presentation may be with an isolated paralysis of vocal folds or as a spectrum of various clinical features. Plott syndrome, described by Plott in 1964 [2], is a rare entity demonstrating X-linked recessive inheritance. Patients usually present with bilateral vocal fold paralysis and mental retardation. Autosomal dominant mode of inheritance has also been reported [3–5]. Other syndromic associations may be Down's syndrome, Moebius syndrome, congenital myasthenic syndrome, 22q deletion syndrome and Goldenhar syndrome [6]. Rarely, it may be an isolated presentation of brainstem discontinuity, for example, medullary defect. This is a very rare congenital abnormality where there is a segmental discontinuity of brainstem [7].

3.1.2 Nongenetic

Several developmental anomalies of brain and brainstem may secondarily present with bilateral abductor palsy. Arnold Chiari malformation, congenital hydrocephalus, meningomyelocele, syringomyelia, syringobulbia, etc. are such examples.

3.2 Acquired causes

Various etiological factors have been mentioned in the literatures so far. Following are the common acquired causes for bilateral abductor palsy.

3.2.1 Idiopathic

In majority of cases with bilateral vocal fold palsy, no aetiological factors can be found. However, 50% these patients tend to recover completely or partially within a period of 1–2 years. The improvement is thought to be a result of delayed maturation of vagal nuclei [8].

3.2.2 Traumatic

Trauma either to the vocal cords and cricoarytenoid joint or to the vagus nerve itself can present with bilateral abductor palsy in neonates. Commonest causes are birth trauma from instrumental delivery, cardiac surgeries, mediastinal surgeries, for example, PDA ligation, etc.

3.2.3 Perinatal encephalopathy

This is another recognized cause for bilateral abductor palsy in neonatal period. It can result from various causes like perinatal hypoxia or ischaemia, birth trauma or infection.

3.2.4 Neurological disorders

Various neurological disorders like Myasthenia Gravis, Charcot-Marie tooth Disease and multiple sclerosis can present with bilateral vocal cord paralysis; however, there are features of other neurological dysfunctions as well. These conditions to present neonatally are also exceedingly rare.

3.2.5 Inflammatory

Neuritis of recurrent laryngeal nerve resulting from bacterial or viral infections can cause bilateral abductor palsy. In the pre-antibiotic era, Syphilis was considered one of the common causes, which now has become very rare. Viruses such as Influenza and Herpes Simplex virus are also reported of causing bilateral abductor palsy [9].

4. Clinical evaluation

A detailed history and a thorough clinical examination will most of the times lead to the inciting cause. Clinical history should focus on any significant perinatal events like maternal infection, maternal drug use, time and mode of delivery, instrumentation during labour, birth weight and neonatal infection. A family history should be taken as there are reported cases of this entity being inherited within the family members.

A complete head to toe examination of the affected child should always be done as there may be signs that can guide towards the aetiological cause. Neurological examination should include motor and sensory evaluation along with examination of cranial nerves specially 9th, 10th and 11th which exit commonly through the jugular foramen. Features of raised ICP such as bulged fontanelle, papilloedema should be sought. Chest and heart should be examined thoroughly. ENT examination should focus on palatal mobility, tongue mobility and presence of gag reflex.

The child may have a wide range of presentations. Most of the cases are asymptomatic until they present with sudden onset stridor preceded by upper respiratory tract infections. Other cases might present with stridor immediately following birth or few days after birth. Stridor is usually during the inspiratory phase and tends to worsen on crying where it is not unusual for a child to become cyanotic. Since the vocal folds are in adducted position change in voice is usually not encountered. Other clinical features may be difficulty in feeding, recurrent pneumonia, O_2 dependence and repeated failure to extubate. Although nonspecific, these clinical features always warrant a laryngeal evaluation.

5. Investigations

5.1 Endoscopic evaluation

An in-office flexible laryngoscopy can be done as an initial diagnostic procedure to evaluate the mobility of bilateral vocal folds, adequacy of glottic chink and to rule out other associated laryngeal anomalies such as laryngomalacia, laryngeal cleft, anterior or posterior glottic stenosis, etc. In addition, it is also important to look for velopharyngeal closure. Functional endoscopic evaluation of swallowing should be done in those who have recurrent aspiration. A rigid endoscopic evaluation under intravenous anaesthesia will also be required to assess the subglottis, trachea and bronchi as it is not uncommon to encounter second laryngeal pathology such as subglottic stenosis and tracheobronchomalacia. Cricoarytenoid joint should also be assessed for its mobility and to rule out any traumatic dislocation.

5.2 Imaging

5.2.1 Ultrasonography

Ultrasound can detect the neurological abnormalities like meningomyelocele, Arnold Chiari malformation, hydrocephalus prenatally which can have associated bilateral abductor palsy. In neonates with significant morbidity, laryngeal ultrasound can also be done to detect vocal fold palsy and any associated pathologies in the neck [10].

5.2.2 Magnetic resonance imaging

MRI scan of brain, brainstem, neck and mediastinum should be done routinely as pathologies like Arnold Chiari malformation, intraventricular hemorrhage, meningomyelocele, brainstem dysgenesis, neck or mediastinal masses can be identified easily.

5.2.3 X-ray

Chest x-ray can give the evidence of aspiration if present as well as any associated cardiac, lungs or mediastinal pathologies.

5.3 Serology

Cases where there are features of viral infection, viral serology should always be done specially for Herpes Simplex and Influenza virus. Anti-viral drugs if started early have good outcome in these cases. Also, serological tests for syphilis may be warranted if there are features of congenital syphilis.

5.4 Laryngeal electromyography

It is usually done to differentiate between vocal cord immobility due to denervation and mechanical fixation, for example, cricoarytenoid joint fixation and posterior glottis stenosis.

6. Management

Primary pathology should always be sought and managed accordingly as in most of the cases correcting the primary pathology reverts the mobility of vocal folds as well, for example in Arnold-Chiari malformation a shunt procedure may lower the intracranial pressure and thus reduce the stretching of the vagus nerve. In idiopathic cases, where no obvious inciting pathology could be found a watchful waiting up to 24 months can be done. Many of these cases gain normal or partial mobility of the cords during this period.

Most of the neonates with bilateral abductor palsy are asymptomatic until they present with an acute respiratory compromise due to upper respiratory tract infection. Management can be broadly discussed under following two headings.

6.1 Medical

It has a very limited role in the management. Corticosteroids can be given in cases presenting with stridor to reduce vocal cord oedema. Antivirals, for example, Acyclovir, have shown to hasten the recovery in cases with suspected viral aetiology.

6.2 Surgical management

There has been a huge advancement in the field of airway surgery in the past century with various surgical modalities coming forth. Here, we discuss various surgical treatment modalities for bilateral vocal cord palsy.

6.2.1 Tracheostomy

Tracheostomy may not always be required. However, in cases presenting with stridor immediate establishment of an alternate airway by tracheostomy is the earliest and safest procedure that can be performed. Tracheostomy provides a secured airway following which a specific management approach can be planned. Following tracheostomy, the tracheostomy tube care also poses a challenge as it is not uncommon for neonatal tracheostomy tube to get easily blocked with tracheal secretions. It is an ideal approach to wait until the child is 2 years old before embarking on other surgical procedures as it will allow a time period for spontaneous recovery.

6.2.2 Lateralization of vocal cord

This is a temporary procedure where the vocal cords are lateralized with a suture. There is a lesser risk of aspiration and this procedure can be reverted once the vocal coed function is back. One of the drawbacks of this procedure is that the suture may give away and the cord may be medialised again. It is reserved for the cases where recovery of vocal cord function is anticipated.

6.2.3 Posterior cordotomy

This is an irreversible procedure. Endoscopic LASER cordotomy was popularized by Dennis and Kashima [11]. In this procedure, a transection is carried out through true vocal fold, ventricle and false vocal fold from the vocal process creating a wedge shaped defect in the posterior glottis. The drawbacks of this surgery are chances of aspiration and change in voice.

6.2.4 Arytenoidectomy

Similar to posterior cordotomy, this is also an irreversible procedure aimed at creating a defect in posterior glottis. However, in this surgery most of the arytenoid is removed. This procedure also carries a risk of change in voice and aspiration. This procedure can be carried out via both open and endoscopic approach.

6.2.5 Combined posterior cordotomy and arytenoidectomy

6.2.6 Posterior cricoid split and grafting

This surgery aims at widening the glottic aperture by expanding the posterior laryngeal commissure with the help of costal cartilage. It can be performed via both open and endoscopic approach. The advantage of this procedure is that integrity of the vocal folds and arytenoids is kept intact and there are also minimal chances of aspiration.

6.2.7 Reinnervation

Reinnervation using ansa cervicalis nerve-muscle pedicle transfer or phrenic nerve transfer to posterior cricoarytenoid muscle can be done. The results are, however, not consistent and more clinical human trails are further needed to draw a definite conclusion.

7. Conclusion

Bilateral abductor palsy in neonates, although the second most common cause for stridor in paediatric population, is still a rare and clinically challenging entity. It can be a presentation of various pathologies, both genetic and non-genetic. Investigations should be guided by the mode of presentation and the possible aetiological factors, however, MRI brain should be done in all cases to rule out anomalies such as Arnold-Chiari malformation. Watchful waiting is always a standard approach until the child is 2 years old in idiopathic cases as significant number of cases tend to improve by 1–2 years.

Author details

Bigyan Raj Gyawali
Institute of medicine, Tribhuvan University Teaching hospital, Kathmandu, Nepal

*Address all correspondence to: bigyan.gyawali@gmail.com

References

[1] Murty GE, Shinkwin C, Gibbin KP. Bilateral vocal fold paralysis in infants: Tracheostomy or not? The Journal of Laryngology and Otology. 1994;**108**:329-331

[2] Plott D. Congenital laryngeal-abductor paralysis due to nucleus ambiguusdysgenesisinthreebrothers. The New England Journal of Medicine. 1964;**271**:593-597

[3] Gacek RR. Hereditary abductor vocal cord paralysis. Annals of Otology, Rhinology, and Laryngology. 1976;**85**:90

[4] Mace M, Williamson E, Worgan D. Autosomal dominantly inherited abductor laryngeal paralysis—A new syndrome with a suggestion of linkage to HLA. Clinical Genetics. 1978;**14**:265-270

[5] Moreili G, Mesolella C, Cavaliere ML, Stabile M, Ventruto V. Autosomal dominant inheritance of Gerhardt's syndrome in three generations of a family. Journal of Medical Genetics. 1980;**17**:325

[6] Hsu AK, Rosow DE, Wallerstein RJ, April MM. Familial congenital bilateralvocal fold paralysis: A novel gene translocation. International Journal of Pediatric Otorhinolaryngology. 2015;**79**:323-327

[7] Brotelande et al. Isolated neonatal bilateral vocal cord paralysis revealing a unilateral medullary defect: A case report. BMC Paediatrics. 2018;**18**:351

[8] Dedo DD. Paediatri vocal cord paralysis. The Laryngoscope. 1979;**89**:1378

[9] Dupuch V, Saroul N, Aumeran C, Pastourel R, Mom T, Gilain L. Bilateral vocal cord abductor paralysis associated with primary herpes simplex infection: A case report. European Annals of Otorhinolaryngology, Head and Neck Diseases. 2012;**129**:272-274

[10] Wang LM, Zhu Q, Ma T, Li JP, Hu R, Rong XY, et al. Value of ultrasonography in diagnosis of pediatric vocal fold paralysis. International Journal of Pediatric Otorhinolaryngology. 2011;**75**:1186-1190

[11] Dennis DP, Kashima H. Carbon dioxide laser posterior cordectomy for treatment of bilateral vocal cord paralysis. The Annals of Otology, Rhinology, and Laryngology. 1989;**98**(12 Pt 1):930-934

Chapter 5

Primary Immunodeficiency

Renfen Chen

Abstract

Primary immunodeficiency (PID) is a large group of rare diseases present with chronic, serious, or life-threatening infections and other immune complications caused by defects or dysfunction of human immune system. Unlike secondary immunodeficiency acquired from an environmental factor or other medical conditions, PIDs are initiated by genetic defects. PIDs are divided into innate/adaptive immunodeficiencies, phagocytic deficiencies, complement deficiencies, and immune dysregulation. Due to the heterogeneous nature of the clinical presentations, diagnosis of PIDs can be of significant challenge. Review of clinical history and physical examination is important for raising initial suspicion of PIDs, whereas laboratory testing is essential to establish a diagnosis. Laboratory investigation includes the assessment of antibody and cellular response, as well as evaluation of the phagocytic and complement system. Flow cytometry and genetic assays are generally served as confirmation tools to validate a diagnosis. The recent exponential increase of genetic analysis has facilitated the identification of known and novel mutations. The advances in understanding of the immune system, development of novel cellular and molecular methodologies, and increased clinical awareness have led to significant improvement of disease management and clinical outcome for these diseases.

Keywords: primary immunodeficiency, innate immunity, adaptive immunity, phenotype, gene defect, infection, autoimmune disorder, classification, clinical awareness, laboratory diagnosis, flow cytometry, genetic testing, treatment, prognosis

1. Introduction

Primary immunodeficiency (PID) is a large group of rare diseases attributed to inborn genetic errors that impair different components of adaptive and innate immune system, resulting in chronic, serious infections, or other complications. The diseases are often accompanied by a predisposition to autoimmune disorders, autoinflammation, atopy, and malignancy [1–4]. Unlike secondary immunodeficiency acquired from other diseases or conditions such as malnutrition, immunosuppression, or HIV infections, PIDs are triggered by genetic defects. Based on the abnormality of one or more components of human immunity, PIDs can be divided into antibody deficiencies, combined T- and B-cell deficiencies, deficiencies in the phagocytic or complement system, and immune dysregulation [1]. Diagnosis of these disorders requires good clinical awareness and specialized laboratory testing. Flow cytometry and genetic testing are essential to identify the phenotypic and genetic defects of the diseases and to confirm the diagnosis. Accurate diagnosis and efficient management are important for reducing morbidity and mortality in patients with PID [2]. The chapter provides an overview of the classification and manifestation as well as the diagnosis and management of these disorders.

2. Prevalence

Individual type of PIDs is considered to be rare in the population; however, recent studies have shown that PIDs may be more common than previously estimated 1% of the population when all varieties are combined [5]. The prevalence of PIDs varies depending on the type of immunodeficiencies and is difficult to be precisely calculated as the number of diagnosed cases is rapidly increasing. A 2018 global survey from the Jeffrey Modell Centers Network (JMCN) reported the case of PID patients followed in the JMCN increased by 35.4% to 102,097, while the case of patients identified with a specific gene defect increased 21.8% to 67,308 during the same period [5]. Up to 2018, 354 distinct disorders with 344 different gene defects were recognized [6]. Of note, most of the cases reported are from developed countries. It is estimated that 70–90% of individuals living with a PID are undiagnosed [7], particularly in the area with poor medical condition and lacking laboratory resources. With the extensive application of exome or whole genome sequencing, it was predicted that the associated PID genetic defects would reach 1000 under current trend in next decade [5]. **Table 1** listed the reported number of 18 most common PID defects among 354 inborn errors of immunity [5]. As shown, antibody deficiencies have much higher occurrence rate against other types of the disorders. Studies also showed that the selective IgA deficiency has the highest prevalence worldwide with a range from 1 in

Rank	PID defects	Global number
1	Predominantly antibody deficiencies, including selective IgA deficiency, unspecified hypogammaglobulinemia, and hyper-IgM syndrome	13,333
2	Common variable immunodeficiency (CVID), AR	11996
3	Chrom 22q11.2 deletion syndrome (de novo HS or AD)	5215
4	IgG subclass deficiency, isolated, AR	4612
5	Specific antibody deficiency (normal Ig and B cells), AR	4072
6	Hypogammaglobulinemia of infancy, transient (normal B cells), AR	4028
7	MEFV deficiency (familial Mediterranean fever (FMF), AD/AR)	2835
8	ATM deficiency (ataxia-telangiectasia (AT)), AR	2514
9	C1QA deficiency (C1 inhibitor), AD	2420
10	BTK deficiency, XL	2486
11	TACI deficiency	2239
12	Immunodeficiencies affecting cellular and humoral immunity, including SCID	2178
13	Autoinflammatory disorders, including PFAPA	1983
14	Complement deficiencies	1629
15	Congenital defects of phagocyte number, function, or both	1563
16	IgA with IgG subclass deficiency, AR	1562
17	CGD, XL (gp91phox deficiency)	1385
18	WAS deficiency (Wiskott-Aldrich syndrome), XL	1258
	Total	67308

AR: autosomal recessive transmission; AD: autosomal dominant transmission; Ig: immunoglobulins; SCID: severe combined immunodeficiency; CGD: Chronic Granulomatous Disease; XL: X-linked transmission; PFAPA: periodic fever with aphthous stomatitis, pharyngitis and adenitis.

Table 1.
Global prevalence of PIDs reported by Jeffrey Modell Centers Network [5].

223 to 1 in 1000 depending on ethnic background [8], while severe combined immunodeficiency (SCID), although fatal, is much rarer (1 in 100,000) [9, 10].

3. Classification

The classification of PIDs is generally based on the defects of the major components of human immunity, such as innate/adaptive immunodeficiencies, phagocytic deficiencies, complement deficiencies, and immune dysregulation. The classification has evolved over time with more phenotypic and genetic defects identified [4, 11].

Major category	Subcategory
1. Immunodeficiencies affecting cellular and humoral immunity	Severe combined immunodeficiencies, defined by CD3 T cell lymphopenia Combined immunodeficiencies generally less profound than severe combined immunodeficiency
2. Combined immunodeficiencies with associated or syndromic features	Immunodeficiency with congenital thrombocytopenia DNA repair defects other than those listed in major category 1 Thymic defects with additional congenital anomalies Immuno-osseous dysplasias Hyper IgE syndromes Dyskeratosis congenita, myelodysplasia, short telomeres Defects of vitamin B12 and folate metabolism Anhidrotic ectodermal dysplasia with immunodeficiency Calcium channel defects Others
3. Predominantly antibody deficiencies	Hypogammaglobulinemia (Severe reduction in all serum immunoglobulin isotypes with profoundly decreased or absent B Cells) Other antibody deficiencies • Severe reduction in at least 2 serum immunoglobulin isotypes with normal or low number of B Cells, CVID phenotype • Severe reduction in serum IgG and IgA with normal/elevated IgM and normal numbers of B cells, hyper IgM • Isotype, light chain, or functional deficiencies with generally normal numbers of B Cells
4. Diseases of immune dysregulation	Hemophagocytic lymphohistocytosis (HLH) & EBV susceptibility Syndromes with autoimmunity and others
5. Congenital defects of phagocyte number or function or both	Congenital neutropenias Functional defects • Defects of respiratory burst • Other non-lymphoid defects
6. Defects in intrinsic and innate immunity	Bacterial and parasitic infections Mendelian susceptibility to mycobacterial disease and viral infection
7. Autoinflammatory disorders	Recurrent inflammation Systemic inflammation on with urticaria rash Sterile inflammation (skin / bone / joints) Type 1 interferonopathies Others
8. Complement deficiencies	Susceptibility to infections (high) • Disseminated neisserial infections • Recurrent pyogenic infections Susceptibility to infections (low) • SLE-like syndrome • Atypical hemolytic uremic syndrome • Others
9. Phenocopies of PID	Associated with somatic mutations Associated with autoantibodies

Table 2.
The 2017 IUIS phenotypic categorization of PIDs [6, 11].

The International Union of Immunological Societies (IUIS) expert committee, currently named as Inborn Errors of Immunity Committee, has been responsible for issuing the classification of PIDs every other year from 1970. The complete catalog of classification has now been widely used as a reference by clinicians and researchers. From 2013, IUIS published more user-friendly phenotypic classification in two formats: one is a pdf file, namely clinically oriented phenotype categorization in the Journal of Clinical Immunology, and the other is a csv file containing a comprehensive list of various disorders that can be downloaded from http://www.iuisonline.org [6, 11]. The phenotypic categorization published in the journal has been well designed for clinical use, while the online list contains the most updated information demonstrated in a digital friendly excel format that can be sorted by phenotypic and genetic features, which are very useful for designing sequencing panels, disease code lists, and diagnostic algorithms.

The major category and subcategory of PIDs from the revised 2017 IUIS phenotypic classification are summarized in **Table 2**.

4. Clinical presentations

Patients with PID present highly heterogeneous clinical symptoms with increased susceptibility to infections and other immune complications [12, 13]. Recurrent infection is the hallmark of the PIDs although a variety of other clinical manifestations may appear before the infection [13, 14]. In fact, noninfectious manifestations, such as gastrointestinal disorders, hematological diseases, autoimmune/autoinflammatory conditions, atopy or malignancy, can be the predominant clinical presentations in some patients with underlying immunodeficiency [3, 15]. Furthermore, patients with PID also demonstrate overlapping symptoms and share similarities with many "routine" diseases.

4.1 Infections

Majority of patients with PID suffer mild to severe or life-threatening infections. The unique clinical characteristics of infections in PIDs are recurring, chronic, and can appear in multiple anatomic sites. Recurrent infections in both the sinuses and the respiratory tract, such as sinusitis, bronchitis, otitis, and pneumonia, are the most frequent symptoms observed in patients with PID [16], while recurrent systemic infections (e.g., meningitis and bacteremia) are also not rare [17, 18]. Patients with SCID may suffer from unusual or opportunistic infections leading to unexpected complications or death [19].

4.2 Autoimmune and autoinflammatory disorders

Autoimmune and autoinflammatory disorders are more frequently seen in some categories of the PIDs than in other diseases [20]. The associated conditions in PID individuals may present in a single tissue or organ, such as autoimmune hemolytic anemia, thrombocytopenia, and autoimmune thyroiditis, or affect multiple organs, exemplified by an related vasculitis, or resemble rheumatic symptoms such as (e.g., dermatomyositis, rheumatoid arthritis, and systemic lupus erythematosus) [3, 20, 21]. To note, family members that carry the same gene mutation may present different types of autoimmune/autoinflammatory symptoms, or without such disorders [22]. In comparison with other types of defects, the autoimmune presentations are relatively common in PIDs with antibody deficiencies (e.g., CVID, selective IgA deficiency), and absence of initial components (C1–C4) of the classical complement system [23, 24].

4.3 Gastrointestinal and hematological disorders

Patients with PID, particularly infants and young children, may manifest chronic diarrhea, malnutrition, and malabsorption. Some individuals may undergo infections in gastrointestinal tract, such as chronic giardiasis and rotavirus [25], while others may experience a variety of autoimmune or autoinflammatory disorders including inflammatory bowel disease, atrophic gastritis with pernicious anemia, or gluten-sensitive enteropathy [20].

Hematological disorders, such as autoimmune hemolytic anemia, and/or neutropenia and/or thrombocytopenia, are also frequently seen in patients with CVID or selective IgA deficiency [26]. Patients with the Wiskott-Aldrich syndrome, a disease characterized by variable defects in B- and T-lymphocyte function, can present with reduced platelet volume and significant thrombocytopenia [27].

4.4 Immunodeficiency syndromes

PID patients may also present with a syndrome complex. For example, recurrent bacterial/fungal infections and chronic inflammation of the gastrointestinal and respiratory tract often present in patients with chronic granulomatous disease, while an individual suffering from Wiskott-Aldrich syndrome may have manifestations of eczema, recurrent bacterial infections, autoimmune disorders, and thrombocytopenia [27]. In addition, congenital heart disease and hypocalcemic tetany frequently appear in a newborn baby with the DiGeorge syndrome [28, 29]. In fact, the investigation of patients with a syndrome derived from immunodeficiency may trigger an early diagnosis of PID before the typical immunodeficiency symptoms appear [4].

4.5 Malignancy

Compared to individuals with a healthy immune system, patients with PID are expected to have higher prevalence and/or broader spectrum of malignancies [30]. A study showed that lymphoma, the most common malignancy seen in PID patients, has increased 10-folds in male and 8.34-folds in female compared to age-matched controls [31]. Other types of cancer with higher frequency in PIDs are leukemia, digestive tract cancers, and virus-induced cancers [30]. Interestingly, the four most common cancers routinely occurred in men and women (lung, colon, breast, and prostate cancers) do not have significant elevation in subjects diagnosed with PID [31]. Evidence also demonstrated that patients with specific forms of immunodeficiency caused by highly penetrant gene defects have higher risk of developing cancer [32].

5. Clinical investigation

Early diagnosis of PID is critical for reducing morbidity or mortality and improving treatment outcomes. Review of clinical and family history and physical examination are the first steps in evaluating the need for further laboratory investigation.

The differentiation of PIDs from other medical conditions can be complicated as the symptoms of infection (e.g., sinusitis, bronchitis, pneumonia, gastroenteritis, meningitis, or sepsis) and other manifestations often present in patients with non-PID. Hence, it is important to delineate the infectious organisms, the pattern of infections, and clinical pictures for guiding the clinical judgment, prior to focusing on laboratory testing.

	Warning signs in children	Warning signs in adults
1	Equal or more than four new ear infections within one year	Equal or more than two new ear infections within one year
2	Equal or more than two serious sinus infections within one year	Equal or more than two new sinus infections within one year without allergy
3	Equal or more than two months on antibiotics with little effect	One pneumonia per year for more than one year
4	Equal or more than two pneumonias within one year	Chronic diarrhea with weight loss
5	Failure of an infant to gain weight or grow normally	Recurrent viral infections (colds, herpes, warts, condyloma)
6	Recurrent, deep skin or organ abscesses	Recurrent need for IV antibiotics to clear infections
7	Persistent thrush in mouth or fungal infection on skin	Recurrent, deep abscesses of the skin or internal organs
8	Need for intravenous antibiotics to clear infections	Persistent thrush or fungal infection on skin or elsewhere
9	Equal or more than two deep-seated infections including septicemia	Infection with normally harmless tuberculosis-like bacteria
10	A family history of PID	A family history of PID

Adapted from Jeffrey Modell Foundation http://www.info4pi.org/library/educational-materials/10-warning-signs. Accessed on 09/Oct/2019.

Table 3.
Clinical warning signs of PIDs.

Due to the highly variable clinical presentations and low frequency of the PIDs, the diagnosis of patients is often delayed for years. To raise clinical awareness, JMCN has promoted 10 warning signs for children and adults (**Table 3**). Patients presenting with two or more of the clinical warning signs should be prompted for further investigation for the possible underlying immunodeficiencies and referred to immunologists for proper disease management.

6. Laboratory diagnosis

The laboratory testing is essential to diagnose and delineate the immunologic defects of PIDs. Patients with clinical suspicion should be further investigated for the response of innate immunity and adaptive immunity [33, 34]. **Table 4** listed the most common tests used for initial screening of PIDs.

6.1 Evaluation of humoral immunity

Measurement of serum immunoglobulins is the first-line test for evaluating B-lymphocyte functions. Quantitative measurements of IgG, IgA, IgM, and IgE will identify either hypogammaglobulinemia or deficiency of an individual class of immunoglobulins. Evaluation of IgG subclasses may be required when a patient has strong implication of humoral immunodeficiency but the total IgG is normal. To be mindful, the results of immunoglobulin quantitation must be interpreted with appropriate age-specific ranges. Assessment of antibody responses to immunization with protein antigens (e.g., tetanus or diphtheria toxoids) and polysaccharide antigens (e.g., pneumococcal capsular) is another way to evaluate humoral immunity,

Suspected immunodeficiency	Laboratory tests
Humoral immunity	Quantitation of immunoglobulins (IgG, IgA, IgM), IgE, IgG subclass Antibody response to immunization (Tetanus/diphtheria toxoids, pneumococcal) B cell (CD19) and subtype enumeration
Cell-mediated immunity	Lymphocyte enumeration T cell and subtype enumeration (CD3,CD4, CD8) T cell functions • Delayed type hypersensitivity skin tests • Vaccine-specific T cell responses • In vitro proliferation to the stimulation of mitogen (e.g. PHA, PMA or specific antigen(candida, tetanus toxoid) • Cytotoxicity • Cytokines in response to stimulation
Complement system	Complement activity for classical pathway (CH50) Complement activity for alternate pathway (AH50) C1 inhibitor (quantitation and function) Individual complement level
Phagocytosis system	Neutrophil enumeration Nitroblue tetrazolium (NBT) dye test Oxidative burst by Dihydrorhodamine 123
NK cells	NK cell enumeration NK cell functions • ^{51}Chromium release assay • CD107 expression • Perforin / granzyme expression

Table 4.
Initial laboratory tests for PIDs.

although note is to be taken that live viral vaccines must be restricted to a patient with underlying immunodeficiency [35].

6.2 Evaluation of cellular immunity

Delayed-type hypersensitivity (DTH) skin test is commonly used to screen whether the patient has intact cell-mediated immune response. A positive DTH skin test generally rules out the possible defect of cellular immunity [36]. Nevertheless, the test requires that individuals must have sufficient prior exposure and sensitization to the testing antigen; therefore, it may not be suitable for infants and young children. Quantitation of T-lymphocytes (CD3, CD4, CD8) in peripheral blood is able to indirectly reflect the aberrant cellular immunity and can be easily performed by flow cytometry. More specialized T-cell function tests would provide in-depth information in immune system, which include the assessment of lymphocyte proliferation in response to stimulus such as mitogens (e.g., phytohemagglutinin, ConA, and PMA), or specific antigens (e.g., candida). Furthermore, in vitro measurements of intra- and/or extracellular cytokine responses (e.g., interleukin 2, interferon-gamma, BAFF, and TNF) are informative for the investigation of T- and B-lymphocyte regulation [37].

6.3 Evaluation of phagocytic function

Leukocyte count and differential can assess the phagocytic disorders such as congenital agranulocytosis or cyclic neutropenia. Phagocytic function can be indirectly assessed by traditional nitroblue tetrazolium (NBT) assay, which measures phagocytic cells' killing capability in response to an oxidative burst. More recently, a simpler dihydrorhodamine 123 (DHR) assay based on flow cytometry has replaced NBT test for assisting the diagnosis of chronic granulomatous disease (CGD), Rac2 deficiency, and complete myeloperoxidase deficiency [38, 39]. Other complicated in-vitro functional methods such as the measurement of directed cell movement (chemotaxis), ingestion (phagocytosis), and intracellular killing (bactericidal activity) are available in some specialized laboratories [40].

6.4 Evaluation of NK function

The importance of evaluating NK cells in human immunity has been previously underscored, and this is supported by two evidences: significantly increased number of patients with reduced NK cells and/or functions, and over 40 genetically defined congenital immunodeficiencies present with impaired NK cell functions [41]. There are several methods utilized for the examination of NK cell functions including ^{51}chromium release assay, flow cytometry-based perforin/granzyme expression and CD107a degranulation. These assays are particularly valuable for the patients suspected of primary hemophagocytic lymphohistiocytosis [42, 43].

6.5 Evaluation of the complement system

The complement system can be evaluated by measuring the level or function of complement proteins that are involved in the classical and alternative activation pathways. C3 and C4 are the complements routinely tested. Quantitative and functional assay of C1 esterase inhibitor is essential for the diagnosis of hereditary angioedema. Assays of CH50 and AH50 are, respectively, used to measure the overall complement activity in the classical or alternative pathway. Combining the results of CH50 and AH50 is indicative for further investigation of individual complement proteins that initiate the classical or alternative pathway or common terminal pathway [44].

6.6 Flow cytometry

As our understanding of the defect or dysfunction of immune system increases, immunophenotypic and functional assays based on flow cytometry have been extensively used in identifying the abnormality of various cell types and their functions associated with certain diseases, including PIDs. Furthermore, flow cytometry is also a favorable technique for the measurement of intra- and extracellular cytokine production (e.g., IL12, IFN, TNF, and TH17), cell surface protein expression (e.g., Foxp3, CTLA-4, and BTK), and cellular signaling pathways (e.g., phosphor-STAT) [45]. The information gained from flow cytometry analysis can assist not only in the diagnosis, monitoring, and treatment of the diseases but also in understanding the influence of immune system associated with genetic defects that are newly identified. **Table 5** lists the flow cytometry assays used for common PID disorders. Most of the tests listed are required to be undertaken in a specialized laboratory, with the exception of TBNK cell populations, memory B cells, and some function assays that can be performed in a routine diagnostic laboratory.

Proper instrument setting, standardized operating procedures, and good quality controls must be exercised when performing flow cytometric analysis, as flow cytometry is susceptible to assay variation,. The reported data must include both percentage and absolute number of specific cell population. Moreover, appropriate age-matched reference ranges should also be provided in the final report [47, 48].

Ideally, each laboratory should establish their own normal ranges, but this is often not feasible; alternatively, published reference ranges may be used if a proper validation has been undertaken.

To date, flow cytometry has also been widely used for evaluating cell functions. Traditionally, lymphocyte functions were tested by radioactive methods, such as cytotoxicity of T and NK cells (chromium release) or proliferation of T cells

Defect of PIDs	Flow cytometric assessment
Combined immunodeficiencies	
SCID	Absent T cells and variable number of B and NK cells, reduced or absent $CD31^+$ recent thymus emigrant, disruptions in naïve and memory T cells[a]
X-SCID	Reduced or absent of CD132 on lymphocytes [a], reduced phosphorylation of STAT5 in response to cytokine stimulation [c]
Omenn Syndrome and leaky SCID	Reduced memory T cells, TCR analysis for oligoclonality[a]
BLS Type 1	Reduced or absent MHC Class I, decreased CD8 T cells [a]
BLS Type 2	Reduced or absent MHC Class II, decreased CD4 T cells[a]
X-linked HIGM	Reduced expression or function of CD40L on activated T cells[c]
Autosomal recessive HIGM	Absent CD40 expression on B cells[a]
Jak-3 mutations	Reduced phosphorylation of STAT5 in response to cytokine stimulation [c]
ZAP-70 deficiency	Decreased CD8 T cells[a], absent ZAP70 in T cells[b]
DOCK8 deficiency	Absent DOCK8 expression in lymphocytes[b]
Combined immunodeficiencies with syndromic or associated features	
Wiskott-Aldrich syndrome (WAS)	Reduced WAS protein in major mature B cell subsets and regulatory B cells [b]
Hyper-IgE Syndrome	Disruptions in T and B cell populations [a], reduced TH17 cells [b,c]
Antibody deficiencies	
X-linked Agammaglobulinemia	Reduced/Absent B cells[a], reduced/absent BTK protein in monocytes[b]
CVID	Absent CD19 and BAFF-R on B cells[a] , disruptions in switched, non-switched, transitional B cells [a], reduced inducible costimulator on activated T cells [c]
Autosomal recessive HIGM (uracil N glycosylase, AICDA)	Reduced memory B cells, disruptions in switched and non-switched memory B cells [a]
Intrinsic and innate immune defects	
Mendelian susceptibility to mycobacterial disease	Reduced IFNγR1 expression on monocyte and IL12Rβ1 expression on activated T cells [a], reduced phosphorylation of STAT1, or STAT4 in monocytes[b,c]
STAT1 GOF	Delayed dephosphorylation of STAT1 in response to IFNγ or IFNα in monocytes[b,c]
IL17 RA deficiency	Reduced IL17 RA expression on lymphocytes and monocytes [a]

IRAK-4 and MyD88 deficiency	Reduced intracellular TNF-α in monocytes in response to LPS[b,c]
Neutrophil defects	
CGD- X-linked	Reduced surface expression of gp91[a], reduced or absent oxidative burst in DHR123 assay[c]
CGD - autosomal recessive	Reduced surface expression of gp22[a], reduced intracellular expression of gp47 or gp67[b], reduced oxidative burst in DHR123 assay[c]
Leukocyte adhesion defect I	Reduced expression of CD18, CD11a, CD11b, and CD11c[a]
Leukocyte adhesion defect II	Reduced CD15s expression[a]
Complement defects	
Atypical hemolytic uremic syndrome	Reduced CD46 (MCP) expression in neutrophils[a]
Immune dysregulation	
Autoimmune lymphoproliferative syndrome	Elevated $CD3^+TCR\alpha\beta^+$ CD4-CD8- T cells [a]
X-linked lymphoproliferative disease type 1	Significantly reduced iNKT cells[a], decreased intracellular SAP in CD8 + T cells[b] and NK cells
X-linked lymphoproliferative disease type 2	Reduced intracellular XIAP in lymphocytes[b]
Immune dysregulation, polyendocrinopathy, X-linked syndrome	Reduced $FoxP3^+$ Treg cells[b]
CTLA-4 haploinsufficiency	Reduced CTLA-4 expression in Treg cells[b]
LRBA deficiency	Reduced intracellular LRBA in stimulated PBMC[b, c] and decreased CTLA-4 in Tregs[b]
STAT3-GOF	Delayed dephosphorylation of STAT3 following stimulation with IL-6[b,c]
Familial HLH3, 4 and 5, Chediak-Higashi, Griscelli or Hermansky-Pudlak Syndromes	Reduced CD107a expression on NK cells in response to target cells[c]
Familial HLH2 (PRF1 mutations)	Reduced intracellular perforin in CD8 T cells and NK cells[b]
IL-10R deficiency	Reduced STAT3 phosphorylation in lymphocytes in response to IL-10[c]
Infantile-onset multisystem autoimmune disease 1 (heterozygous GOF mutation in STAT 3)	Enhanced STAT3 phosphorylation[c]
Phenocopies of PIDs	
Autoantibodies to IFNγ	Inhibition of IFNγ-induced phosphorylation of STAT1 with patient's serum [b,c]
Autoantibodies to GMCSF	Inhibition of GMCSF-induced phosphorylation of STAT5 with patient's serum [b,c]

SCID: severe combined immunodeficiency; STAT: signal transducer and activator of transcription; BLS: bare lymphocyte syndrome; HIGM: hyper-IgM syndrome; BTK: Bruton's tyrosine kinase; CVID: common variable immunodeficiency; CGD: chronic granulomatous disease; DHR: dihydrorhodamine; HLH: hemophagocytic lymphohistiocytosis; CTLA-4: cytotoxic T-lymphocyte associated protein-4; LRBA: LPS responsive Beige-like anchor protein; GOF: gain-of-function; GMCSF: granulocyte macrophage colony stimulating factor.
[a] Detection of surface molecules. [b] Detection of intracellular or intranuclear molecules. [c] Detection of cellular function.

Table 5.
Phenotypic and functional assessment for PIDs by flow cytometry [45, 46].

(tritiated thymidine uptake). These approaches are still recognized as gold standard by some clinicians. However, radioactive methods have the following intrinsic limitations: involvement of radioactivity, labor intensive, high expertise required, and poor result reproducibility. Additionally, seeking for a consistent healthy

Method	Advantages	Limitations	Recommendations by Immunology Society
Chromosomal microarray	Detection of CNVs and majority of structural variations Greater analytical sensitivity than conventional cytogenetics Fast result TAT	Unable to detect SNVs and very small deletions/duplications (<100kb) or chromosomal rearrangements that do not affect the nucleotide copy number	Use as initial screening test to narrow the list of genetic candidates in an undetermined phenotype Complement each other with WES
Sanger sequencing	Detection of noncoding variants Lowest overall cost Fast result TAT High accuracy	Unable to detect CNVs and structural variations Inability to detect portions not included in the assay	Use for the detection of monogenetic PID for patient and family members Technical confirmation of genetic mutations detected by other approaches
Gene panel by massively parallel sequencing	High throughput Increased depth of sequencing coverage in target genes with fewer regions missed Higher accuracy and sensitivity versus NGS Detection of mosaicism Less expensive than WES or GS	Unable to detect non-targeted variants Newly defined variants/genes need to be constantly updated in the testing panel Inability to detect novel disease-causing genes Only very small gene (1-25 nucleotide) insertions and deletions can reliably be detected	Use as rapid testing for limited gene candidates
Whole exome sequencing (WES)	Covers all known coding regions of all genes. High diagnostic yield with the detection of the majority of important pathogenic variants in only 1% of the genome Capable of discovering new pathogenic genes Identification of defects in multiple genes	Poor coverage of noncoding, novel exons or poorly understood regions Unreliable detection of copy number, structural variations and insertions or deletions more than 25 nucleotides More expensive than Sanger and panel sequencing Detection of variants of unclear significance Baits cannot be optimized for all target genes	Use in individuals with complicated manifestations or phenotypes with significant locus heterogeneity Use in conjunction with chromosomal microarray when a genetic diagnosis cannot be secure after Sanger or gene panel testing
Genome sequencing (GS)	More consistent coverage across all genes Identification of variants in coding, noncoding, regulatory regions and duplications and deletions not covered by WES. Detect CNVs and structural variations and large deletions Discover new pathogenic genes	Highest cost Slowest result TAT Detection of variants of unclear significance Labor and knowledge -intensive in the interpretation of large volume of data (around 3 billion base pairs of DNA)	Use when other genomic methods can not discover the genetic variations or secure the genetic diagnosis

CNVs: copy-number variations; SNV: single-nucleotide variant; TAT: turn around time; NGS: Next generation sequencing.

Table 6.
The advantages, limitations and recommendations of genetic technologies [50, 53].

fresh blood as assay normal control and obtaining a proper reference range can be challenging in routine laboratory practice. Therefore, they have been gradually replaced by other methodologies, such as bioluminescence-based assay or flow cytometry–based assay, which use specific dye for the detection of cell proliferation (e.g., CFSE, PKH-2, or PKH-26) or cell death (e.g., 7AAD and Annexing V) [49]. Many assays based on flow cytometry have been increasingly popular as they are easier to perform, have quicker turnaround time, are nonradioactive, are capable of using whole blood, and are more robust compared to the traditional radioactive assays.

6.7 Genetic testing

Genetic testing plays a critical role in patients with PID in confirming diagnosis, predicting the prognosis, assessing the influences of genotype-phenotype associations, and family planning [50, 51]. Besides, early and accurate molecular diagnosis is vital for guiding the selection of appropriate treatment including genetic therapy. Several molecular tests are available in identifying the genetic defects of PIDs, such as chromosomal analysis, fluorescence in situ hybridization, chromosomal microarray, single gene by Sanger sequencing, gene panels by massively parallel, whole exome, and genome by next-generation sequencing [52]. The selection of these assays should consider their inherent advantages and limitations [50, 53]. The summary of these tests is shown in **Table 6**. Recent emerged simple molecular assays for measuring circular DNA segments namely T-cell receptor excision circles and kappa-deleting recombination excision circles, based on quantitative PCR amplification of DNA extracted from dried blood spots, enable for a quick screening of newborn SCID [54].

The choice of specific gene(s) for examination is suggested by the patient's clinical history and phenotypical and functional results. Clinicians are required to have a basic understanding of the utility, accessibility of different genetic approaches. The selection criteria of molecular methodology should be based on the greatest odds of achieving the diagnosis within an acceptable time frame with the most cost-effective test. There is no specific algorithm for genetic testing in patients with PID as individual's genetic mutation is often unique, the technology, cost, and the assay turnaround time are constantly changing, and each molecular method has inherent advantages and limitations. Practically, two or more approaches are often used together to achieve an optimal diagnosis [50]. For example, single gene Sanger sequencing is considered to be not only a simple and reliable assay for testing patients with known monogenic mutations of PID or their family members, but it can also serve as a tool for confirming the genetic variants detected by whole exome sequencing. When assessing large numbers of mutations, gene panels or whole genome/exome approach may be more cost-effective and faster than single gene analysis. Since genetic testing in primary immunodeficiency is highly personalized, and a specific genetic mutation does not always translate into a disease, test results must be interpreted with caution by genetic consultants and immunologists.

The recent advances of sequencing technologies have facilitated the genomic assays to become the standard of care in some hospitals although these techniques may face the challenges of cost, accessibility, and interpretation issues. The exponential growth of genetic analysis by next-generation sequencing and other novel molecular technologies has enabled quick identification of known and novel mutations, which contributed to a dramatic expansion of the number and types of PIDs [16, 53, 55].

7. Treatment

Treatments for PIDs involve preventing and controlling recurrent infections, treating symptoms, strengthening the immunity, and treating the underlying cause of the immune defects. Illness associated with PIDs such as autoimmune disorders or malignancies should also be managed [1, 13].

More aggressive and/or longer course of antibiotics than "normal infections" is usually prescribed in patients with PID, in order to control the infections caused by bacteria or fungi. Some patients may require prolonged antibiotic therapy to prevent infections and permanent damage to organs [13]. Routine immunizations can also provide protective immunity to those at risk of infections, but the attenuated vaccines such as oral polio and measles-mumps-rubella might not be suitable for children with PIDs. For viral infection, interferon-gamma therapy may be of choice besides other antiviral drugs routinely used (e.g., amantadine and acyclovir) [13]. In patients with chronic granulomatous disease, using granulocyte colony–stimulating factor, a glycoprotein that is able to stimulate the proliferation/differentiation and improve the functions of neutrophil, can help increase the levels of immune-strengthening leukocytes to control the infections [56].

Immunoglobulin replacement has been the pillar of therapy for recurrent infections of PIDs, since around 60% of PID cases have impaired antibody production [57]. In fact, most of these patients will require life-time immunoglobulin replacement therapy. Immunoglobulin can be delivered either intravenously (abbreviated IVIG) or subcutaneously (abbreviated SCIG). The choice of which route depends on the circumstance although both of them have been demonstrated to be effective. Because higher IgG levels can be obtained through intravenous administration, IVIG has been routinely used for preventing serious/recurrent infections [58]; however, SCIG has recently emerged as a popular route for delivery due to its fewer side effects and greater flexibility [57, 59]. Future research direction is focusing on more precise IgG replacement in PIDs, such as the development of IgG subclass-specific enriched preparation and microbe-specific IgG [58].

Defects	Supportive treatment	Definitive treatment
CIDs/SCID	Ig replacement (IV or SC) Enzyme replacement Antibiotic prophylaxis Antifungal prophylaxis Aggressive prevention and management of infections Immunosuppressants for autoinflammation	Thymus transplantation [66] Stem cell transplant Gene therapy
Antibody deficiencies	Ig replacement therapy (IV or SC) Antibiotic prophylaxis Antifungal prophylaxis Biological agents or immunosuppressants for autoinflammation	Stem cell transplant Gene therapy
Innate immunodeficiencies	Antibiotic prophylaxis Antifungal prophylaxis Cytokine replacement Granulocyte colony stimulating factor Immunizations Ig replacement if indicated	Stem cell transplant Gene therapy
Autoimmune/autoinflammatory disorders	Corticosteroids Other immunosuppressants Biological agents	Stem cell transplant Gene therapy
Immune dysregulation disorders	Antibiotic prophylaxis Antifungal prophylaxis Immunizations Immunosuppressants Biological agents	Stem cell transplant Gene therapy

Ig: immunoglobulin; IV: intravenous; SC: subcutaneous; CID: combined immunodeficiency; SCID: severe combined immunodeficiency.

Table 7.
Current strategies for the treatment of PIDs [1, 13, 66].

Apart from controlling infections, the considerable morbidity and mortality caused by noninfectious complications of PIDs can also be troublesome to clinicians. To standardize clinical practices and improve treatment outcome, British Society of Immunology has recently published the first set of recommendations for monitoring and managing the noninfectious complications of CVID [60].

Bone marrow transplantation (BMT) and hematopoietic stem cell transplantation (HSCT) are feasible options for a permanent cure for several types of life-threatening immunodeficiency, with SCID in particular [61, 62]. Immune system can reconstitute when stem cells harvested from bone marrow or cord blood are transferred to the patients with PID. However, the successful rate of biological match, possibility of life-threatening graft-versus-host-disease, and the risk of uncontrolled infections following the destruction of the patient's own immune system prior to the transplant should be well evaluated.

The technical advances of genetic engineering provide another hope to cure PIDs. Substantial progress has been made in the past decade in treating several types of PIDs (e.g., adenosine deaminase-SCID, SCID-X1, chronic granulomatous disorder, and Wiskott-Aldrich syndrome) with gene therapy [63–65]. Current treatment scenario is mostly based on ex-vivo deliver of therapeutic transgene through viral vectors to autologous stem cells, followed by transplantation back to the same patient. Although the overall outcome from all the clinical trials targeting different PIDs has been extremely promising, however, serious adverse events (e.g., vector-mediated oncogenesis) and high cost may be a hindrance to clinical trials and promotion of gene therapy [63, 65]. A summary of current strategies for treatment and management of PIDs is shown in **Table 7**.

8. Prognosis

The prognosis of patients with PID is extremely variable depending on the type of immune defects. Infants with SCID will die in the first 2 years of life without HSCT/BMT or gene therapy. Individuals who obtained stem cell transplantation in early childhood (before 3.5 months) have better prognosis [67]. Many PID patients who received proper medical care and treatments are able to live healthy and independent life for a long term. With the enhancement in managing infections and other complications and growing application of definitive therapies, the outcomes and long-term survival of PIDs have improved dramatically since the 1970s [13].

9. Conclusion

The investigation of PIDs has provided valuable insights to understand the specific gene defect that impairs the immune system. Flow cytometry and genetic testing enable to identify existing and novel phenotypes and genotypes as well as their impact on PIDs. The applications of flow cytometry and genetic technologies have expanded dramatically with more types of PID is defined, and the use of mass sequencing technologies has accelerated the identification of novel disorders. To efficiently use these complex assays, clinicians should have a good understanding of these methods and know how to interpret the results for diagnosis and disease management [33].

The management of patients with PID is based on three aspects of diagnosis: suspicious clinical manifestations, aberrant results of immune response, and the underlying genetic defect [4]. However, the diagnosis of PIDs may confront significant challenges: there are large numbers of variable types of PIDs to be recognized and most of them have alike clinical presentations with common diseases; immunodeficiencies derived from multiple gene defects can share similar symptoms, and a defect in the same gene may have various clinical manifestations [1]. While severe forms of PIDs are relatively easier to be recognized, milder immunodeficiencies may not raise alertness until typical presentation occurs [68, 69]. Additionally, the criteria for constituting a PID diagnosis are subjective, for example, the degree of frequency and the severity of the infections for establishing the diagnosis are unclear, the association of PIDs with autoimmune disorder or malignancy is ambiguous, and some individuals may not have noticeable symptoms apart from laboratory findings. Furthermore, advanced laboratory examination such as specialized flow cytometric and genetic analysis is not always easy to access. All these factors may contribute to delayed or missed diagnosis of the diseases.

To combat the challenges, clinical warning signs of PIDs should be disseminated to all clinicians for raising earlier recognition of the diseases, and an immunologist must be consulted for proper diagnosis and management. Due to the complexity of clinical presentations and large number of disease types, the use of scoring system based on the codes of the international classification of PIDs [69] assisted by artificial intelligence may be beneficial for clinicians to differentiate these disorders from other diseases and raise initial recognition. The recent advances in understanding the human immune system, development of novel cellular and molecular assays, and collaborations from the international/national organizations have led to significant increase of clinical awareness and cases diagnosed and improvement of disease management and treatment outcomes for PIDs.

Acknowledgements

The author thanks Dr. Alexander Richardson from the Royal College of Pathologists of Australasia for assisting the references work and Mrs. Xiumei Wei from the Sutherland Centre of Immunology in NSW, Australia, for valuable opinions.

Conflict of interest

The author declares that there is no conflict of interest.

Author details

Renfen Chen
Central Sydney Immunology Laboratory, Royal Prince Alfred Hospital, NSW Health Pathology, Camperdown, NSW, Australia

*Address all correspondence to: ren.chen@health.nsw.gov.au

References

[1] Raje N, Dinakar C. Overview of immunodeficiency disorders. Immunology and Allergy Clinics of North America. 2015;**35**(4):599-623. DOI: 10.1016/j.iac.2015.07.001

[2] Condino-Neto A, Espinosa-Rosales FJ. Changing the lives of people with primary immunodeficiencies (PI) with early testing and diagnosis. Frontiers in Immunology. 2018;**9**:1439. DOI: 10.3389/fimmu.2018.01439

[3] Amaya-Uribe L et al. Primary immunodeficiency and autoimmunity: A comprehensive review. Journal of Autoimmunity. 2019;**99**:52-72. DOI: 10.1016/j.jaut.2019.01.011

[4] Mahlaoui N et al. Advances in the care of primary immunodeficiencies (PIDs): From birth to adulthood. Journal of Clinical Immunology. 2017;**37**(5):452-460. DOI: 10.1007/s10875-017-0401-y

[5] Modell V et al. Global report on primary immunodeficiencies: 2018 update from the Jeffrey Modell Centers Network on disease classification, regional trends, treatment modalities, and physician reported outcomes. Immunologic Research. 2018;**66**(3):367-380. DOI: 10.1007/s12026-018-8996-5

[6] Picard C et al. International Union of Immunological Societies: 2017 primary immunodeficiency diseases committee report on inborn errors of immunity. Journal of Clinical Immunology. 2018;**38**(1):96-128. DOI: 10.1007/s10875-017-0464-9

[7] Primary Immunodeficiencies (PID). Driving Diagnosis for Optimal Care in Europe, European Reference Paper. Available from: http://worldpiweek.org/sites/default/files/basic_page_documents/PI_European_Reference_Paper.pdf

[8] Yel L. Selective IgA deficiency. Journal of Clinical Immunology. 2010;**30**(1):10-16. DOI: 10.1007/s10875-009-9357-x

[9] Kwan A et al. Newborn screening for severe combined immunodeficiency in 11 screening programs in the United States. JAMA. 2014;**312**(7):729-738. DOI: 10.1001/jama.2014.9132

[10] Rivers L, Gaspar HB. Severe combined immunodeficiency: Recent developments and guidance on clinical management. Archives of Disease in Childhood. 2015;**100**(7):667-672. DOI: 10.1136/archdischild-2014-306425

[11] Bousfiha A et al. The 2017 IUIS phenotypic classification for primary immunodeficiencies. Journal of Clinical Immunology. 2018;**38**(1):129-143. DOI: 10.1007/s10875-017-0465-8

[12] Carneiro-Sampaio M, Coutinho A. Immunity to microbes: Lessons from primary immunodeficiencies. Infection and Immunity. 2007;**75**(4):1545-1555. DOI: 10.1128/IAI.00787-06

[13] McCusker C, Upton J, Warrington R. Primary immunodeficiency. Allergy, Asthma and Clinical Immunology. 2018;**14**(Suppl 2):61. DOI: 10.1186/s13223-018-0290-5

[14] Bazregari S et al. Evaluation of infectious and non-infectious complications in patients with primary immunodeficiency. Central European Journal of Immunology. 2017;**42**(4):336-341. DOI: 10.5114/ceji.2017.72825

[15] Guffroy A et al. Primary immunodeficiency and autoimmunity. La Revue de Médecine Interne. 2017;**38**(6):383-392. DOI: 10.1016/j.revmed.2016.10.388

[16] Jesenak M et al. Pulmonary manifestations of primary

immunodeficiency disorders in children. Frontiers in Pediatrics. 2014;**2**:77. DOI: 10.3389/fped.2014.00077

[17] Ruffner MA, Sullivan KE, Henrickson SE. Recurrent and sustained viral infections in primary immunodeficiencies. Frontiers in Immunology. 2017;**8**:665. DOI: 10.3389/fimmu.2017.00665

[18] Sanges S et al. Diagnosis of primary antibody and complement deficiencies in young adults after a first invasive bacterial infection. Clinical Microbiology and Infection. 2017;**23**(8):576-576. DOI: 10.1016/j.cmi.2017.02.005

[19] Burg M, Gennery AR. Educational paper. The expanding clinical and immunological spectrum of severe combined immunodeficiency. European Journal of Pediatrics. 2011;**170**(5):561-571. DOI: 10.1007/s00431-011-1452-3

[20] Fischer A et al. Autoimmune and inflammatory manifestations occur frequently in patients with primary immunodeficiencies. The Journal of Allergy and Clinical Immunology. 2017;**140**(5):1388-1393. DOI: 10.1016/j.jaci.2016.12.978

[21] Arakelyan A et al. Autoimmunity and autoinflammation: A systems view on signaling pathway dysregulation profiles. PLoS One. 2017;**12**(11):e0187572. DOI: 10.1371/journal.pone.0187572

[22] Martorana D et al. Monogenic autoinflammatory diseases with Mendelian inheritance: Genes, mutations, and genotype/phenotype correlations. Frontiers in Immunology. 2017;**8**:344. DOI: 10.3389/fimmu.2017.00344

[23] Sarmiento E et al. Autoimmune disease in primary antibody deficiencies. Allergologia et Immunopathologia. 2005;**33**(2):69-73

[24] Sparchez M et al. Primary complement and antibody deficiencies in autoimmune rheumatologic diseases with juvenile onset: A prospective study at two centers. Pediatric Rheumatology Online Journal. 2015;**13**:51. DOI: 10.1186/s12969-015-0050-8

[25] Agarwal S, Cunningham-Rundles C. Gastrointestinal manifestations and complications of primary immunodeficiency disorders. Immunology and Allergy Clinics of North America. 2019;**39**(1):81-94. DOI: 10.1016/j.iac.2018.08.006

[26] Azizi G et al. Autoimmunity in primary T-cell immunodeficiencies. Expert Review of Clinical Immunology. 2016;**12**(9):989-1006. DOI: 10.1080/1744666X.2016.1177458

[27] Park JY et al. Early deficit of lymphocytes in Wiskott-Aldrich syndrome: Possible role of WASP in human lymphocyte maturation. Clinical and Experimental Immunology. 2004;**136**(1):104-110. DOI: 10.1111/j.1365-2249.2004.02409.x

[28] Grassi MS et al. Congenital heart disease as a warning sign for the diagnosis of the 22q11.2 deletion. Arquivos Brasileiros de Cardiologia. 2014;**103**(5):382-390. DOI: 10.5935/abc.20140145

[29] Rayannavar A et al. Association of hypocalcemia with congenital heart disease in 22q11.2 deletion syndrome. American Journal of Medical Genetics. Part A. 2018;**176**(10):2099-2103. DOI: 10.1002/ajmg.a.40495

[30] Satge D. A tumor profile in primary immune deficiencies challenges the cancer immune surveillance concept. Frontiers in Immunology. 2018;**9**:1149. DOI: 10.3389/fimmu.2018.01149

[31] Mayor PC et al. Cancer in primary immunodeficiency diseases: Cancer incidence in the United States immune

deficiency network registry. The Journal of Allergy and Clinical Immunology. 2018;**141**(3):1028-1035. DOI: 10.1016/j.jaci.2017.05.024

[32] Haas OA. Primary immunodeficiency and cancer predisposition revisited: Embedding two closely related concepts into an integrative conceptual framework. Frontiers in Immunology. 2018;**9**:3136. DOI: 10.3389/fimmu.2018.03136

[33] Locke BA, Dasu T, Verbsky JW. Laboratory diagnosis of primary immunodeficiencies. Clinical Reviews in Allergy and Immunology. 2014;**46**(2):154-168. DOI: 10.1007/s12016-014-8412-4

[34] Nagy G. Laboratory evaluation of immunological dysfunctions in primary immunodeficiency diseases. Orvosi Hetilap. 2018;**159**(49):2087-2094. DOI: 10.1556/650.2018.31261

[35] Eibl MM, Wolf HM. Vaccination in patients with primary immune deficiency, secondary immune deficiency and autoimmunity with immune regulatory abnormalities. Immunotherapy. 2015;**7**(12):1273-1292. DOI: 10.2217/IMT.15.74

[36] Folds JD, Schmitz JL. 24. Clinical and laboratory assessment of immunity. The Journal of Allergy and Clinical Immunology. 2003;**111**(2 Suppl):S702-S711. DOI: 10.1067/mai.2003.122

[37] Varzaneh FN et al. Cytokines in common variable immunodeficiency as signs of immune dysregulation and potential therapeutic targets: A review of the current knowledge. Journal of Clinical Immunology. 2014;**34**(5):524-543. DOI: 10.1007/s10875-014-0053-0

[38] Abraham RS, Aubert G. Flow cytometry, a versatile tool for diagnosis and monitoring of primary immunodeficiencies. Clinical and Vaccine Immunology. 2016;**23**(4):254-271. DOI: 10.1128/CVI.00001-16

[39] Milligan KL et al. Complete myeloperoxidase deficiency: Beware the "false-positive" dihydrorhodamine oxidation. The Journal of Pediatrics. 2016;**176**:204-206. DOI: 10.1016/j.jpeds.2016.05.047

[40] Dinauer MC. Disorders of neutrophil function: An overview. Methods in Molecular Biology. 2007;**412**:489-504. DOI: 10.1007/978-1-59745-467-4_30

[41] Orange JS. Natural killer cell deficiency. The Journal of Allergy and Clinical Immunology. 2013;**132**(3):515-525. DOI: 10.1016/j.jaci.2013.07.020

[42] Rubin TS et al. Perforin and CD107a testing is superior to NK cell function testing for screening patients for genetic HLH. Blood. 2017;**129**(22):2993-2999. DOI: 10.1182/blood-2016-12-753830

[43] Chiang SCC, Bleesing JJ, Marsh RA. Current flow cytometric assays for the screening and diagnosis of primary HLH. Frontiers in Immunology. 2019;**10**:1740. DOI: 10.3389/fimmu.2019.01740

[44] Nilsson B, Ekdahl KN. Complement diagnostics: Concepts, indications, and practical guidelines. Clinical & Developmental Immunology. 2012;**2012**:962702. DOI: 10.1155/2012/962702

[45] Kanegane H, et al. Flow cytometry-based diagnosis of primary immunodeficiency diseases. Allergology International. 2018;**67**(1):43-54. DOI: 10.1016/j.alit.2017.06.003

[46] Knight V. The utility of flow cytometry for the diagnosis of primary immunodeficiencies. International Journal of Laboratory Hematology. 2019;**41**(Suppl 1):63-72. DOI: 10.1111/ijlh.13010

[47] Piatosa B et al. B cell subsets in healthy children: Reference values for evaluation of B cell maturation process in peripheral blood. Cytometry. Part B, Clinical Cytometry. 2010;**78**(6):372-381. DOI: 10.1002/cyto.b.20536

[48] Schatorje EJ et al. Age-matched reference values for B-lymphocyte subpopulations and CVID classifications in children. Scandinavian Journal of Immunology. 2011;**74**(5):502-510. DOI: 10.1111/j.1365-3083.2011.02609.x

[49] Karimi MA et al. Measuring cytotoxicity by bioluminescence imaging outperforms the standard chromium-51 release assay. PLoS One. 2014;**9**(2):e89357. DOI: 10.1371/journal.pone.0089357

[50] Heimall JR et al. Use of genetic testing for primary immunodeficiency patients. Journal of Clinical Immunology. 2018;**38**(3):320-329. DOI: 10.1007/s10875-018-0489-8

[51] Ameratunga R et al. The clinical utility of molecular diagnostic testing for primary immune deficiency disorders: A case based review. Allergy, Asthma and Clinical Immunology. 2010;**6**(1):12. DOI: 10.1186/1710-1492-6-12

[52] Zheng X et al. The effects of cryoprotectants on sperm motility of the Chinese pearl oyster, *Pinctada fucata* martensii. Cryobiology. 2018;**82**:64-69. DOI: 10.1016/j.cryobiol.2018.04.007

[53] Chinn IK, Bostwick BL. The role of genomic approaches in diagnosis and management of primary immunodeficiency. Current Opinion in Pediatrics. 2018;**30**(6):791-797. DOI: 10.1097/MOP.0000000000000695

[54] Barbaro M et al. Newborn screening for severe primary immunodeficiency diseases in Sweden-a 2-year pilot TREC and KREC screening study. Journal of Clinical Immunology. 2017;**37**(1):51-60. DOI: 10.1007/s10875-016-0347-5

[55] Raje N et al. Utility of next generation sequencing in clinical primary immunodeficiencies. Current Allergy and Asthma Reports. 2014;**14**(10):468. DOI: 10.1007/s11882-014-0468-y

[56] Dinauer MC. Primary immune deficiencies with defects in neutrophil function. Hematology. American Society of Hematology. Education Program. 2016;**2016**(1):43-50. DOI: 10.1182/asheducation-2016.1.43

[57] Krivan G et al. New insights in the use of immunoglobulins for the management of immune deficiency (PID) patients. American Journal of Clinical and Experimental Immunology. 2017;**6**(5):76-83

[58] Bonagura VR. Using intravenous immunoglobulin (IVIG) to treat patients with primary immune deficiency disease. Journal of Clinical Immunology. 2013;**33**(Suppl 2):S90-S94. DOI: 10.1007/s10875-012-9838-1

[59] Shapiro RS et al. Emerging paradigm of primary immunodeficiency disease: Individualizing immunoglobulin dose and delivery to enhance outcomes. Journal of Clinical Immunology. 2017;**37**(2):190-196. DOI: 10.1007/s10875-014-9990-x

[60] Bethune C et al. British Society for Immunology/United Kingdom Primary Immunodeficiency Network consensus statement on managing non-infectious complications of common variable immunodeficiency disorders. Clinical and Experimental Immunology. 2019;**196**(3):328-335. DOI: 10.1111/cei.13272

[61] Heimall J et al. Current knowledge and priorities for future research in late effects after hematopoietic stem cell transplantation (HCT) for severe

combined immunodeficiency patients: A consensus statement from the second pediatric blood and marrow transplant consortium international conference on late effects after pediatric HCT. Biology of Blood and Marrow Transplantation. 2017;**23**(3):379-387. DOI: 10.1016/j.bbmt.2016.12.619

[62] Castagnoli R et al. Hematopoietic stem cell transplantation in primary immunodeficiency diseases: Current status and future perspectives. Frontiers in Pediatrics. 2019;**7**:295. DOI: 10.3389/fped.2019.00295

[63] Chinen J, Puck JM. Successes and risks of gene therapy in primary immunodeficiencies. The Journal of Allergy and Clinical Immunology. 2004;**113**(4):595-603. DOI: 10.1016/j.jaci.2004.01.765

[64] Booth C et al. Gene therapy for primary immunodeficiency. Human Molecular Genetics. 2019. DOI: 10.1093/hmg/ddz170. [Epub ahead of print]

[65] Mukherjee S, Thrasher AJ. Gene therapy for PIDs: Progress, pitfalls and prospects. Gene. 2013;**525**(2):174-181. DOI: 10.1016/j.gene.2013.03.098

[66] Markert ML, Devlin BH, McCarthy EA. Thymus transplantation. Clinical Immunology. 2010;**135**(2):236-246. DOI: 10.1016/j.clim.2010.02.007

[67] Wahlstrom JT, Dvorak CC, Cowan MJ. Hematopoietic stem cell transplantation for severe combined immunodeficiency. Current Pediatrics Reports. 2015;**3**(1):1-10. DOI: 10.1007/s40124-014-0071-7

[68] Starr SP. Immunology update: Primary immunodeficiency diseases. FP Essentials. 2016;**450**:35-53

[69] Yarmohammadi H et al. Recognizing primary immune deficiency in clinical practice. Clinical and Vaccine Immunology. 2006;**13**(3):329-332. DOI: 10.1128/CVI.13.3.329-332.2006

Chapter 6

Cerebral Autosomal Dominant Arteriopathy with Subcortical Infarcts and Leukoencephalopathy (CADASIL)

Carmine Ungaro and Teresa Sprovieri

Abstract

Cerebral autosomal dominant arteriopathy with subcortical infarcts and leukoencephalopathy (CADASIL) is an inherited cerebrovascular disease whose key features are recurrent transient ischemic attacks (TIA), strokes, migraine with aura, vascular dementia, and diffuse white matter abnormalities detectable through neuroimaging. The disease results from mutations in the NOTCH3 gene, encoding a transmembrane receptor involved in cellular signaling and fate during embryonic development. Genetic testing is the gold standard for diagnosing this condition, but the syndrome can be suspected clinically based on family history and characteristic findings of white matter changes. Nevertheless, different individual symptom types, onset, and disease severity, even among individuals in the same family, have been increasingly recognized. The molecular mechanisms by which NOTCH3 mutations lead to vascular degeneration remain unclear. Most CADASIL-associated mutations result in either a gain or loss of cysteine residue in one of the 34 EGF-like repeats in the extracellular domain of the Notch3 protein, thus sparing the number of cysteine residues. More than 200 different mutations in the NOTCH3 gene have been reported in CADASIL patients, of which 95% are missense point mutations. Although it has been suggested that some mutations may be associated with a milder or more severe phenotype, so far no clear genotype-phenotype correlation has been found. To date, no disease-modifying treatment is available for this condition.

Keywords: arteriopathy, leukoencephalopathy, cerebrovascular disease, NOTCH3 gene, Notch3 protein

1. Introduction

CADASIL (MIM 125310) is the acronym for cerebral autosomal dominant arteriopathy with subcortical infarcts and leukoencephalopathy, coined in 1993 to define a hereditary small vessel disease of the brain affecting middle-aged adults and leading to disability and dementia [1, 2]. The disease was first described in 1955 by Van Bogaert as "Binswanger's disease with a rapid course in two sisters" [3]. Before 1993, a number of families with an apparently hereditary vascular dementia accompanied by a Binswanger-like arteriopathy were described [3–5], but only in 1991, Tournier-Lasserve et al. [6] described nine patients of a single family, with recurrent cerebrovascular ischemic events and dementia, variably associated with migraine headaches and epilepsy, suggesting the term "autosomal dominant syndrome with stroke-like episodes and leukoencephalopathy." In 1993, a linkage analysis of two unrelated European families led to the mapping of the defective gene to chromosome 19q12, and the syndrome was renamed CADASIL [1]. Compared with other inherited brain disorders such as Huntington's disease or inherited early-onset Alzheimer's dementia, CADASIL is still relatively unknown in the medical community. This is not so much due to the fact that it is a rare disease but more to the fact that there is only a short history of recognition of the disease [7].

2. Clinical picture

CADASIL is an inherited cerebrovascular disorder, whose main clinical features are migraine with aura, recurrent subcortical ischemic attacks, strokes, vascular dementia, cognitive impairment, psychiatric disturbances, and apathy [8–16]. Due to the rarity of the disease, CADASIL is often overlooked and misdiagnosed; nevertheless, the combined symptomatic and asymptomatic prevalence of CADASIL is estimated at least 10.7 per 100,000 adults [11, 12, 17–20]. Migraine with aura is an early sign, with average onset in the third decade of life, and it is typically reported to occur in 20–40% of patients [9, 21]. Transient ischemic attacks (TIA) or lacunar ischemic strokes are the most common signs, occurring in up to 85% of individuals with a mean onset in the fifth or sixth decade; usually they take the form of clinical lacunar syndromes [21, 22]. The second most frequent clinical manifestation is cognitive impairment, often leading to dementia, which occurs in a very high proportion of patients by the age of 50 years. Mood disturbances are reported in 20% of CADASIL patients, presenting as severe depressive episodes [21]. Moreover, researchers recognize apathy, which is independent from depression, as a major clinical manifestation, affecting about 40% of patients [23]. Patients with CADASIL exhibit, even more rarely, other clinical manifestations such as seizures in 5–10% of cases [22]; intracerebral hemorrhages [24], mostly in hypertensive patients, in 16–25% of cases [25, 26]; and, in a few cases, territorial infarcts [27], deafness [6], and parkinsonism [28]. All symptomatic patients present typical magnetic resonance imaging (MRI) findings, including noticeable signal abnormalities with hyperintense lesions on the T2-weighted images in the subcortical white matter, basal ganglia, and thalamus (a crucial difference from multiple sclerosis, a frequent mimic of CADASIL) [1, 6, 29–33]. Anterior temporal lobe hyperintensities may be more specific than external capsule changes and appear in young presymptomatic subjects [34]. In the vast majority of patients, brain MRI abnormalities precede the onset of symptoms by 10–15 years; thus, brain MRI is crucial for the diagnosis of CADASIL. Although marked population differences in the clinical and radiological manifestation of CADASIL have been recognized, potentially due to differences in underlying genetic mutations [21, 35–37], in the proper clinical evaluation based on symptoms suggestive of CADASIL, confluent anterior temporal pole white matter changes show sensitivity and specificity of 89 and 86%, respectively, based on case series. From a pathological point of view, CADASIL patients have a systemic non-amyloid, non-atherosclerotic angiopathy affecting the walls of small blood vessels [38, 39]. The accumulation of granular osmiophilic material (GOM) within the smooth muscle cell basement membrane and the surrounding extracellular matrix is pathognomonic [40–42]. Because the arteriopathy in CADASIL is systemic, GOM deposits, which contain Notch3 proteins, among other poorly defined components [40, 43, 44], can be detected in arteries of many different organs, including dermal arterioles. In fact, actually GOMs are detected in skin biopsies, but the reported sensitivity is variable [45, 46]. CADASIL is inherited dominantly, with over 500 families detected worldwide and de novo cases observed sporadically [47].

3. Genetics

NOTCH3 gene mutations are causative of the disease. This gene, consisting of 33 exons spanning roughly 7 kb and located on chromosome 19p13 [48], encodes a single-pass transmembrane heterodimer receptor Notch3 of 2321 amino acids involved in cellular signaling and fate during embryonic development [49, 50]. Notch3 protein comprising an N-terminal extracellular domain (NECD) involved in ligand binding, a transmembrane domain (NTMD), and an intracellular domain (NICD), which contains seven ankyrin repeats is required for downstream signal transduction (**Figure 1**) [51, 52]. More specifically, the NECD is non-covalently associated with the membrane-tethered intracellular domain, and it is composed of 34 epidermal growth factor (EGF)-like repeats, followed by 3 Notch/lin12 repeats [53]. Each EGF-like repeat encompasses six cysteine residues, forming three pairs of disulfide bonds [54, 55]. The receptor is synthesized as single precursor protein which is cleaved during transport to the cell surface (S1 cleavage), where it is expressed as heterodimer. Upon binding of its ligand (a protein of the delta/jagged family) [56] at EGF repeats 10–11, Notch3 receptor undergoes two other proteolytic cleavages: at first, N3 is cleaved (S2 cleavage) in its extracellular domain by a TNF-α-converting enzyme (TACE), subsequently in its transmembrane domain (S3 cleavage) in a presenilin-dependent manner. These proteolytic events, mutually dependent, generate the NICD fragment, which released from the NTMD enters the nucleus for activating the transcription of its target genes [53, 57–59]. Although the mutations are highly stereotyped, atypical phenotypes have been recognized, and the disease is probably underdiagnosed in most of the stroke population. Most CADASIL-associated mutations result in a gain or loss of cysteine residue in one of the 34 EGF-like repeats in the extracellular domain of the Notch3 protein, thus sparing the number of cysteine residues within the domain [60–62]. The alteration of the 3-D structure of the Notch3 protein, which is due to an aberrant dimerization of Notch3 through an abnormal disulfide bridging with another Notch3 molecule or with another protein, may play a central role in the pathogenesis of CADASIL [63–65]. A founder effect has been documented for the Finnish population but

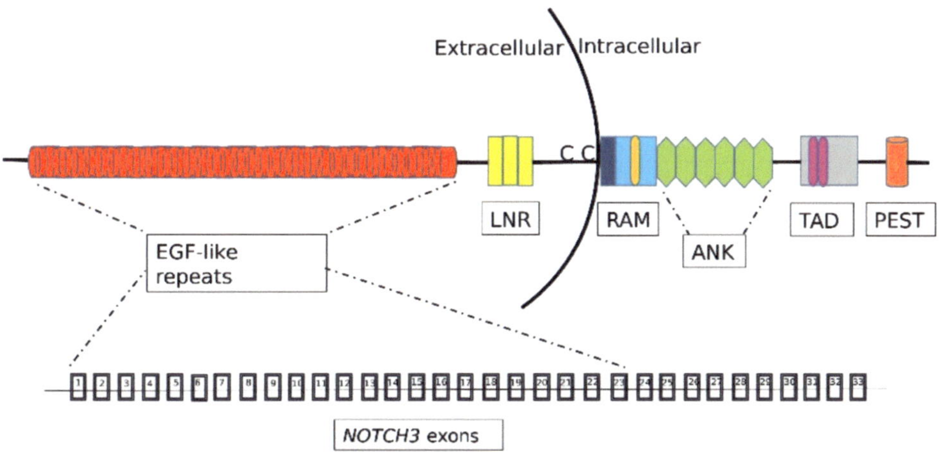

Figure 1.
Schematic structure of Notch3 protein: Notch3 domains are differently colored.

not for other countries [66]. To date, more than 200 different mutations in the NOTCH3 gene have been reported in CADASIL patients, of which 95% are heterozygous missense point mutations [67]. The remaining consist of small deletions, duplications, in frame [68–71] and frame shift mutations, splice site mutations [36], and a small deletion not directly involving a cysteine residue [72]. Moreover, a three-nucleotide insertion has been described as the first pathogenic insertion [73]. Recent studies have found that mutations that do not affect the number of cysteines (unlike the typical mutations) seem to be associated with clinical CADASIL syndrome. However, the pathogenic role of these mutations is uncertain. Although it has been suggested that some mutations may be associated with a milder or more severe phenotype, so far no clear genotype-phenotype correlation has been found [7]. Moreover, only a few cases in the literature reported homozygous mutations of NOTCH3 [74–78]. Many polymorphisms have also been identified in the NOTCH3 coding sequence [67], some of them leading to amino acid substitutions [79]. However, it is unknown whether these polymorphisms affect Notch signaling or whether they are involved in cerebrovascular disease.

4. Diagnosis

The pathology should be suspected in all cases with unexplained white matter hyperintensities and a family history of stroke and/or vascular dementia, consistent with an autosomal dominant inheritance. However, because affected family members may have been misdiagnosed [80] and de novo cases have been described [69, 81], the lack of an apparent family history of CADASIL does not preclude the diagnosis. Several groups of clinicians [13, 14, 82] proposed suitable diagnostic strategies to be used in the clinical setting for the selection of patients to be subjected to NOTCH3 gene analysis. In fact, in order to establish a correct diagnosis, clinical signs, neuroimaging findings, and family history need to be evaluated. Molecular screening is the gold standard for the diagnosis and is based on the identification in a proband of a pathogenic variation in the NOTCH3 coding sequence [36, 83]. With a suggestive diagnosis of CADASIL, a single-gene testing or a multigene panel could be applied; if NOTCH3 screening is unavailable or gives a negative result in a patient with convincing clinical and MRI findings highly suggestive of CADASIL, a skin biopsy analysis using both Notch3 immunostaining and electron microscopy should be recommended to confirm or reject the diagnosis [21, 84]. If CADASIL phenotype overlaps with other inherited cerebrovascular diseases, a comprehensive genomic testing, such as exome sequencing, should be recommended in evaluating different genes involved.

5. Therapeutic approach and outlooks

CADASIL is one of the most monogenic causes of stroke. No disease-modifying treatment is available. Being a genetic disease, two possible gene therapeutic approaches have been highlighted [85, 86], but, to date, only a symptomatic therapy focused on mitigating symptoms and management of the patient's vascular risk factor can be applied [87, 88], beginning as immediate action to promote healthy individual behaviors, i.e., to refrain from smoking. Anyway, it is important that patients be referred to multidisciplinary and specialized centers, not only providing genetic counseling but also integrating the clinical and neuroimaging follow-up with neuropsychiatric, psychologic, and physical rehabilitation consultations.

Acknowledgements

Authors gratefully acknowledge Ariangela Belvedere, Walter Carpino, Patrizia Rizzuto, Tiziana Martire, Benedetto Bruno, and Angelo Bagalà for their administrative and technical support.

Conflict of interest

The authors declare no conflict of interest.

Author details

Carmine Ungaro* and Teresa Sprovieri
Institute for Research and Biomedical Innovation, National Research Council, Mangone (CS), Italy

*Address all correspondence to: carmine.ungaro@cnr.it

References

[1] Tournier-Lasserve E, Joutel A, Melki J, Weissenbach J, Lathrop GM, Chabriat H, et al. Cerebral autosomal dominant arteriopathy with subcortical infarcts and leukoencephalopathy maps on chromosome 19q12. Nature Genetics. 1993;**3**:256-259. DOI: 10.1038/ng0393-256

[2] Bousser MG, Tournier-Lasserve E. Summary of the proceedings of the first international workshop on CADASIL. Stroke. 1994;**25**:704-707

[3] Van Bogaert L. Encéphalopathie sous-corticale progressive (Binswanger) à évolution rapide chez deux soeurs. Médecine Hellénique. 1955;**24**:961-972

[4] Stevens DL, Hewlett RH, Brownell B. Chronic familial vascular encephalopathy. The Lancet. 1977;**1**(8026):1364-1365

[5] Sourander P, Wålinder J. Hereditary multi-infarct dementia. Morphological and clinical studies of a new disease. Acta Neuropathologica. 1977;**39**(3):247-254

[6] Tournier-Lasserve E, Iba-Zizen MT, Romero N, Bousser MG. Autosomal dominant syndrome with strokelike episodes and leukoencephalopathy. Stroke. 1991;**22**(10):1297-1302

[7] Rutten JW, Haan J, Terwindt GM, van Duinen SG, Boon EM, Lesnik Oberstein SA. Interpretation of NOTCH3 mutations in the diagnosis of CADASIL. Expert Review of Molecular Diagnostics. 2014;**14**(5):593-603. DOI: 10.1586/14737159.2014.922880

[8] Majersik JJ. Single gene causes of stroke. Seminars in Neurology. 2017;**37**(3):351-365. DOI: 10.1055/s-0037-1603952

[9] Majersik JJ. Inherited and uncommon causes of stroke. Continuum (Minneap Minn). 2017;**23**(1, Cerebrovascular Disease):211-237. DOI: 10.1212/CON.0000000000000432

[10] Bersano A, Bedini G, Oskam J, Mariotti C, Taroni F, Baratta S, et al. CADASIL: Treatment and management options. Current Treatment Options in Neurology. 2017;**19**(9):31. DOI: 10.1007/s11940-017-0468-z

[11] Chabriat H, Vahedi K, Iba-Zizen MT, Joutel A, Nibbio A, Nagy TG, et al. Clinical spectrum of CADASIL: A study of 7 families. Cerebral autosomal dominant arteriopathy with subcortical infarcts and leukoencephalopathy. The Lancet. 1995;**346**:934-939

[12] Opherk C, Peters N, Herzog J, Luedtke R, Dichgans M. Long-term prognosis and causes of death in CADASIL: A retrospective study in 411 patients. Brain. 2004;**127**:2533-2539. DOI: 10.1093/brain/awh282

[13] Mizuta I, Watanabe-Hosomi A, Koizumi T, Mukai M, Hamano A, Tomii Y, et al. New diagnostic criteria for cerebral autosomal dominant arteriopathy with subcortical infarcts and leukoencephalopathy in Japan. Journal of the Neurological Sciences. 2017;**381**:62-67. DOI: 10.1016/j.jns.2017.08.009

[14] Bersano A, Bedini G, Markus HS, Vitali P, Colli-Tibaldi E, Taroni F, et al. Lombardia GENS-group. The role of clinical and neuroimaging features in the diagnosis of CADASIL. Journal of Neurology. 2018;**265**(12):2934-2943. DOI: 10.1007/s00415-018-9072-8

[15] Vahedi K, Chabriat H, Levy C, Joutel A, Tournier-Lasserve E, Bousser MG. Migraine with aura and brain magnetic resonance imaging abnormalities in patients with CADASIL. Archives of Neurology. 2004;**61**:1237-1240. DOI: 10.1001/archneur.61.8.1237

[16] Rhea YYT, Markus HS. CADASIL: Migraine, encephalopathy, stroke and their inter-relationships. PLoS One. 2016;**11**(6):e0157613. DOI: 10.1371/journal.pone.0157613

[17] Moreton FC, Razvi SS, Davidson R, Muir KW. Changing clinical patterns and increasing prevalence in CADASIL. Acta Neurologica Scandinavica. 2014;**130**(3):197-203. DOI: 10.1111/ane.12266

[18] Portegies MLP, Koudstaal PJ, Ikram MA. Cerebrovascular Disease. In: Rosano C, Ikram MA, Ganguli M, editors. Handbook of Clinical Neurology. 3rd Series: Neuroepidemiology. Vol. 138. Amsterdam: Elsevier BV; 2016. p. 239-261. DOI: 10.1016/B978-0-12-802973-2.00014-8

[19] Narayan SK, Gorman G, Kalaria RN, Ford GA, Chinnery PF. The minimum prevalence of CADASIL in Northeast England. Neurology. 2012;**78**(13):1025-1027. DOI: 10.1212/WNL.0b013e31824d586c

[20] Adib-Samii P, Brice G, Martin RJ, Markus HS. Clinical spectrum of CADASIL and the effect of cardiovascular risk factors on phenotype: Study in 200 consecutively recruited individuals. Stroke. 2010;**41**:630-634. DOI: 10.1161/STROKEAHA.109.568402

[21] Chabriat H, Joutel A, Dichgans M, Tournier-Lasserve E, Bousser MG. Cadasil. Lancet Neurology. 2009;**8**(7):643-653. DOI: 10.1016/S1474-4422(09)70127-9

[22] Dichgans M, Mayer M, Uttner I, Brüning R, Müller-Höcker J, Rungger G, et al. The phenotypic spectrum of CADASIL: Clinical findings in 102 cases. Annals of Neurology. 1998;**44**(5):731-739. DOI: 10.1002/ana.410440506

[23] Reyes S, Viswanathan A, Godin O, Dufouil C, Benisty S, Hernandez K, et al. Apathy: A major symptom in CADASIL. Neurology. 2009;**72**(10):905-910. DOI: 10.1212/01.wnl.0000344166.03470.f8

[24] Ragoschke-Schumm A, Axer H, Witte O, Isenmann S, Fitzek C, Dichgans M, et al. Intracerebral haemorrhage in CADASIL. Journal of Neurology, Neurosurgery, and Psychiatry. 2005;**76**(11):1606-1607. DOI: 10.1136/jnnp.2004.059212. Correction in: Journal of Neurology, Neurosurgery, and Psychiatry. 2006;**77**(1):125

[25] Choi JC, Kang SY, Kang JH, Park JK. Intracerebral hemorrhages in CADASIL. Neurology. 2006;**67**(11):2042-2044. DOI: 10.1212/01.wnl.0000246601.70918.06

[26] Liao YC, Hsiao CT, Fuh JL, Chern CM, Lee WJ, Guo YC, et al. Characterization of CADASIL among the Han Chinese in Taiwan: Distinct genotypic and phenotypic profiles. PLoS One. 2015;**10**(8):e0136501. DOI: 10.1371/journal.pone.0136501

[27] Choi EJ, Choi CG, Kim JS. Large cerebral artery involvement in CADASIL. Neurology. 2005;**65**(8):1322-1324. DOI: 10.1212/01.wnl.0000180965.79209.50

[28] Van Gerpen JA, Ahlskog JE, Petty GW. Progressive supranuclear palsy phenotype secondary to CADASIL. Parkinsonism & Related Disorders. 2003;**9**(6):367-369

[29] Chabriat H, Mrissa R, Levy C, Vahedi K, Taillia H, Iba-Zizen MT, et al. Brain stem MRI signal abnormalities in CADASIL. Stroke. 1999;**30**(2):457-459

[30] Chabriat H, Pappata S, Poupon C, Clark CA, Vahedi K, Poupon F, et al. Clinical severity in CADASIL related to ultrastructural damage in white matter: in vivo study with diffusion tensor MRI. Stroke. 1999;**30**(12):2637-2643

[31] Chabriat H, Levy C, Taillia H, Iba-Zizen MT, Vahedi K, Joutel A, et al. Patterns of MRI lesions in CADASIL. Neurology. 1998;**51**(2): 452-457. DOI: 10.1212/wnl.51.2.452

[32] Dichgans M, Holtmannspötter M, Herzog J, Peters N, Bergmann M, Yousry TA. Cerebral microbleeds in CADASIL: A gradient-echo magnetic resonance imaging and autopsy study. Stroke. 2002;**33**(1):67-71

[33] van Den Boom R, Lesnik Oberstein SA, van Duinen SG, Bornebroek M, Ferrari MD, Haan J, et al. Subcortical lacunar lesions: An MR imaging finding in patients with cerebral autosomal dominant arteriopathy with subcortical infarcts and leukoencephalopathy. Radiology. 2002;**224**(3):791-796. DOI: 10.1148/radiol.2243011123

[34] Wang MM. CADASIL. Handbook of Clinical Neurology. 2018;**148**:733-743. DOI: 10.1016/B978-0-444-64076-5.00047-8

[35] Zhu S, Nahas SJ. CADASIL: Imaging characteristics and clinical correlation. Current Pain and Headache Reports. 2016;**20**(10):57. DOI: 10.1007/s11916-016-0584-6

[36] Markus HS, Martin RJ, Simpson MA, Dong YB, Ali N, Crosby AH, et al. Diagnostic strategies in CADASIL. Neurology. 2002;**59**(8): 1134-1138. DOI: 10.1212/wnl.59.8.1134

[37] Singhal S, Rich P, Markus HS. The spatial distribution of MR imaging abnormalities in cerebral autosomal dominant arteriopathy with subcortical infarcts and leukoencephalopathy and their relationship to age and clinical features. American Journal of Neuroradiology. 2005;**26**(10):2481-2487

[38] Ruchoux MM, Guerouaou D, Vandenhaute B, Pruvo JP, Vermersch P, Leys D. Systemic vascular smooth muscle cell impairment in cerebral autosomal dominant arteriopathy with subcortical infarcts and leukoencephalopathy. Acta Neuropathologica. 1995;**89**(6):500-512

[39] Schröder JM, Züchner S, Dichgans M, Nagy Z, Molnar MJ. Peripheral nerve and skeletal muscle involvement in CADASIL. Acta Neuropathologica. 2005;**110**(6):587-599. DOI: 10.1007/s00401-005-1082-9

[40] Lorenzi T, Ragno M, Paolinelli F, Castellucci C, Scarpelli M, Morroni M. CADASIL: Ultrastructural insights into the morphology of granular osmiophilic material. Brain and Behavior: A Cognitive Neuroscience Perspective. 2017;**7**(3):e00624. DOI: 10.1002/brb3.624

[41] Lewandowska E, Dziewulska D, Parys M, Pasennik E. Ultrastructure of granular osmiophilic material deposits (GOM) in arterioles of CADASIL patients. Folia Neuropathologica. 2011;**49**(3):174-180

[42] Gridley T. Notch signaling in the vasculature. Current Topics in Developmental Biology. 2010;**92**:277-309. DOI: 10.1016/S0070-2153(10)92009-7

[43] Ishiko A, Shimizu A, Nagata E, Takahashi K, Tabira T, Suzuki N. Notch3 ectodomain is a major component of granular osmiophilic material (GOM) in CADASIL. Acta Neuropathologica. 2006;**112**(3):333-339. DOI: 10.1007/s00401-006-0116-2

[44] Yamamoto Y, Craggs LJ, Watanabe A, Booth T, Attems J, Low RW, et al. Brain microvascular accumulation and distribution of the NOTCH3 ectodomain and granular osmiophilic material in CADASIL. Journal of Neuropathology and Experimental Neurology. 2013;**72**(5):416-431. DOI: 10.1097/NEN.0b013e31829020b5

[45] Tikka S, Mykkänen K, Ruchoux MM, Bergholm R, Junna M, Pöyhönen M, et al. Congruence between NOTCH3 mutations and GOM in 131 CADASIL patients. Brain. 2009;**132**(Pt 4):933-939. DOI: 10.1093/brain/awn364

[46] Morroni M, Marzioni D, Ragno M, Di Bella P, Cartechini E, Pianese L, et al. Role of electron microscopy in the diagnosis of cadasil syndrome: A study of 32 patients. PLoS One. 2013;**8**(6):e65482. DOI: 10.1371/journal.pone.0065482

[47] Pippucci T, Maresca A, Magini P, Cenacchi G, Donadio V, Palombo F, et al. Homozygous NOTCH3 null mutation and impaired NOTCH3 signaling in recessive early-onset arteriopathy and cavitating leukoencephalopathy. EMBO Molecular Medicine. 2015;**7**(6):848-858. DOI: 10.15252/emmm.201404399

[48] Joutel A, Corpechot C, Ducros A, Vahedi K, Chabriat H, Mouton P, et al. Notch3 mutations in CADASIL, a hereditary adult-onset condition causing stroke and dementia. Nature. 1996;**383**(6602):707-710. DOI: 10.1038/383707a0

[49] Xu X, Choi SH, Hu T, Tiyanont K, Habets R, Groot AJ, et al. Insights into autoregulation of Notch3 from structural and functional studies of its negative regulatory region. Structure. 2015;**23**(7):1227-1235. DOI: 10.1016/j.str.2015.05.001

[50] Domenga V, Fardoux P, Lacombe P, Monet M, Maciazek J, Krebs LT, et al. Notch3 is required for arterial identity and maturation of vascular smooth muscle cells. Genes & Development. 2004;**18**:2730-2735. DOI: 10.1101/gad.308904

[51] Weinmaster G. The ins and outs of notch signaling. Molecular and Cellular Neurosciences. 1997;**9**(2):91-102. DOI: 10.1006/mcne.1997.0612

[52] Monet M, Domenga V, Lemaire B, Souilhol C, Langa F, Babinet C, et al. The archetypal R90C CADASIL-NOTCH3 mutation retains NOTCH3 function in vivo. Human Molecular Genetics. 2007;**16**(8):982-992. DOI: 10.1093/hmg/ddm042

[53] Tikka S, Baumann M, Siitonen M, Pasanen P, Pöyhönen M, Myllykangas L, et al. CADASIL and CARASIL. Brain Pathology. 2014;**24**(5):525-544. DOI: 10.1111/bpa.12181

[54] Hiruma-Shimizu K, Hosoguchi K, Liu Y, Fujitani N, Ohta T, Hinou H, et al. Chemical synthesis, folding, and structural insights into O-fucosylated epidermal growth factor-like repeat 12 of mouse Notch-1 receptor. Journal of The American Chemical Society. 2010;**132**(42):14857-14865. DOI: 10.1021/ja105216u

[55] Hambleton S, Valeyev NV, Muranyi A, Knott V, Werner JM, McMichael AJ, et al. Structural and functional properties of the human notch-1 ligand binding region. Structure. 2004;**12**(12):2173-2183. DOI: 10.1016/j.str.2004.09.012

[56] Artavanis-Tsakonas S, Muskavitch MA. Notch: The past, the present, and the future. Current Topics in Developmental Biology. 2010;**92**:1-29. DOI: 10.1016/S0070-2153(10)92001-2

[57] Belin de Chantemèle EJ, Retailleau K, Pinaud F, Vessières E, Bocquet A, Guihot AL, et al. Notch3 is a major regulator of vascular tone in cerebral and tail resistance arteries. Arteriosclerosis, Thrombosis, and Vascular Biology. 2008;**28**:2216-2224. DOI: 10.1161/ATVBAHA.108.171751

[58] Guruharsha KG, Kankel MW, Artavanis-Tsakonas S. The notch signalling system: Recent insights into the complexity of a conserved pathway. Nature Reviews. Genetics. 2012;**13**(9):654-666. DOI: 10.1038/nrg3272

[59] Boucher J, Gridley T, Liaw L. Molecular pathways of notch signaling in vascular smooth muscle cells. Frontiers in Physiology. 2012;**3**:81. DOI: 10.3389/fphys.2012.00081

[60] Dichgans M, Herzog J, Gasser T. NOTCH3 mutation involving three cysteine residues in a family with typical CADASIL. Neurology. 2001;**57**(9): 1714-1717. DOI: 10.1212/wnl.57.9.1714

[61] Rutten JV, Dauwerse HG, Gravesteijn G, van Belzen MJ, van der Grond J, Polke JM, et al. Archetypal NOTCH3 mutations frequent in public exome: Implications for CADASIL. Annals of Clinical Translational Neurology. 2016;**3**(11):844-853. DOI: 10.1002/acn3.344

[62] Muiño E, Gallego-Fabrega C, Cullell N, Carrera C, Torres N, Krupinski J, et al. Systematic review of cysteine-sparing NOTCH3 missense mutations in patients with clinical suspicion of CADASIL. International Journal of Molecular Sciences. 2017;**18**(9):1964. DOI: 10.3390/ijms18091964

[63] Duering M, Karpinska A, Rosner S, Hopfner F, Zechmeister M, Peters N, et al. Co-aggregate formation of CADASIL-mutant NOTCH3: A single-particle analysis. Human Molecular Genetics. 2011;**20**(16):3256-3265. DOI: 10.1093/hmg/ddr237

[64] Meng H, Zhang X, Yu G, Lee SJ, Chen YE, Prudovsky I, et al. Biochemical characterization and cellular effects of CADASIL mutants of NOTCH3. PLoS One. 2012;**7**(9):e44964. DOI: 10.1371/journal.pone.0044964

[65] Opherk C, Duering M, Peters N, Karpinska A, Rosner S, Schneider E, et al. CADASIL mutations enhance spontaneous multimerization of NOTCH3. Human Molecular Genetics. 2009;**18**(15):2761-2767. DOI: 10.1093/hmg/ddp211

[66] Mykkänen K, Savontaus ML, Juvonen V, Sistonen P, Tuisku S, Tuominen S, et al. Detection of the founder effect in Finnish CADASIL families. European Journal of Human Genetics. 2004;**12**(10):813-819. DOI: 10.1038/sj.ejhg.5201221

[67] Federico A, Bianchi S, Dotti MT. The spectrum of mutations for CADASIL diagnosis. Neurological Sciences. 2005;**26**(2):117-124. DOI: 10.1007/s10072-005-0444-3

[68] Dichgans M, Ludwig H, Müller-Höcker J, Messerschmidt A, Gasser T. Small in-frame deletions and missense mutations in CADASIL: 3D models predict misfolding of Notch3 EGF-like repeat domains. European Journal of Human Genetics. 2000;**8**(4):280-285. DOI: 10.1038/sj.ejhg.5200460

[69] Joutel A, Chabriat H, Vahedi K, Domenga V, Vayssière C, Ruchoux MM, et al. Splice site mutation causing a seven amino acid Notch3 in-frame deletion in CADASIL. Neurology. 2000;**54**(9):1874-1875. DOI: 10.1212/wnl.54.9.1874

[70] Joutel A, Dodick DD, Parisi JE, Cecillon M, Tournier-Lasserve E, Bousser MG. De novo mutation in the Notch3 gene causing CADASIL. Annals of Neurology. 2000;**47**(3):388-391

[71] Dotti MT, De Stefano N, Bianchi S, Malandrini A, Battisti C, Cardaioli E, et al. A novel NOTCH3 frameshift deletion and mitochondrial abnormalities in a patient with CADASIL. Archives of Neurology. 2004;**61**(6):942-945. DOI: 10.1001/archneur.61.6.942

[72] Mazzei R, Conforti FL, Lanza PL, Sprovieri T, Lupo MR, Gallo O, et al. A novel Notch3 gene mutation not involving a cysteine residue in an Italian family with CADASIL. Neurology. 2004;**63**(3):561-564. DOI: 10.1212/01.wnl.0000133399.37716.84

[73] Mazzei R, Guidetti D, Ungaro C, Conforti FL, Muglia M, Cenacchi G, et al. First evidence of a pathogenic insertion in the NOTCH3 gene causing CADASIL. Journal of Neurology, Neurosurgery, and Psychiatry. 2008;**79**(1):108-110. DOI: 10.1136/jnnp.2007.128009

[74] Tuominen S, Juvonen V, Amberla K, Jolma T, Rinne JO, Tuisku S, et al. Phenotype of a homozygous CADASIL patient in comparison to 9 age-matched heterozygous patients with the same R133C Notch3 mutation. Stroke. 2001;**32**(8):1767-1774

[75] Liem MK, Lesnik Oberstein SA, Vollebregt MJ, Middelkoop HA, van der Grond J. Helderman-van den Enden AT. Journal of Neurology. 2008;**255**(12):1978-1980. DOI: 10.1007/s00415-009-0036-x

[76] Soong BW, Liao YC, Tu PH, Tsai PC, Lee IH, Chung CP, et al. A homozygous NOTCH3 mutation p.R544C and a heterozygous TREX1 variant p.C99MfsX3 in a family with hereditary small vessel disease of the brain. Journal of the Chinese Medical Association. 2013;**76**(6):319-324. DOI: 10.1016/j.jcma.2013.03.002

[77] Ragno M, Pianese L, Morroni M, Cacchiò G, Manca A, Di Marzio F, et al. "CADASIL coma" in an Italian homozygous CADASIL patient: Comparison with clinical and MRI findings in age-matched heterozygous patients with the same G528C NOTCH3 mutation. Neurological Sciences. 2013;**34**(11):1947-1953. DOI: 10.1007/s10072-013-1418-5

[78] Vinciguerra C, Rufa A, Bianchi S, Sperduto A, De Santis M, Malandrini A, et al. Homozygosity and severity of phenotypic presentation in a CADASIL family. Neurological Sciences. 2014;**35**(1):91-93. DOI: 10.1007/s10072-013-1580-9

[79] Joutel A, Vahedi K, Corpechot C, Troesch A, Chabriat H, Vayssière C, et al. Strong clustering and stereotyped nature of Notch3 mutations in CADASIL patients. The Lancet. 1997;**350**(9090):1511-1515. DOI: 10.1016/S0140-6736(97)08083-5

[80] Razvi SS, Davidson R, Bone I, Muir KW. Is inadequate family history a barrier to diagnosis in CADASIL? Acta Neurologica Scandinavica. 2005;**112**(5):323-326. DOI: 10.1111/j.1600-0404.2005.00495.x

[81] Coto E, Menéndez M, Navarro R, García-Castro M, Alvarez V. A new de novo Notch3 mutation causing CADASIL. European Journal of Neurology. 2006;**13**(6):628-631. DOI: 10.1111/j.1468-1331.2006.01337.x

[82] Pescini F, Nannucci S, Bertaccini B, Salvadori E, Bianchi S, Ragno M, et al. The cerebral autosomal-dominant arteriopathy with subcortical infarcts and leukoencephalopathy (CADASIL) scale: A screening tool to select patients for NOTCH3 gene analysis. Stroke. 2012;**43**(11):2871-2876. DOI: 10.1161/STROKEAHA.112.665927

[83] Peters N, Opherk C, Bergmann T, Castro M, Herzog J, Dichgans M. Spectrum of mutations in biopsy-proven CADASIL: Implications for diagnostic strategies. Archives of Neurology. 2005;**62**(7):1091-1094. DOI: 10.1001/archneur.62.7.1091

[84] Hack R, Rutten J, Lesnik Oberstein SAJ. CADASIL. In: Adam MP, Ardinger HH, Pagon RA, Wallace SE, LJH B, Stephens K, Amemiya A, editors. Source GeneReviews® 1993-2019. Seattle, WA: University of Washington; 2000 [Updated March 14, 2019]

[85] Koutsilieri E, Rethwilm A, Scheller C. The therapeutic potential of siRNA in gene therapy of neurodegenerative disorders. Journal of

Neural Transmission. Supplementum. 2007;**72**:43-49

[86] Scholefield J, Watson L, Smith D, Greenberg J, Wood MJ. Allele-specific silencing of mutant Ataxin-7 in SCA7 patient-derived fibroblasts. European Journal of Human Genetics. 2014;**22**(12):1369-1375. DOI: 10.1038/ejhg.2014.39

[87] Di Donato I, Bianchi S, De Stefano N, Dichgans M, Dotti MT, Duering M, et al. Cerebral autosomal dominant Arteriopathy with subcortical infarcts and leukoencephalopathy (CADASIL) as a model of small vessel disease: Update on clinical, diagnostic, and management aspects. BMC Medicine. 2017;**15**(1):41. DOI: 10.1186/s12916-017-0778-8

[88] del Río-Espínola A, Mendióroz M, Domingues-Montanari S, Pozo-Rosich P, Solé E, Fernández-Morales J, et al. CADASIL management or what to do when there is little one can do. Expert Review of Neurotherapeutics. 2009;**9**(2):197-210. DOI: 10.1586/14737175.9.2.197

Chapter 7

The Research Progress of Monogenic Inherited Hypertension

Wenxiu Liu and Xinhua Yin

Abstract

Monogenic inherited hypertension, which is caused by a single gene mutation, generally conforms to the Mendel's law, but its phenotype is affected by environmental factors as well. This type of hypertension is characterized by early onset (more common in adolescents), family history, severe hypertension, or refractory hypertension. It is often accompanied by abnormal hormone level and biochemical indicators, including low activity of plasma renin, abnormal potassium, and acid-base metabolization disorder. For adolescents with a family history of moderate to severe hypertension, hormone level (including plasma renin-angiotensin-aldosterone, cortisol, and sex hormone) and blood electrolytes should be measured and the detailed diagnosis should be determined according to medical history, physical signs, and test results. Currently, 17 kinds of monogenic hereditary hypertension have been clearly determined. Thanks to the development of gene detection technology, the diagnostic level of monogenic inherited hypertension has greatly improved and the pathogenesis has been gradually clarified. Our review mainly discussed the research progress in this field.

Keywords: monogenic hereditary disease, hypertension, rennin, potassium, gene detection

1. Introduction

Monogenic inherited hypertension, which was caused by a single gene mutation, generally conforms to the Mendel's law, but the phenotype is also affected by environmental factors. It can be identified in a large and heterogeneous family of hypertensive patients with highly specific etiologies and similar clinical manifestations [1]. It is characterized by early onset (more common in adolescents), familial aggregation, and refractory hypertension and the renin-angiotensin-aldosterone system features typical changes in almost every case. In the following report, we will review some well-characterized disorders.

1.1 Liddle syndrome

Liddle syndrome (LS), known as pseudohypoaldosteronism type I, which was firstly reported by Liddle in 1963 [2], is an autosomal dominant genetic form of low renin arterial hypertension caused by germline mutations in the SCNN1A, SCNN1B, and SCNN1G genes that encode the α, β, and γ subunits of the epithelial sodium channel (ENaC), respectively. The prevalence of LS across the general hypertensive population still remains unknown. Three small single-center studies have estimated the prevalence to be about 0.91 [3], 1.52 [4], and 6% [5] among hypertensive patients with genetic testing and phenotypical LS, respectively.

The mutation gene was the nonsense p.Agr566* substitution of the β subunit, firstly described in the large kindred by Liddle et al. and subsequently Botero-Velez et al. [6] found that the mutation causes a truncation of the C-terminus of the β subunit with a loss of the PY motif. The first germinal mutation of SCNN1G gene, resulting in the nonsense substitution p.Trp573*, was identified by Hansson et al. in 1995 [7], the mutation erases the γ subunit's C-terminus, causing the loss of the PY motif. Different rare variants of SCNN1A have also been associated with pseudohypoaldosteronism type I, with the possibility of the compound heterozygotes in different ENaC subunits contributing to its phenotype in a digenic manner.

Recently, a germline mutation in the α subunit (p.Cys479Arg) was identified in a Caucasian family suffering from LS [8]. This missense mutation increases the open conformation of the channel, resulting in a two-fold increase in Na^+ current, without affecting channel density at the plasma membrane. It has been reported that there are 31 different mutations responsible for LS in 72 families so far [9].

Most of these mutations are frameshift, missense, or nonsense, impairing the PY motif and increasing ENaC expression at the distal nephron apical membrane, following a subsequent increase in Na^+ reabsorption. LS is characterized by resistant and early onset salt-sensitive arterial hypertension clinically, often associated with a family history of early onset hypertension and sudden death.

On average, hypertension develops around the second decade of life (15.5 ± 3.3 years) [10], with variation in the age of onset and severity of hypertension [6]. Without treatment, subjects will present with complications of severe hypertension during the third or fourth decade of life. Despite the typical phenotype presenting with severe hypertension and hypokalemia, the disease can be clinically heterogeneous, even with mild phenotypes.

Biochemically, the characteristic findings are hypokalemia, metabolic alkalosis, suppressed plasma renin activity (PRA), and low serum aldosterone levels. The diagnosis of LS is based on gene sequencing of SCNN1A, SCNN1B, and SCNN1G. Considering the autosomal dominant inheritance (50% risk of transmission) and the variable phenotype reported in some families, genetic screening also has to be performed in first-degree relatives of a mutation carrier.

As for the treatment of LS, amiloride which is a potassium-sparing diuretics, or triamterene which a direct ENaC inhibitor, combined with a low sodium diet, mitigate sodium-sensitive hypertension by inhibiting sodium transport through ENaC. The drug effect is rapid and exceptionally good. While spironolactone, another potassium-sparing diuretics, has no therapeutic effect on LS.

1.2 Gordon syndrome

Gordon syndrome (GS), also known as pseudohypoaldosteronism type II or familial hyperkalemia hypertension, is a rare form of monogenic hypertension characterized by low renin, hyperkalemia, hyperchloremic metabolic acidosis, and normal glomerular filtration rate [11].

This phenotype was first discovered in 1964 by Paver and Pauline [12], and Gordon [13] identified the phenotype to be an inheritable disorder based on a study of several pedigrees later in the 1980s. The hyperkalemia is a useful discriminator, distinguishing GS from other forms of monogenic hypertension which present with normokalemia or hypokalemia [14].

Although GS is considered to be an autosomal dominant inherited disease, new molecular studies reported some recessive cases [15]. Mutations in four genes such as WNK1 (pseudohypoaldosteronism type IIC), WNK4 (pseudohypoaldosteronism type IIB) [16], CUL3 (pseudohypoaldosteronism type IIE), and KLHL3 (pseudohypoaldosteronism type IID) [17] have been identified to be responsible for GS.

WNKs belong to a large family of serine-threonine protein kinases with pleiotropic effects. The WNK kinases (encoded by the WNK1 and WNK4 genes) regulate the expression of the Na^+/Cl^--cotransporter (NCC) in the distal nephron and the Na^+-K^+-$2Cl^-$-cotransporter (NKCC2) in the thick ascending limb of Henle's loop, which play an important role in the development of hypertension in patients with GS.

However, WNKs phosphorylate these transporters indirectly, and it is controversial how WNKs regulate the transporters and how mutations of WNKs cause activation of the transporters.

Recently, it has been discovered that STE20/SPS1-related proline/alanine-rich kinase and oxidative stress-responsive kinase 1 which are two other serine/threonine kinases downstream of WNKs, phosphorylate and activate NCC and NKCC2 actually [18–20]. While the scaffold protein Cullin3 and the adaptor protein Kelch3 (encoded by the CUL3 and KLHL3 genes, respectively), which accounted for the majority of pathogenic mutations [18], are involved in the ubiquitination and proteasomal degradation of the WNK kinases [21].

Therefore, loss-of-function mutations in these genes result in inhibited degradation of WNKs in the distal nephron and thus upregulation of NCC activity. Different mutant genes are significantly correlated with the clinical manifestations of GS, which can be sorted as CLU3 > KLHL3 > WNK4 > WNK1 according to the age of onset and clinical manifestations.

CLU3 mutants develop early onset, most of them present hypertension when they are minors, and show severe hyperkalemia and metabolic acidosis. Patients with WNK1 may not develop hypertension until late adulthood, and the clinical symptoms are relatively mild, but occasionally they are severe accompanied by periodic paralysis.

Affected subjects have suppressed renin levels consistent with salt-loaded state, while the aldosterone levels are typically low despite their hyperkalemia. Dietary sodium restriction (20 mmol/day) and/or low doses of thiazide diuretics can reverse hypertension and hyperkalemia of patients with GS [13, 22].

1.3 Apparent mineralocorticoid excess syndrome

Apparent mineralocorticoid excess (AME) syndrome is an autosomal recessive disorder due to the loss of functional mutations in HSD11B2 gene on chromosome 16q22, and it is first described in the late 1970s [23].

Approximately 40 causative mutations in HSD11B2 have been identified in 100 AME patients worldwide [24]. In AME syndrome, the function of 11β-HSD2 with a potential age-dependent decline in the activity [25] is impaired, and therefore the MR, which has the same affinity for both aldosterone and cortisol, is protected from cortisol activation by 11β-HSD2 activity under physiological conditions, is occupied and activated by cortisol, resulting in hypertension.

Affected patients display low birth weight, severe hypertension, polyuria and polydipsia, hypokalemia, low PRA, and low aldosterone in the classical AME syndrome which is caused by absolutely or essentially absent of the 11β-HSD2 activity.

While it may be mild when the mutant enzyme retains some activity [26], patients in this type present adult onset, mild-to-moderate hypertension, and normal potassium. The diagnosis of AME is usually suspected in the setting on non-aldosterone dependent low-renin hypertension (LRH) with classic features of MR activation and confirmed by a high cortisol/cortisone (F/E) ratio in the serum or urine, and/or genetic sequencing of HSD11B2 [27, 28].

It is notable that both glycyrrhizic acid and grapefruit juice are HSD11B2 inhibitors and an excessive intake can induce clinical symptoms and laboratory findings of AME syndrome [29]. Baudrand and Vaidya conceived that lower cortisone levels (in combination with higher F/E ratio) were strongly associated with higher MR activity (lower renin activity and higher urinary potassium excretion) in patients suspected to have mild or non-classical AME [30].

The treatment for classic AME is low-dose dexamethasone in combination with MRAs or renal transplantation in extreme cases.

1.4 Congenital adrenal hyperplasia

Congenital adrenal hyperplasia (CAH) is an autosomal recessive disorder caused by defects in different enzymes involved in adrenal steroid production. Among them, the deficiency of 21-hydroxylase caused by CYP21A2 gene mutation is the most frequent cause of CAH (90–95%).

Affected patients present sodium loss but normal blood pressure, followed by 11β-hydroxylase deficiency which is caused by gene mutation of CYP11β1 (5–8%), while the other defects are rare, including CYP17α1 gene mutation caused 17α-hydroxylase (CYP17) deficiency [31].

The 11β-hydroxylase catalyzes the 11-deoxycortisol and 11-deoxycorticosterone (DOC) to cortisol and corticosterone, CYP11B1 deficiency impairs above function and results in low levels of cortisol and high levels of 11-deoxycortisol and 11-DOC and a shunting of metabolites into the androgen synthesis pathway.

Due to the mineralocorticoid function of DOC, two-thirds of the affected subjects display hypertension at diagnosis, together with suppressed renin, low aldosterone levels, and hypokalemia [32]. Due to the excessive androgens, patients present various degrees of virilization of female external genitalia and pseudo-precocious pubertal development in males, together with accelerated somatic growth, but premature closure of growth plates resulting in short stature in adulthood.

The diagnosis can be confirmed via elevated DOC and androgen levels and/or genetic sequencing of 11β-hydroxylase. 17α-hydroxylase deficiency present a clinical phenotype sustained by a reduction in cortisol and adrenal and gonadal sex steroids production associated with an increase in DOC levels, featuring a clinical phenotype of mineralocorticoid excess. The deficiency of sex hormones results in hypogonadism in men and infantilism in women.

High levels of DOC result in MR activation, hypertension, and hypokalemia. Clinical examination of plasma cortisol, sex hormone precursors, and DOC is helpful for diagnosis, and ultrasound examination of genitals is helpful to understand the development of uterus, gonadal, and vagina.

Treatment involves glucocorticoid and MR antagonists to normalize blood pressure and sex hormone replacement therapy [33].

1.5 Mineralocorticoid receptor activating mutations

In 2000, Geller et al. [34] first reported the single-gene genetic hypertension caused by the active mutation of mineralocorticoid receptor (MR), an autosomal dominant genetic disease, also known as the pregnancy aggravated hypertension.

Functional mutation is achieved through a substitution of leucine for serine at codon 810 (abbreviated as S810L) in the MR gene. The worsening in pregnancy is explained by the theory that progesterone activates the mutant S810L MR, where progesterone typically antagonizes wild-type MR. So termination of pregnancy is a must for pregnant women to lower blood pressure.

While in males and non-pregnant females, cortisone and DOC activate the mutant MR and result in increased sodium reabsorption [35]. Surprisingly, spironolactone is ineffective since its agonist effect on the mutant MR and it can increase MR activation paradoxically.

Treatment with sodium channel blockers such as amiloride to inhibit ENaC may be effective, the novel and potent nonsteroidal selective MR antagonist-finerenone may also be a useful option [36].

1.6 Glucocorticoid resistance syndrome

Glucocorticoid resistance syndrome (GRS) is an autosomal recessive or dominant disease, caused by glucocorticoid receptor gene NR3C1 point mutation or deletion in the chromosome 5q31-q32 [37, 38].

Affected patients are characterized by a various degree of end-organ insensitivity to glucocorticoids, compensatory ACTH hypersecretion, excessive production of cortisol, adrenal androgens, and other adrenal steroids displaying mineralocorticoid activity. The classic phenotype of GRS is chronic fatigue and malaise, low renin hypertension, hypokalemia, and metabolic alkalosis.

Although female fetus virilization is extremely rare, affected children can display precocious puberty and premature adrenarche, and female patients can display acne, hirsutism, male pattern alopecia, and infertility.

The therapy is using overnight low-dose dexamethasone to suppress ACTH secretion, which improves ACTH-induced symptoms, and spironolactone can further help to control hypertension and female hirsutism.

1.6.1 Glucocorticoid remediable aldosteronism

Glucocorticoid remediable aldosteronism (GRA) is an autosomal dominant genetic disease [39], also known as familial hyperaldosteremia type I (FH-I), is the first identified monogenic hypertension.

CYP11B1 and CYP11B2 genes were identified as the culprit of FH-1 [40]. FH-I is a low renin hypertension characterized by severe early onset hypertension which is remediable by glucocorticoid, and is at high risk of experiencing cerebrovascular events at a young age, however milder phenotypes can coexist.

Stowasser et al. described the severity of the hypertension correlates with the sex: female subjects show a less-severe phenotype and a better prognosis [41].

GRA should be suspected when CT and other imaging examinations do not reveal adrenal cortical hyperplasia or tumor. Selective screening of GRA patients combined with typical clinical features can improve diagnostic level.

According to the Endocrine Society guideline, the diagnosis of FH-I should be pursued in patients younger than 20 years old with an onset of confirmed PA and in those who have a family history of primary aldosteronism or stroke at a young age (<40 years).

On the basis of positive dexamethasone suppression test as well as the 18-hydroxycortisol >2 times the normal limit of 24 h urine or > 10 nmol/L, GRA may be considered; and if the chimeric genes of CYP11B2 and CYP11B1 were screened, the definite diagnosis can be made.

The first-line therapy is low doses of glucocorticoid, administered at bedtime to suppress the early morning ACTH. Treatment with mineralocorticoid receptor antagonist is the second line therapy, which may have same effect and avoids side effects of corticoid iatrogenic.

1.6.2 Familial hyperaldosteremia type II

This type may be the most common form of familial hyperaldosteremia, and was first reported in 1991 by Gordon et al. [42].

Familial hyperaldosteremia type II (FH-II) is an autosomal dominant genetic disease with incomplete penetrance in which the pathogenic gene is located on chromosome 7p22, and the genetic basis has been very recently identified in germline mutations in the CLCN2 gene, encoding Cl^- channel ClC-2, which is expressed in adrenal zona glomerulosa [43].

Further studies are needed to establish the impact (in term of prevalence) of CLCN2 mutations on FH-II. Unlike FH-I, FH-II is not a glucocorticoid remediable form of primary aldosteronism, traditionally considered clinically and biochemically indistinguishable in a sporadic form. Some patients with FH-II had unilateral primary aldosteronism caused by aldosterone-producing adenomas and were surgically curable by unilateral adrenalectomy.

1.6.3 Familial hyperaldosteremia type III

Familial hyperaldosteremia type III (FH-III) was reported as a novel form of primary aldosteronism in 2008 [44] and the molecular basis is a germline mutation of the KCNJ5 gene, which is located on chromosome 11q24 and encodes for a K^+ channel, GIRK4, also known as Kir3.4.

The prevalence of this disease is low, it was reported to be about 0.3% of all patients with primary aldosteronism. So far, 12 families and 6 germline mutations have been reported, most affected patients display extremely severe primary aldosteronism (type A) that requires bilateral adrenalectomy to control drug-resistant hypertension.

In 2012, 2 studies independently reported the G151E germline mutation in patients with milder hyperaldosteronism (type B), who had no adrenal hyperplasia and responded well to antihypertensive therapy.

The endocrine society guidelines recommend FH-III genetic testing (KCNJ5 target gene sequencing) for all patients who have early onset of primary aldosteronism.

1.6.4 Familial hyperaldosteremia type IV

Familial hyperaldosteremia type IV (FH-IV) described by Scholl et al. [45] recently, is a rare form of familial primary aldosteronism. It is an autosomal dominant disease and caused by a germline mutation of CACNA1H, which locates on chromosome 16p13 and encodes for a T-type calcium channel, Cav3.2.

Mutations in CACNA1H showed drastically impaired channel inactivation and activation at more hyperpolarized potentials, increased intracellular Ca^{2+}, and aldosterone production. Compared to FH-II patients affected in a sporadic form, this disease displays an incomplete penetrance and the affected patients did not display any peculiar biochemical characteristics.

1.7 Hypertension and brachydactyly syndrome

Hypertension and brachydactyly syndrome (HTNB), also named Bilginturan syndrome, is reported in a Turkish family by Bilginturan et al. [46] in 1973, which is characterized by severe salt-independent hypertension, a short stature, brachydactyly, and death from stroke before the age of 50 years when untreated.

It is autosomal dominant inheritance and full penetrance, and pathogenic genes at 12p12.2-p11.2 [47]. In 2015, Maass et al. [48] identified mutations in the PDE3A gene at 12p12.2 from 6 families with HTNB, which were heterozygous missense mutation.

These mutations were suggested to cause hypertension in the HTNB patients by increasing peripheral vascular resistance. HTNB is less reactive to β blockers, CCB, α blockers, and ACEI, combination therapy maybe more effective.

2. Conclusion

The disorders described above highlight the importance of the identification and diagnosis of monogenic hereditary hypertension. The gold standard for the diagnosis of monogenic forms of hypertension is gene detection. It attaches great significance to carry out gene detection for patients with hypertension who are clinically suspected.

Genetic testing can not only screen pathogenic genes to guide targeted therapy, but also screen the genes of the proband's family to detect all individuals carrying pathogenic genes, which is conducive to early detection, early treatment, and prenatal diagnosis of the disease.

Meanwhile, monogenic hypertension is a hereditary rare disease with relatively definite genes. The study on its genetic mechanism has greatly extended the understanding about the pathologic molecular mechanism of hypertension, which will help us to learn the correlation between hypertension and heredity more deeply.

Acknowledgements

We thank Dr Yue Liu and Dr Wenjia Chen for their efforts on the article topic selecting, and Jiaxing Sun for the modifying English language. This article was supported by the National Natural Science Foundation of China (Grant No. 81700318 and 81570437).

Conflict of interest

The authors declare no conflict of interest.

Author details

Wenxiu Liu and Xinhua Yin*
Department of Cardiology, First Affiliated Hospital of Harbin Medical University, Harbin, Heilongjiang Province, China

*Address all correspondence to: yinxinhua5063@163.com

References

[1] New MI, Geller DS, Fallo F, et al. Monogenic low renin hypertension. Trends in Endocrinology and Metabolism. 2005;**16**(3):92-97. DOI: 10.1016/j.tem.2005.02.011

[2] Liddle GW, Bledsoe T, Coppage WS. A familial renal disorder simulating primary aldosteronism but with negligible aldosterone secretion. Proceedings of the Association of American Physicians. 1963;**76**:199-213

[3] Liu K, Qin F, Sun X, et al. Analysis of the genes involved in Mendelian forms of low-renin hypertension in Chinese early-onset hypertensive patients. Journal of Hypertension. 2018;**36**(3):502-509. DOI: 10.1097/HJH.0000000000001556

[4] Wang LP, Yang KQ, Jiang XJ, et al. Prevalence of Liddle syndrome among young hypertension patients of undetermined cause in a Chinese population. Journal of Clinical Hypertension. 2015;**17**:902-907. DOI: 10.1111/jch.12598

[5] Tapolyai M, Uysal A, Dossabhoy NR, et al. High prevalence of Liddle syndrome phenotype among hypertensive US veterans in Northwest Louisiana. Journal of Clinical Hypertension (Greenwich, Conn.). 2010;**12**:856-860. DOI: 10.1111/j.1751-7176.2010.00359.x

[6] Botero-Velez M, Curtis JJ, Warnock DG. Brief report: Liddle's syndrome revisited-A disorder of sodium reabsorption in the distal tubule. The New England Journal of Medicine. 1994;**330**:178-181. DOI: 10.1056/NEJM199401203300305

[7] Hansson JH, Nelson-Williams C, Suzuki H, et al. Hypertension caused by a truncated epithelial sodium channel γ subunit: Genetic heterogeneity of Liddle syndrome. Nature Genetics. 1995;**11**: 76-82. DOI: 10.1038/ng0995-76

[8] Salih M, Gautschi I, van Bemmelen MX, et al. A missense mutation in the extracellular domain of αENaC causes Liddle syndrome. Journal of the American Society of Nephrology. 2017;**28**:3291-3299. DOI: 10.1681/ASN.2016111163

[9] Tetti M, Monticone S, Burrello J, et al. Liddle syndrome: Review of the literature and description of a new case. International Journal of Molecular Sciences. 2018;**19**(3):812. DOI: 10.3390/ijms19030812

[10] Cui Y, Tong A, Jiang J, et al. Liddle syndrome: Clinical and genetic profiles. Journal of Clinical Hypertension (Greenwich, Conn.). 2017;**19**(5):524-529. DOI: 10.1111/jch.12949

[11] Gordon RD, Geddes RA, Pawsey CG, et al. Hypertension and severe hyperkalaemia associated with suppression of renin and aldosterone and completely reversed by dietary sodium restriction. Australasian Annals of Medicine. 1970;**19**:287-294

[12] Paver WK, Pauline GJ. Hypertension and hyperpotassaemia without renal disease in a young male. The Medical Journal of Australia. 1964;**2**:305-306

[13] Gordon RD. The syndrome of hypertension and hyperkalemia with normal glomerular filtration rate: Gordon's syndrome. Australian and New Zealand Journal of Medicine. 1986;**16**:183-184

[14] Toka HR, Koshy JM, Hariri A. The molecular basis of blood pressure variation. Pediatric Nephrology. 2013;**28**:387-399. DOI: 10.1007/s00467-012-2206-9

[15] Park JS, Park E, Hyun HS, et al. Three cases of Gordon syndrome with dominant KLHL3 mutations. Journal of Pediatric Endocrinology & Metabolism.

2017;**30**:361-364. DOI: 10.1515/jpem-2016-0309

[16] Wilson FH, Disse-Nicodeme S, Choate KA, et al. Human hypertension caused by mutations in WNK kinases. Science. 2001;**293**:1107-1112

[17] Boyden LM, Choi M, Choate KA, et al. Mutations in kelch-like 3 and cullin 3 cause hypertensionnand electrolyte abnormalities. Nature. 2012;**482**:98-102. DOI: 10.1038/nature10814

[18] Vitari AC, Deak M, Morrice NA, et al. The WNK1 and WNK4 protein kinases that are mutated in Gordon's hypertension syndrome phosphorylate and activate SPAK and OSR1 protein kinases. The Biochemical Journal. 2005;**391**(Pt 1):17-24. DOI: 10.1042/BJ20051180

[19] Alessi DR, Zhang J, Khanna A, et al. The WNK-SPAK/OSR1 pathway: Master regulator of cation-chloride cotransporters. Science Signaling. 2014;7(334):re3. DOI: 10.1126/scisignal.2005365

[20] Yang SS, Fang YW, Tseng MH, et al. Phosphorylation regulates NCC stability and transporter activity in vivo. Journal of the American Society of Nephrology. 2013;**24**:1587-1597. DOI: 10.1681/ASN.2012070742

[21] O'Shaughnessy KM. Gordon syndrome: A continuing story. Pediatric Nephrology. 2015;**30**:1903-1908. DOI: 10.1007/s00467-014-2956-7

[22] Mayan H, Vered I, Mouallem M, et al. Pseudohypoaldosteronism type II: Marked sensitivity to thiazides, hypercalciuria, normomagnesemia, and low bone mineral density. The Journal of Clinical Endocrinology and Metabolism. 2002;**87**:3248-3254. DOI: 10.1210/jcem.87.7.8449

[23] Ulick S, Levine LS, Gunczler P, et al. A syndrome of apparent mineralocorticoid excess associated with defects in the peripheral metabolism of cortisol. The Journal of Clinical Endocrinology and Metabolism. 1979;**49**:757-764. DOI: 10.1210/jcem-49-5-757

[24] Yau M, Al Azkawi HS, Haider S, et al. A novel mutation in HSD11B2 causes apparent mineralocorticoid excess in an Omani kindred. Annals of the New York Academy of Sciences. 2016;**1376**(1):65-71. DOI: 10.1111/nyas.13162

[25] Campino C, Martinez-Aguayo A, Baudrand R, et al. Age-related changes in 11β-hydroxysteroid dehydrogenase type 2 activity innormotensive subjects. American Journal of Hypertension. 2013;**26**:481-487. DOI: 10.1093/ajh/hps080

[26] Wilson RC, Dave-Sharma S, Wei JQ, et al. A genetic defect resulting in mild low-renin hypertension. Proceedings of the National Academy of Sciences of the United States of America. 1998;**95**:10200-10205. DOI: 10.1073/pnas.95.17.10200

[27] Funder JW. Apparent mineralocorticoid excess. The Journal of Steroid Biochemistry and Molecular Biology. 2017;**165**:151-153. DOI: 10.1016/j.jsbmb.2016.03.010

[28] Carvajal CA, Romero DG, Mosso LM, et al. Biochemical and genetic characterization of 11 β-hydroxysteroid dehydrogenase type 2 in low-renin essential hypertensives. Journal of Hypertension. 2005;**23**:71-77

[29] Karl M, Lamberts SW, Detera-Wadleigh SD, et al. Familial glucocorticoid resistance caused by a splice site deletion in the human glucocorticoid receptor gene. The Journal of Clinical Endocrinology and Metabolism. 1993;**76**:683-689. DOI: 10.1210/jcem.76.3.8445027

[30] Baudrand R, Vaidya A. The low-renin hypertension phenotype: Genetics and the role of the mineralocorticoid receptor. International Journal of Molecular Sciences. 2018;**19**(2):546. DOI: 10.3390/ijms19020546

[31] El-Maouche D, Arlt W, Merke DP. Congenital adrenal hyperplasia. Lancet. 2017;**390**:2194-2210. DOI: 10.1016/S0140-6736(17)31431-9

[32] Khattab A, Haider S, Kumar A, et al. Clinical, genetic, and structural basis of congenital adrenal hyperplasia due to 11 β-hydroxylase deficiency. Proceedings of the National Academy of Sciences of the United States of America. 2017;**114**:E1933-E1940. DOI: 10.1073/pnas.1621082114

[33] Auchus RJ. Steroid 17-hydroxylase and 17, 20-lyase deficiencies, genetic and pharmacologic. The Journal of Steroid Biochemistry and Molecular Biology. 2017;**165**:71-78. DOI: 10.1016/j.jsbmb.2016.02.002

[34] Geller DS, Farhi A, Pinkerton N, et al. Activating mineralocorticoid receptor mutation in hypertension exacerbated by pregnancy. Science. 2000;**289**:119-123

[35] Rafestin-Oblin ME, Souque A, Bocchi B, et al. The severe form of hypertension caused by the activating S810L mutation in the mineralocorticoid receptor is cortisone related. Endocrinology. 2003;**144**:528-533. DOI: 10.1210/en.2002-220708

[36] Amazit L, Le Billan F, Kolkhof P, et al. Finerenone impedes aldosterone-dependent nuclear import of the mineralocorticoid receptor and prevents genomic recruitment of steroid receptor coactivator-1. The Journal of Biological Chemistry. 2015;**290**:21876-21889. DOI: 10.1074/jbc.M115.657957

[37] Chrousos GP, Vingerhoeds A, Brandon D, et al. Primary cortisol resistance in man. A glucocorticoid receptor mediated disease. The Journal of Clinical Investigation. 1982;**69**:1261-1269

[38] Nicolaides NC, Charmandari E. Chrousos syndrome: From molecular pathogenesis to therapeutic management. European Journal of Clinical Investigation. 2015;**45**:504-514. DOI: 10.1111/eci.12426

[39] Sutherland DJ, Ruse JL, Laidlaw JC. Hypertension, increased aldosterone secretion and low plasma renin activity relieved by dexamethasone. Canadian Medical Association Journal. 1966;**95**(22):1109-1119

[40] Lifton RP, Dluhy RG, Powers M, et al. A chimaeric 11 beta-hydroxylase/aldosterone synthase gene causes glucocorticoid-remediable aldosteronism and human hypertension. Nature. 1992;**355**:262-265. DOI: 10.1038/355262a0

[41] Stowasser M, Bachmann AW, Huggard PR, et al. Severity of hypertension in familial hyperaldosteronism type I: Relationship to gender and degree of biochemical disturbance. The Journal of Clinical Endocrinology and Metabolism. 2000;**85**:2160-2166. DOI: 10.1210/jcem.85.6.6651

[42] Gordon RD, Stowasser M, Tunny TJ, et al. Clinical and pathological diversity of primary aldosteronism, including a new familial variety. Clinical and Experimental Pharmacology & Physiology. 1991;**18**:283-286

[43] Fernandes-Rosa FL, Daniil G, Orozco IJ, et al. A gain-of-function mutation in the CLCN2 chloride channel gene causes primary aldosteronism. Nature Genetics. 2018;**50**:355-361. DOI: 10.1038/s41588-018-0053-8

[44] Geller DS, Zhang J, Wisgerhof MV, et al. A novel form of human

mendelian hypertension featuring nonglucocorticoid-remediable aldosteronism. The Journal of Clinical Endocrinology and Metabolism. 2008;**93**(8):3117-3123. DOI: 10.1210/jc.2008-0594

[45] Scholl UI, Stölting G, Nelson-Williams C, et al. Recurrent gain of function mutation in calcium channel CACNA1H causes early-onset hypertension with primary aldosteronism. eLife. 2015;**4**:e06315. DOI: 10.7554/eLife.06315

[46] Bilginturan N, Zileli S, Karacadag S, et al. Hereditary brachydactyly associated with hypertension. Journal of Medical Genetics. 1973;**10**:253-259. DOI: 10.1136/jmg.10.3.253

[47] Schuster H, Wienker TE, Bähring S, et al. Severe autosomal dominant hypertension and brachydactyly in a unique Turkish kindred maps to human chromosome 12. Nature Genetics. 1996;**13**:98-100. DOI: 10.1038/ng0596-98

[48] Maass PG, Aydin A, Luft FC, et al. PDE3A mutations cause autosomal dominant hypertension with brachydactyly. Nature Genetics. 2015;**47**:647-653. DOI: 10.1038/ng.3302

Section 3

Benign and Malignant Hematological Rare Diseases

Chapter 8

The Rare Anaemias

Joan-Lluis Vives-Corrons

Abstract

Anaemia is a common worldwide disorder mainly due to iron or vitamins deficiency. However, among the rare diseases (RD), there is a group associated with anaemia as main clinical manifestation or rare anaemias (RA). RA are mostly hereditary, and since they are little known, even for professionals, they remain undiagnosed, or misdiagnosed, for very long periods of time. This creates in patients, or, in their parents (if they are children) a permanent situation of stress due to the absence of a diagnosis, the impossibility to predict the course of the disease, and to the impossibility to perform, genetic counselling for future pregnancies. About 83 different RA have been described and their mechanism is in general a bone marrow or a red blood cell (RBC) defect. The most well-known RA are Fanconi anaemia, the thalassemia syndromes, sickle cell disease, hereditary haemolytic anaemias and paroxysmal nocturnal haemoglobinuria (PNH). The main objective of this chapter is to offer a review of the state of the art of RA knowledge and a way to facilitate their identification and final diagnosis through clinical manifestations and laboratory diagnostic tests.

Keywords: anaemia, red blood cell erythropoiesis, haemoglobin, haemolysis, haemoglobins, enzymes, membrane

1. Introduction

Anaemia is very common condition in human pathology that may result from a wide variety of causes, either congenital or acquired. It is always the manifestation of an underlying disease, and never a disease by itself. Haemoglobin concentration (Hb) is the most reliable indicator of anaemia, but since its normal distribution at population level varies with age, sex, and physiological status, the Word Health Organization (WHO) has defined the existence of anaemia when Hb is less than 110 g/L in children and pregnant women, 120 g/L in non-pregnant women and 130 g/L in men. Moreover, measuring Hb is relatively easy and inexpensive, and currently, all automated and semi-automated haematology analysers measure Hb with great precision and accuracy. It is well known that iron deficiency in children and women and chronic diseases in adults and elderly, is the most frequent cause of mild to moderate anaemia worldwide [1, 2].

In general, there are three primary causes of anaemia: (1) Bone marrow erythropoietic defects associated with or without reduced haemoglobin synthesis. (2) Haemolysis or excessive destruction of mature red blood cells (RBCs), and (3) blood loss or bleeding. Anaemia can be the consequence of a single disease (e.g. haemoglobinopathy, enzyme deficiency, etc.), but it can be also the expression of external factors such as nutritional deficiencies, parasitic or viral infection, and other. However, there is a group of anaemias that is considered rare because their frequency in our population is less than 5 cases for 10,000 individuals. These are the so-called rare anaemias (RA), mostly of congenital origin [3]. RA are an important, and relatively homogeneous group of rare diseases (RD), where anaemia is the first and most relevant clinical manifestation of the disease. This importance was recognized, for first time, by the European Commission (EC) that in 2002 approved the co-financing of the DG-SANCO Project: "European Network for rare and congenital diseases" (ENERCA; www.enerca.org). Interestingly, this Project started shortly before the creation of the High Level Group (HLG) in 2004 that brought together experts from all the Member States (MS) in several areas of RD expertise. For RA, this was a great advantage, because it facilitated the progressive development of ENERCA Project in parallel to the development of the different HLG areas of action: (a) Patient safety and quality of care, (b) Health impact assessment and health systems, (c) Health technology assessment, (d) European workforce for health professionals, e) European reference networks, (f) Information and e-health and more recently, (g) Cross-border healthcare purchasing and provision [4].

Before ENERCA, RA were almost unknown in Europe, including some health professionals, because in many cases, the cause of the anaemia was not known and/or there is no treatment available. Moreover, for many years, anaemias, in general, have been underestimated by public health providers, due to its frequent misdiagnosis with iron deficiency anaemia, the most frequent cause of anaemia worldwide. ENERCA changed definitively this situation by developing three consecutive phases with a total duration of 15 years (www.enerca.org). The first ENERCA Project (ENERCA 1), starting in 2003, dedicated to congenital RA, only, allowed the establishment of the necessary background for a sustainable coordination in the area of health information, collection of epidemiological data, comparability issues, exchange of data and information within and between MS. At this time, it also facilitated a rapid reaction to RA diagnosis and treatment. The second ENERCA Project (ENERCA 2) starting in 2005, covered, in addition, to congenital anaemias, other rare causes of anaemia, either hereditary or acquired, and dedicated more and stronger activities to health Information, patient's data collection, education and training and quality assessment for special RA diagnostic procedures. This has provided a first and unique approach for prevention, diagnosis and treatment of RA in the word. The third ENERCA Project (ENERCA 3), starting in 2009, was co-financed by the EC through its Executive Agency for Health and Consumers (EAHC) and its objectives were parallel to the strategic objectives of the EU Health Programme 2008–2013 consistent in the creation of a *European Reference Network (ERN) of Centres of Expertise (CEs) in Rare Anaemias* (**Figure 1**).

After 2013, the EC has approved co-financing ENERCA Project for an additional 3 years period (2014–2016), with the aim of developing and implementing the new e-health information and communication technologies (ICT) for assuring the same access to health services in RAs across Europe, independently from the place of residence. This new and last, but not least, ENERCA Project, called e-ENERCA, was based, in part, on previous ENERCA projects achievements, but adapted to the Directive 2011/24/EU of 9 March 2011 on the *application of patients' rights in cross-border healthcare has* become a very important tool for the promotion of Rare Diseases (RD) European Reference Networks (ERN) that, within that general framework, have provided the following benefits:

- Access to experts and expertise throughout the European MS for both patients and health professionals, independently of the country of origin or practice, reduce inequalities and maximize the cost-effective use of resources;

- Epidemiological surveillance throughout EU by gathering comparable data on patients affected by RAs and allowing the implementation of preventive programmes for tackling RAs;

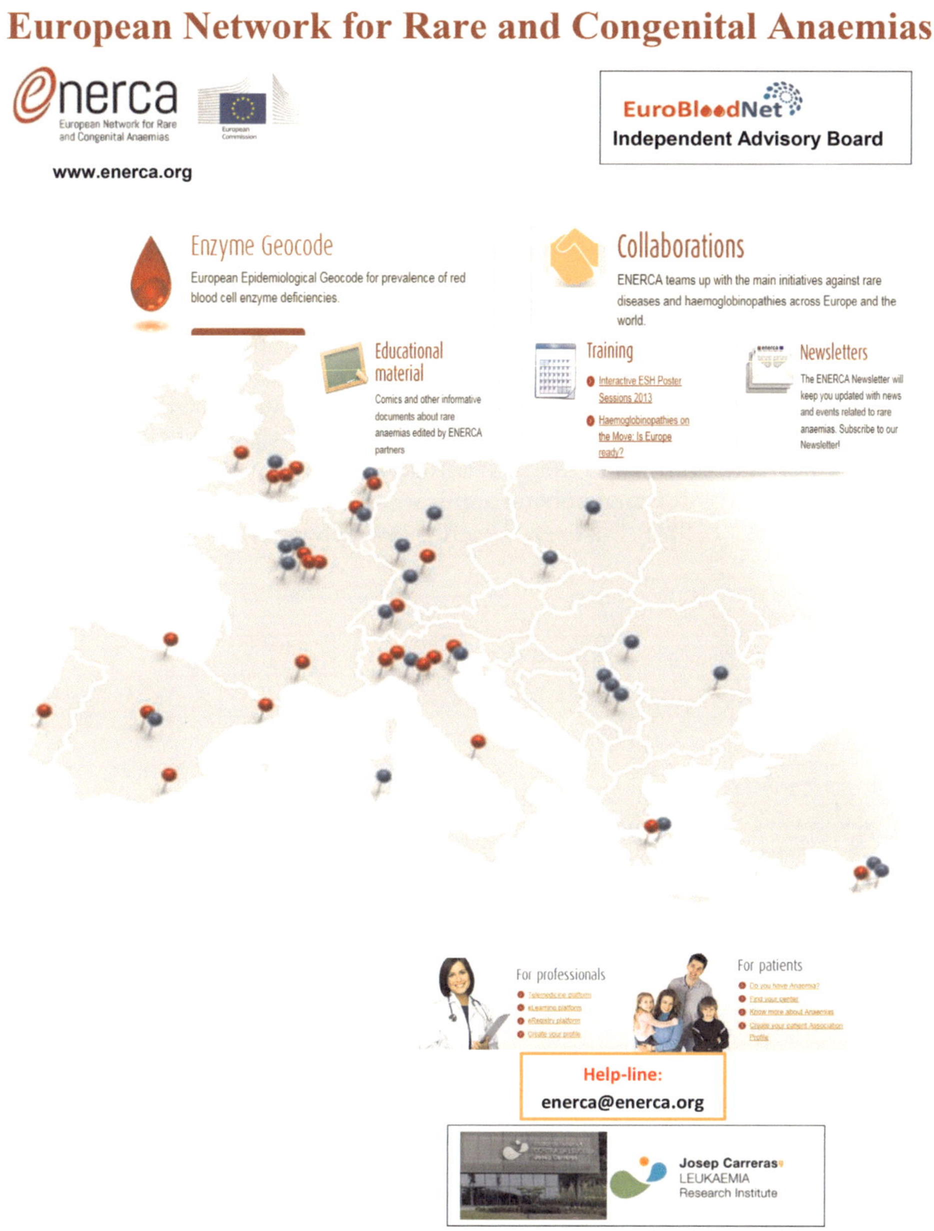

Figure 1.
European Network for Rare and Congenital Anaemias Map.

- Fostering of best practices for prevention, diagnosis and clinical management;
- Promotion of knowledge dissemination of share of expertise and support of research, and increase awareness about RAs;
- Facilitate the transposition of the Directive 2011/24/EU of 9 March 2011 on the application of patients' rights in cross-border healthcare.

For maintaining its sustainability, in March 2016, ENERCA applied for the ERN European Commission (EC) Call, by expanding the rare anaemias to all the other rare haematological diseases (RHD), including oncological and non-oncological diseases [5].

Currently, the ERN for Rare Haematological Diseases (RHD), called EuroBloodNet (www.eurobloodnet.eu), is one of the 24 recognized ERNs, and after its second year of life, can be considered an acceptable tool for the improvement RHD diagnosis and for the provision of high-quality healthcare to all patients who have conditions requiring a particular concentration of resources or expertise. In brief, EuroBloodNet will also provide focal points for medical training and research, information dissemination and evaluation, and will contribute to the establishment of national contact points for RHD. Up to now, however, only 66 Centres in Europe are recognized as Health Care Providers (HCP) for RHD, a situation created by the extremely different endorsement decisions of individual Members States (MS). So, we have arrived to the astonishing situation in that many of the ENERCA experts, well recognized by the state of the art and ENERCA White Book recommendations, are not included as EuroBloodNet experts because they do not belong to an national recognized Healthcare Provider (HCP) and cannot take participate in the Network activities and/or take profit from their advantages. In order to overcome this restraint, a new EC call for membership application to the existing European Reference Networks (ERNs) has been launched on September 30, 2019.

Hereditary (>80%)
Erythropoietic defects (non-regenerative anaemias)
• Fanconi anaemia (FA) • Diamond-Blackfan anaemia (DBA) • Congenital dyserytropoietic anaemia (CDA)
RBC defects (regenerative anaemias)
• Thalassaemia syndromes (Cooley anaemia) • Sickle-cell disease (SCD) • Hereditary membranopathies o Hereditary spherocytosis (HS) o Hereditary elliptocytosis (HE) o Hereditary stomatocytosis (HSt) • Erythroenzymopathies o Glucose-6-phosphate dehydrogenase deficiency (Favism) o Pyruvate kinase deficiency (PKD) o Ultra-rare erythroenzymopathies associated with or without muscular or neurological disease
Iron metabolism defects (non regenerative anaemias)
• Congenital sideroblastic anaemia (CSA) • Non-sideroblastic anaemias with microcytosis (IRIDA)*
Acquired (<20%)
Erythropoietic defects (non-regenerative anaemias)
• Bone marrow aplasia (BMA) • Pure red cell aplasia (PRCA) • Myelodysplastic syndromes (MDS)
RBC defects (regenerative anaemia)
• Paroxysmal nocturnal hemogobinuria (HPN)
Blood plasma abnormalities (regenerative anaemias)
• Autoimmune haemolytic anaemia (AIHA)
Microcirculation defects (regenerative anaemias)
• Haemolytic uremic syndrome (HUS)
**Iron refractory iron deficiency anaemia.*

Table 1.
General classification of rare anaemias.

2. Classification

The RA are classified into two main groups: Hereditary and acquired, and in these groups, the mechanism of the anaemia can be sub classified into five different defects: (1) bone marrow (erythropoietic), (2) peripheral blood (red blood cell), (3) iron metabolism (sideroblastic and non-sideroblastic), (4) blood plasma (autoimmune haemolytic anaemia and related syndromes) and (5) microcirculation (haemolytic uremic syndrome and other microangiopathic disorders). This means that all RA are the consequence of haematopoietic system defects leading to a low RBC production (erythropoietic defects), or of RBC defects, either intrinsic or associated to plasma or microcirculation disorders, leading to low RBC survival or haemolysis (**Table 1**).

ENERCA is actively contributing to the WHO Update Platform ICD-10 of blood and blood forming organs. In this platform, anaemias, are classified into three main groups: D50-D53 (nutritional anaemias), D54-D59 (haemolytic anaemias), and D60-D64 (aplastic and other anaemias). This ICD classification includes all kind of anaemias, hereditary, acquired, common and rare, and ENERCA has extracted the RA group that has been individually listed in the *ENERCA Web page (www.enerca.org).*

For practical purposes, according to their mechanism, prevalence and/or relevant clinical and/or social impact in the European population, ENERCA has classified the Rare Anaemias into 10 different groups [6]:

Group 1. Haemoglobin disorders: Haemoglobinopathies and Thalassaemias.

Group 2. Hereditary Haemolytic Anaemias (HHA): Red blood cell enzymopathies and membrane defects.

Group 3. Hereditary erythropoietic failure or aplasia: Diamond-Blackfan anaemia (DBA) and Fanconi anaemia (FA),

Group 4. Congenital dyserythropoietic anaemias (CDA),

Group 5. Hereditary sideroblastic anaemias,

Group 6. Hereditary non-sideroblastic anaemias due to iron metabolism defects,

Group 7: Hereditary disorders of folic acid and cobalamin defects.

Group 8: Paroxysmal nocturnal haemoglobinuria (PNH),

Group 9: Anaemias due to rare complex mechanisms and.

Group 10: Anaemias of unknown origin (AUO).

The underlying cause of rare anaemias remains still unexplained in about 20% of patients, almost one third of which might be accounted for myelodysplastic syndromes. AUO can be also due to complex clinical situations and multifactorial mechanisms, in general associated with systemic, non-haematological, hereditary or acquired diseases. Their existence is a very important tackling exercise for clinical and biological research.

3. Diagnostic approach

More than 80% of RA are hereditary and, therefore, have no curative treatment, exception made of palliative therapies such as blood transfusions or erythropoietic stimulating drugs (Erythropoietin). In clinical practice they may be some confusion between RA and the anaemias that appear in the course of non-haematological or systemic diseases, also called secondary anaemias. This confusion is due to the fact that anaemia is not a disease, but a clinical manifestation, and some Rare Diseases (RD) are associated with anaemia, moderate or severe. One example of this is the Rendu-Osler disease (hereditary telangiectasia), a relatively well known RD where anaemia, due to iron deficiency, is very common, and sometimes the first clinical manifestation of the disease. Furthermore, the anaemias due to rare chronic inflammatory diseases, vitamin deficiencies, immune diseases, malignancy, or other rare disorders, may probably be also considered RA, although they have not yet been included in this group.

Hereditary RA, as in other RD, the low number of patients creates the need to mobilize resources and their study can be efficient only if done in a coordinated European scene of action level. Among hereditary anaemias, haemoglobinopathies are the commonest genetic defect worldwide with an estimated 269 million carriers [7]. They are the consequence of mutations in the globin genes, which are responsible for the synthesis of haemoglobin, the main component of RBCs. These mutations are leading to abnormal proteins (haemoglobin variants) or to a decreased synthesis of globin chains (thalassaemias). In Europe, certain populations are particularly at risk of having a haemoglobinopathy. In Southern countries, their prevalence is higher than in central or northern Europe, but in all cases the prevalence is less than 1 per 2000 individuals. For this reason, in Europe, haemoglobinopathies and thalassaemias are considered a particular group of RD or RA. Whereas thalassaemia syndromes are inherent in the autochthonous European at risk groups (Mediterranean anaemia), other haemoglobinopathies have been imported by migration (Sickle-cell anaemia).

In general, the diagnosis of a RA is often prompted by pallor, noticed by the patient, the family, and/or the General Practitioner (GP). Severity of clinical manifestations is directly proportional to the acuteness of onset, and many patients do not notice any symptoms when anaemia occurs insidiously. At the laboratory level, the diagnosis of anaemia includes two main steps:

3.1 General diagnostic tests

General diagnostic tests always include a Complete Blood Count (CBC), the reticulocyte count and the peripheral blood cell morphology examination. The CBC includes four main parameters: (a) haemoglobin concentration (Hb), the key for anaemia diagnosis, (b) RBC count or concentration of RBCs, given as number of cells per litre of blood, (c) haematocrit or packed cell volume (PCV), given as the percentage of blood by volume that is occupied by the RBCs and (d) RBC indices or calculations derived from (a), (b), and (c), of great help for the diagnosis and classification of anaemias. These indices are automatically measured by modern haematology full automated or semi-automated, analysers, and are mainly three: (1) the mean corpuscular volume (MCV) or average size of the RBCs expressed in femtolitres (fl), (2) the mean corpuscular haemoglobin (MCH) or average amount of haemoglobin inside a single RBC expressed in picograms (pg) and (3) the mean corpuscular haemoglobin concentration (MCHC) or average concentration of haemoglobin in the RBC expressed as a percent. Sometimes the RBC distribution width (RDW), a measure of the variation of RBC size, can be also used for anaemia classification. Usually RBCs have a standard size of about 6–8 μm, but in certain disorders, a significant variation in RBC size can be present. Here the RDW value is a relatively good indicator of RBC size heterogeneity. RDW is especially useful to differentiate iron deficiency (increased value) from thalassemia (normal value). Reticulocyte count or number of circulating young RBCs (reticulocytes) is an important complementary test which indicates the bone marrow capacity to overcome the severity of anaemia [8]. Accordingly, anaemias due to RBC destruction (haemolysis) are characterized by increased reticulocyte count (*regenerative* anaemias), whereas anaemias due to erythropoietic insufficiency (aplasia or dyserythropoiesis) are characterized by a lower than expected reticulocyte count from the severity of the anaemia (*Non-regenerative* anaemias). In thalassaemias, where erythropoietic insufficiency coexists with some degree of haemolysis, the reticulocyte count may be variable.

The reticulocyte count and MCV are, up to now, the most useful criteria for anaemia classification. According to MCV, anaemias are classified into microcytic (low MCV), macrocytic (high MCV) and normocytic (normal MCV). The two main causes of microcytic anaemias are iron deficiency and thalassaemia and the two main causes of macrocytic anaemias are cobalamin (vitamin B12) and folic acid deficiencies. Normocytic anaemias can be due to several different causes, not related with nutritional defects or thalassaemia, being the most frequent haemolysis and erythropoietic failure. Here, the reticulocyte count is the most useful test to differentiate these two conditions. In clinical practice, the most frequent cause of anaemia is iron deficiency (ID), characterized by a low MCV (microcytic anaemia). In southern Europe countries with higher "at risk" thalassaemia population (Mediterranean basin), this hereditary disorder can be misdiagnosed as iron deficiency anaemia (IDA) because of the low MCV (<82 fL) or microcytosis. Accordingly, in a patient with microcytosis the first step is always to exclude ID. If present, iron supplementation has to be given until the MCV recovers its normal value. However, if after treatment, the MCV remains low, the coexistence of a thalassemic gene has to be investigated. It should be mentioned that there are a number of conditions where the MCV can falsely rose masking the main clue of thalassaemia diagnosis. This is the case in some patients with thalassaemia who co-inherit another cause of haemolytic anaemia leading to an increased reticulocyte count. This can falsely increase the value of MCV and masking the diagnosis of thalassemia if only the MCV is used for initial screening.

As part of the CBC, the blood film examination is sometimes very useful because it may provide a clue to the diagnosis of a particular RBC defect [9]. Despite the advances in automated blood cell counting, the blood film examination retains a crucial role in the diagnosis of RBC disorders. This is particularly important in haemolytic anaemias and in the differential diagnosis of macrocytic anaemias. RBC morphology examination provides in some cases (e.g. red blood cell membrane disorders, sickle-cell anaemia), a definitive diagnosis, but, more often, it suggests a differential diagnosis that indicates further study. Morphological changes such as basophilic stippling and target cells in the blood film are not definitively associated with a haemoglobinopathy, but would be helpful findings in patients with moderate or severe anaemia associated with low MCV (Thalassaemia intermedia, or Thalassaemia major). Finally, RBC morphology examination has also the advantage of speed that may be important in severe anaemias such as those mentioned before.

3.2 Cause-oriented specific diagnostic tests

These tests are the next step for the identification of the cause of the anaemia or of its mechanism. They include a group of laboratory procedures depending on clinical or laboratory diagnostic orientation of the anaemia [8] and, when necessary, a final genetic identification of the cause of the disease [10]. In order to provide a first approach to the cause of the anaemia, several diagnosis oriented flowcharts can be found in the literature, mainly based on the morphological classification of the anaemia (microcytic, macrocytic and normocytic).

ENERCA website (www.enerca.org) provides practical flowcharts for the diagnostic orientation of anaemia. For this, three patient's data have to be provided: sex, Hb and MCV. If anaemia is detected, one of the three available flowcharts will appear, depending on the MCV value: low (microcytic anaemia), high (macrocytic anaemia) and normal (normocytic anaemia). These flowcharts are not exhaustive and the final diagnosis always requires the advice of a health professional, but they provide the basic information on how the investigation of anaemia causes can be undertaken in routine clinical practice. Using these flowcharts the most frequent RAs (haemoglobinopathies, thalassaemias and haemolytic anaemias) can be easily recognized. Depending on the results of the recommended basic tests, more specific tests (including molecular biology) can be performed. Some of these specific tests can also be performed in general haematology laboratories but other tests require to be undertaken in specialized laboratories. In all the cases External Quality Assessment Schemes (EQAS) are necessary for assessing the quality of practice or for obtaining a technical qualification. Since the most specific tests are performed in few specialized laboratories, local (national or regional) EQAS organizations cannot establish a specific EQAS for these procedures due to its high cost. Accordingly, the EQAS for these procedures have to be promoted at European level as ENERCA 3 has done with some rare diagnostic tests for RA such as Pyruvate-kinase deficiency (PKD).

4. Rare Anaemias due to bone marrow defects

Bone marrow failure syndromes (BMFS) are multisystem diseases that are characterized by varying degrees of deficiency in the production of haematopoietic cells, which can range from the depletion of a single cell lineage (cytopenia) to that of multiple lineages or even of all lineages (pancytopenia). The most well-known acquired BMFS is aplastic anaemia (AA).This causes a deficiency of all three blood cell types (pancytopenia): red blood cells (anaemia), white blood cells (leukopenia), and platelets (thrombocytopenia) and aplastic refers to the inability of stem cells to generate mature blood cells. It is more frequent in people in their teens and twenties, but is also common among the elderly [11]. It can be caused by heredity, immune disease, or exposure to chemicals, drugs, or radiation. However, in about half the cases, the cause is unknown. The definitive diagnosis is by bone marrow biopsy; normal bone marrow has 30–70% blood stem cells, but in aplastic anaemia, these cells are mostly gone and replaced by fat. First line treatment for aplastic anaemia consists of immunosuppressive drugs, typically either anti-lymphocyte globulin or anti-thymocyte globulin, combined with corticosteroids and cyclosporine. Haematopoietic stem cell transplantation is also used, especially for patients under 30 years of age with a related matched marrow donor [11]. Congenital BMFS are, as AA, multisystem diseases characterized by varying degrees of deficiency in the production of haematopoietic cells, which can range from the depletion of a single cell lineage (cytopenia) to that of multiple lineages or even of all lineages (pancytopenia). In general they are monogenic diseases with high genetic heterogeneity and phenotypic overlapping, so a bone marrow and genetic analysis is required to reach a correct diagnosis [12]. They are ultra-rare diseases with a usual presentation during childhood and with an incidence of one to two cases per one million individuals. In almost all cases they are associated with morbidity and mortality, requiring lifelong blood transfusions, treatment of infections, growth factors and transplantation of haematopoietic progenitors. Likewise, they present a high risk of developing haematologic cancer or solid tumours and a high toxicity to treatment, which leads to a lower life expectancy. The most relevant aspects of some of these syndromes are the following:

4.1 Fanconi anaemia (FA)

FA (OMIM 227650) is a hereditary disease with a predominantly autosomal recessive pattern and in one case linked to chromosome X. Its prevalence in the general population is estimated at two to five cases per one million individuals, with an estimated incidence of 1/131,000 births. 21 different gene mutations have been identified so far to be a cause of congenital aplasia [13]. In most cases, each of the parents carries one of the pathogenic variants, with three exceptions: male patients of the FA-B subtype (FANCB gene), patients of the FA-R subtype (RAD51 gene), and the cases in which one of the two variants is de novo (not present in the parents or present in only some of the gametes of one of the parents). The gene FANCB is a gene linked to the X chromosome, so that women are asymptomatic carriers of the pathogenic variant. From the clinical point of view, FA is considered as a syndrome of chromosomal instability with a high spectrum of clinical manifestations that can be grouped into congenital malformations, endocrine dysfunction, haematological abnormalities such as severe cytopenias, myelodysplastic syndrome (MDS) or acute myeloid leukaemia (AML) Moreover, a predisposition to develop tumours and chromosomal fragility has been noted and in about 30% of the patients do not present congenital malformations and are only diagnosed at the time when the disease debuts with the haematological abnormalities [13]. To make a diagnosis, it is necessary to confirm the chromosomal fragility by cytogenetics [14] and until a few years ago, genetic testing was not part of the routine clinical analysis of AF patients, partly because it was considered sufficient with the cytogenetic confirmation of the diagnosis (chromosomal fragility) and the subtype of the patient, and on the other hand, because the mutational analysis was boring. However, with the implementation of new high-throughput sequencing technologies [15], subtyping and mutational study are now achieved at the same time, sequencing all AF genes in the same assay, and even identifying new genes involved (**Table 2**). However, this approach

FA Subtype	FA mutated Gen	Chromosome location	Protein
A	*FANCA*	16q24.3	FANCA
B	*FANCB*	Xp22.31	FANCB
C	*FANCC*	9q22.3	FANCC
D1	*FANCD1/BRCA2*[*]	13q12.13	BRCA2
D2	*FANCD2*	3p25.3	FANCD2
E	*FANCE*	6p21–22	FANCE
F	*FANCF*	11p15	FANCF
G	*FANCG*	9p13	FANCG
I	*FANCI*	15q25-26	FANCI
J	*FANCJ/BRIP1*[*]	17q22-24	BRIP1
L	*FANCL*	2p16.1	FANCL
M	*FANCM*	14q21.3	FANCM
N	*FANCN/PALB2*[*]	16p12.2	PALB2
O	*FANCO/RAD51C*[*]	17q25.1	RAD51C
P	*FANCP/SLX4*	16p13.3	SLX4
Q	*FANCQ/ERCC4*	16q24.3	XPF
R	*FANCR/RAD51*	15q15.1	RAD51
S	*FANCS/BRCA1*	17q21.31	BRCA1
T	*FANCT/UBE2T*	7q36.1	UBE2T
U	*FANCU/XRCC2*	7q36.1	XRCC2
V	*FANCV/REV7*	1p36.22	MAD2L2
W	*FANCW/RFWD3*	16q23.1	FANCW

[*]*Gene defects that predispose to the development of cancer in FA carriers.*

Table 2.
Genetic subtypes and genes which mutation are implicated in the development of Fanconi anaemia.

can cause errors in these patients, due to the broad mutational spectrum of the disease and because all the genes related to the disease have not yet been described. For this reason, it is advisable to always start the diagnosis by the mutational study in patients with a positive chromosomal fragility for AF. With regard to treatment, in addition to correcting, as far as possible, some of the congenital malformations, it is essential to carry out a haematological follow-up in order to identify early signs and symptoms of bone marrow (BM) failure. Current guidelines recommend tracking blood counts every three to four months, and an annual bone marrow aspirate. Treatment should be initiated depending on the patient's clinical commitment and continue with it in accordance with the response to it. Support measures include transfusions of red blood cells or platelet concentrates, or the use of colony / cytokine stimulating factors. Currently, the only curative treatment for bone marrow failure in these patients is the allogeneic haematopoietic stem cell transplant (HSCT) from suitable donors. Finally, the correct and early diagnosis of AF does not only allow the discarding of other diseases, but fundamentally enables the proper management of their haematological alterations and genetic counselling to the individual and his family in case of successive pregnancies. In addition, in families with mutations in genes predisposing to cancer, it allows adequate monitoring and risk assessment in family members.

4.2 Diamond-Blackfan anaemia (DBA)

DBA (OMIM 105650), is a rare disease with a dominant autosomal inheritance pattern. No differences were observed between men and women (ratio 1:1) and the short stature is the most frequent anomaly followed by alterations in the thumb. Other less frequent anomalies have been described, such as craniofacial alterations, cleft lip, cleft palate and short neck. In DBA, the first description was a pure neonatal anaemia that required transfusion support. At present, about 1000 cases have already been described in the literature, and approximately 25% of them have at least one congenital anomaly. The average age for diagnosis is 3 months, ranging from birth to 64 years of age, with 98% of cases diagnosed in the first year of life. DBA has its molecular basis in heterozygous mutations in the genes encoding the components of either the small 40S or the large 60S ribosomal subunits that affect the processing of ribosomal RNA. Recently, DBA has also been related to mutations in the GATA-1

DBS Subtypes	% of patients	*Locus*	Mutated Gene	Protein
AD	25	19q13.2	*RPS19*	RPS19
AD	2	10q22–23	*RPS24*	RPS24
AD	1	15q25.2	*RPS17*	RPS17
AD	7	1p22.1	*RPL5*	RPL5
AD	5	1p36.11	*RPL11*	RPL11
AD	3	3q29	*RPL35A*	RPL35A
AD	1	2p25.3	*RPS7*	RPS7
AD	7	6p21.31	*RPS10*	RPS10
AD	3	12q13	*RPS26*	RPS26
AD	<1	17p13.1	*RPL26*	RPL26
AD	<1	14q21.3	*RPS29*	RPS29
AD	<1	18q21.1	*RPL17*	RPL17
AD	<1	3p24.2	*RPL15*	RPL15

DBS Subtypes	% of patients	*Locus*	Mutated Gene	Protein
AD	<1	17p13.1	*RPL26*	RPL26
AD	<1	17q12	*RPL19*	RPL19
AD	<1	2q11.2	*RPL31*	RPL31
AD	<1	8q12.1	*RPS20*	RPS20
AD	<1	19p13.2	*RPS28*	RPS28
LX	<1	Xp11.23	*GATA-1*	GATA1
Unkown	40	—	—	—

Source: [35].

Table 3.
Genetic subtypes and genes implicated in Diamond-Blackfan anaemia (DBA).

transcription factor [16], but about 45% of patients with ADB lack mutations in these identified genes, as shown in **Table 3**. It is likely that the genetic defects in this pathology accelerate the apoptosis of erythroid progenitor cells, since it has been shown that MDM2, a central regulator of p53, that acts as a ubiquitin ligase that leads to the degradation of p53, binds specifically to several free ribosomal proteins. From the clinical point of view, the diagnosis of DBA is complex. Blood counts generally show a macrocytic anaemia with reticulocytopenia, as well as elevated Hb F and RBC adenosine deaminase (ADA) in more than 85% of patients. In the bone marrow, a pure erythroblastopenia without abnormalities in the other haematopoietic cell lines is characteristic. The cumulative incidence for MDS, AML, and some solid tumours (osteosarcoma, Hodgkin's lymphoma) has been estimated at 20% at 46 years, which implies an increased risk of developing cancer. The treatment is based on the response of a large number of patients to steroids. However, it is advised not to perform this treatment until after the first year of age. Until then, and in those patients who do not respond to steroids, or who require them at very high doses, the only treatment will be adequate transfusion support with packed red blood cells. The only curative treatment for the disease is the HSCT, provided the existence of an identical HLA family donor [11].

4.3 Congenital dyserythropoetic anaemia (CDA)

CDA is, in fact, a heterogeneous group of defects of erythropoiesis with medullary abortion of the erythroblasts before maturing to reticulocytes (dyserythropoiesis), and important erythrocyte morphology abnormalities. Clinically, CDA is characterized by anaemia, usually macrocytic, and iron overload. To date, five clinical forms of CDA have been described: CDA I, CDA II, CDA III, CDA IV and CDA with thrombocytopenia [17]. The first two (CDA I and CDA II) have an autosomal recessive hereditary pattern and the other two (CDA III and CDA IV) are autosomal dominant. Thrombocytopenia with CDA has an inheritance linked to the X chromosome. The two best known CDAs are CDA I (OMIM 224120) characterized by a marked dyserythropoiesis and frequent inter nuclear chromatin bridges and CDA II (OMIM 224100), characterized by marked dyserythropoiesis associated with erythroblastic binuclearity or multinuclearity, and the presence of erythroblasts with double cell membrane (**Figure 2**). CDA III (OMIM 105600) is a ultra-rare disease where the marked dyserythropoiesis is associated with severe nuclear size and chromatin morphological abnormalities that resemble an erythroleukemia or Di-Guglielmo disease.

CDA I is due to mutations of the CDAN1 gene or less frequently to mutations of the C15ORF41 gene, In a small percentage of cases the mutation is unknown.

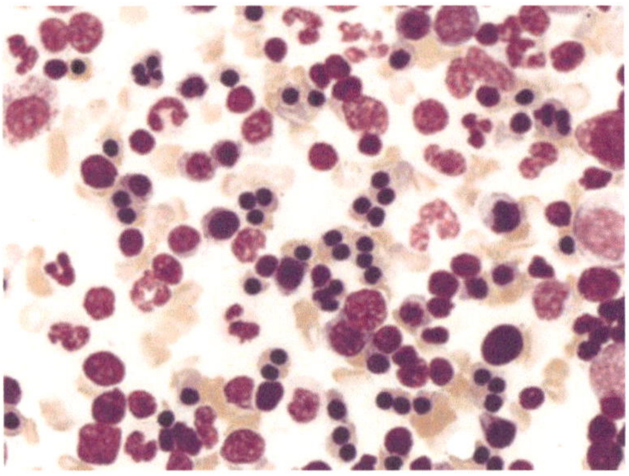

Figure 2.
Typical bone marrow picture of Congenital Dyserythropoietic Anaemia type II also known by hereditary erythroblastic multinuclearity with positive acidified serum lysis (HEMPAS) test.

In CDA II, the disease is due to mutations of the SEC23B gene and in CDA III, its most frequent gene mutation is the KIF23 gene.

5. Rare Anaemias due to red blood cell defects

RBC defects can be classified into two main groups: (a) Hereditary or intrinsic defects due to structural or functional abnormalities of RBC components haemoglobin (haemoglobinopathies), membrane (membranopathies) and enzymes of metabolism (enzymopathies), and (b) Acquired or extrinsic defects due to blood plasma or vascular abnormalities. In both cases the consequence is a haemolytic syndrome characterized by anaemia of variable severity associated with a compensatory increase of bone marrow erythropoiesis and of circulating reticulocytes. In addition to anaemia, the haemolytic syndrome is characterized by three main clinical manifestations 1. reticulocytosis, 2. splenomegaly and 3. jaundice [18].

5.1 Haemoglobinopathies

Haemoglobinopathies are the most frequent RBC defects in comparison with membranopathies and erythroenzymopathies that in many cases can be considered ultra-rare anaemias (prevalence <1 case per 10^6 inhabitants). All these diseases are more frequent in Southern Europe than in Central or Northern Europe, and their clinical expression is always an hereditary haemolytic anaemia [19, 20]. Haemoglobinopathies are the consequence of globin gene mutations that can alter the synthesis (thalassaemias) or the structure of haemoglobin (structural haemoglobinopathies). Its worldwide prevalence is around 269 million carriers, and in Europe there are risk populations, especially for thalassemia, which are located in the geographical regions surrounding the Mediterranean basin (Mediterranean Anaemia).

The most frequent haemoglobinopathy is HbS (OMIM 603903), prevalent in African populations due to the protection that it has offered against malaria. HbS is the result of substitution of valine for glutamic acid in the sixth position of the globin beta chain and in its homozygous form or combined with other haemoglobinopathies, is responsible for sickle cell disease (SCD) that consists in haemolytic anaemia associated with severe vaso-occlusive crises and pain due to multiple micro-infarcts [21]. These crises are triggered by hypoxia that decreases HbS

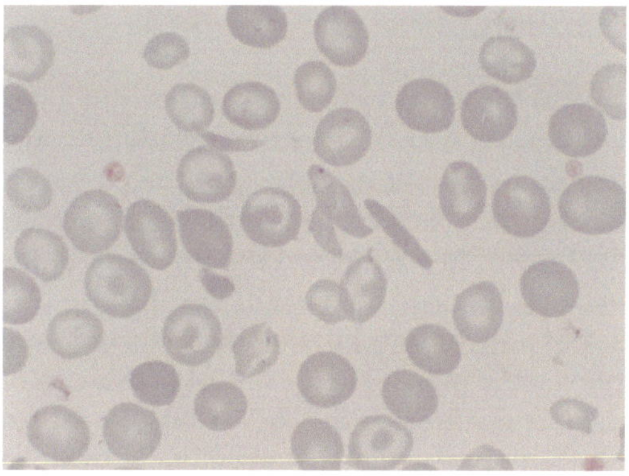

Figure 3.
Sickle-cells in a SCD patient with vaso-occlusive crisis.

solubility leading to a characteristic RBC shape distortion (sickle cell) and to a drastic decrease of deformability (**Figure 3**) Over the last 30 years, it has been observed a significant increase due to the immigration impact of populations from other geographical areas, mainly from Sub-Saharan African regions but also from Asia and Central America, where this disease is very prevalent. Currently, the neonatal screening programs allow an early diagnosis of the disease and its preventive treatment from the first years of life and, as a consequence, the frequency of complications have significantly reduced, and mortality during early childhood dramatically decreased [22]. There is no specific treatment for SCD, although in severe cases, the administration of hydroxyurea (HU) is recommended since, as the concentration of HbF increases, the frequency of vaso-occlusive crises, the need for transfusions, and especially the onset of the acute thoracic syndrome decrease. In addition to HbS, there are other structural haemoglobinopathies of clinical interest such as HbS, HbJ HbD and unstable haemoglobins that precipitate, and inclusion bodies or Heinz bodies are formed (**Figure 4**). Clinically, they present with a chronic haemolytic syndrome of variable severity and unlike the SCD, patients presents an autosomal dominant pattern of inheritance.

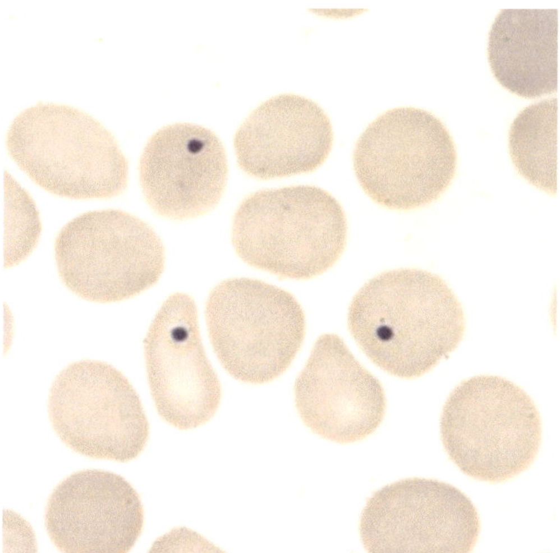

Figure 4.
Howell Jolly bodies in a patient with unstable haemoglobin.

5.2 Thalassaemias

Thalasaemias are due to the decrease in the synthesis of a globin chain (alpha or beta), due to absence, diminution or defective translation of specific messenger RNA (mRNA) caused by deletions or point mutations of the globin genes. While point mutations predominate in beta genes, large deletions are more frequent in alpha genes. According to the type of mutation and the intensity of the synthesis decrease, the severity of the clinical picture can be more or less intense [23]. In beta thalassemia the milder forms consist of a slight or moderate hypochromic and microcytic anaemia (thalassemia trait) whereas the more severe clinical forms can be classified as "thalassemia major" or "thalassemia intermedia" depending on the severity of the anaemia and the periodic transfusion requirements, respectively. In alpha thalassemia, as the genetic cluster has two genes, the mutation of a single allele, relatively common in Southern Europe in characterized by a moderate microcytosis (MCV around 80 fl) without anaemia alpha thalassemia trait, whereas if more than one allele is affected more severe forms of alpha-thalassemia occur The mutation of three alleles gives rise to the so-called haemoglobinopathy H, a clinical form very similar to intermediate beta thalassemia but with the presence of HbH or beta-globin tetramers, a result of the excess or imbalance of beta chains due to the decrease of alpha chains. The complete loss of the four alleles (homozygous alpha-thalassemia) is incompatible with life (hydrops faetalis).

Diagnosis of both forms of thalassemia is based on the data provided by the CBC and the study of haemoglobins by electrophoresis or high-performance liquid chromatography (HPLC). In the case of beta thalassemia trait an increase in the HbA2 fraction is always observed, whereas in alpha thalassaemia trait the haemoglobin pattern is normal and a molecular study is mandatory. An accurate family study is also very important to prevent diagnostic errors and the application of unnecessary treatments. In addition, an appropriate identification of the carrier condition allows the identification of couples at risk.

The treatment of severe clinical forms of β-thalassemias has been historically based on blood transfusions and iron chelation therapy. The only curative therapy currently available is allogeneic haematopoietic stem cell transplant (HSCT) from suitable donors. However, with the limited pool of suitable donors, HSCT remains unavailable for many thalassemic patients. They may instead benefit from globin gene therapy and other modalities, which exploit recent advances in understanding of globin gene regulation [24].

5.3 Membranopathies

Membranopathies are due to structural or functional defects of the RBC membrane proteins. In general, they are inherited as autosomal dominant pattern but transmitted with a recessive character. Hereditary spherocytosis (HS; OMIM 182870, 182,900, 270,970, 612,653, 612,690) is the most frequent cause of HHA in Caucasians due to a defect of membrane skeletal proteins that cause vesiculation and partial loss of the same with the decrease in surface/volume ratio and formation of spherocytes (**Figure 5**). Proteins affected in HS are beta-Spectrin (SPTB-1) Ankyrin and Band 3, and haemolysis occurs almost exclusively in the spleen, leading to frequent severe splenomegaly. Along with splenomegaly, several complications of HHA can be frequently observed in HS such as, intermittent jaundice and increased bilirubin pigments leading to premature gallstone formation, transient erythroblastopenia crisis due to parvovirus B19 infection, folic acid deficiency and torpid malleolar ulcers [25]. In general, physicians become more familiar with diagnosing HS in the newborn period, fewer neonates with HS will develop

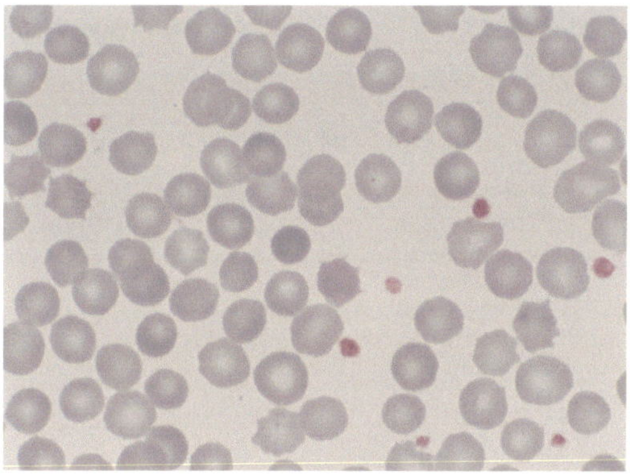

Figure 5.
Circulating peripheral blood spherocytes in a patient with hereditary spherocytosis.

hazardous hyperbilirubinemia or present to emergency departments with unanticipated symptomatic anaemia. The early suspicion, prompt diagnosis and treatment, using anticipatory guidance, will prevent adverse outcomes in neonates with HS [26].

The diagnosis of HS is based on the triad: (1) anaemia with jaundice, (2) severe splenomegaly and (3) spherocytosis, easily demonstrated by the peripheral blood morphological examination (**Figure 5**). Currently the diagnosis of HS can be easily performed by measuring RBC deformability and osmotic gradient ektacytometry (OGE) using the new generation LoRRca Osmoscan from Mechatronics [27]. Curves obtained with this device allow a clear distinction between hereditary spherocytosis and the other RBC hereditary membranopathies, elliptocytosis and xerocytosis (**Figure 6**). The implementation of the automated haematological analysers that determine the CCMH by means of a direct system, allows us to use this magnitude as a criterion of HS when it is increased in the presence of an elevated reticulocyte count. Finally, the use of the EMA-binding test technique is currently being implemented as a reference technique, especially in the diagnosis of HS, together with ektacytometry. This test is based on the measurement of the fluorescence intensity in RBCs after incubation with a fluorochrome, eosin-5-maleimide (EMA) that binds specifically to the anion transporter (Band 3) and decreases when Band 3 decreases.

Another hereditary membranopathy is hereditary elliptocytosis (HE, OMIM 109270, 130,600, 179,650, 225,450, 611,804), with milder clinical expression when compared to HS, but with the presence of more than 30% of circulating elliptocytes in peripheral blood (**Figure 7**). Like HS, HE is due to a skeletal protein defect, mainly alpha-Spectrin (SPTA-1) and Band 4.1 that alters the elasticity of the membrane preventing its recovery after elongation [28]. There is no loss of membrane and, therefore, CCMH is normal. OGE profile (Osmoscan) shows here a characteristic curve that is different from HS (**Figure 6**). In severe clinical forms of HE known as hereditary pyropoikilocytosis (HPP) the SPTA-1 gene mutation in heterozygous state is associated "in trans" with a SPTA-1 "Lely" mutation leading to severe HHA with markedly abnormal RBC morphology and decreased heat stability (**Figure 8**).

Finally, there is a very rare form of membrane disease called hereditary stomatocytosis (OMIM 194380, 185,000) which most relevant characteristic is the presence of RBC with an elongated central pallor instead of a round one (**Figure 9**). Its genetic and molecular mechanism is poorly understood, although it is known that in all forms there is a disorder of the permeability to sodium or potassium ions by which the RBC can be hydrated or dehydrated. These disorders of erythrocyte

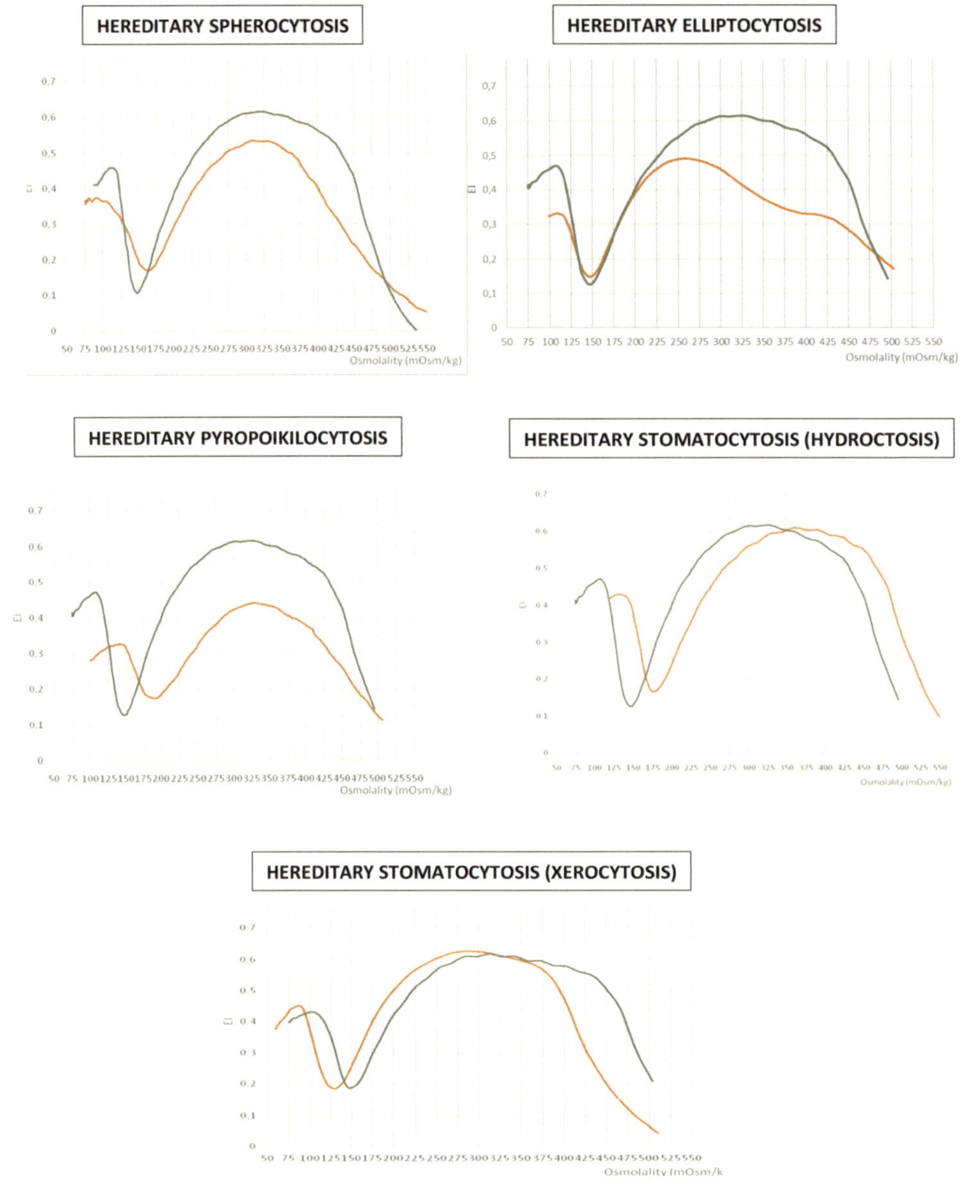

Figure 6.
Osmotic gradient ektacytometry (OGE) profiles from Osmoscan (LoRRca) in different hereditary membranopathies. EI: Elongation Index.

hydration are classified as primary, due to inherent disorders of erythrocyte volume regulation, and secondary, due to other disorders affecting the erythrocyte that secondarily influence cell hydration. In general, the degree of perturbation of water and ion content parallels the degree of haemolytic anaemia [29].

Overhydrated stomatocytosis (OHSt) or hereditary hydrocytosis refers to a rare, heterogeneous group of disorders with haemolytic anaemia and large numbers of stomatocytes on peripheral blood smear (**Figure 9**). OHSt is associated with markedly increased sodium permeability of the membrane from 10 to 40 times normal. This leads to a significant increase in intracellular sodium with a lesser decrease in intracellular potassium, resulting in increased total mono-valent cation content and increased intracellular water. Erythrocyte membranes from many OHSt patients

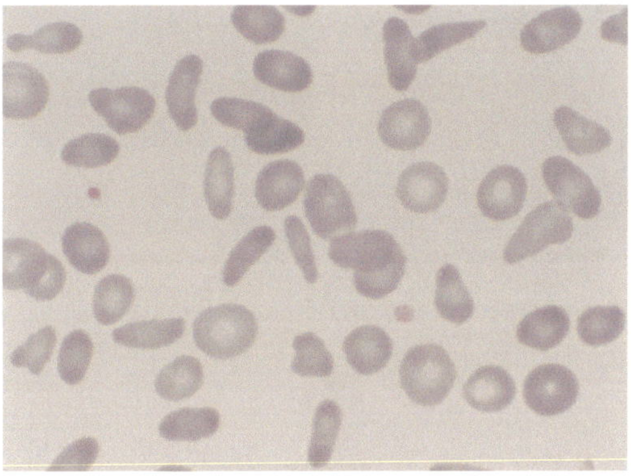

Figure 7.
Ellyptocytes in a patient with hereditary elliptocytosis.

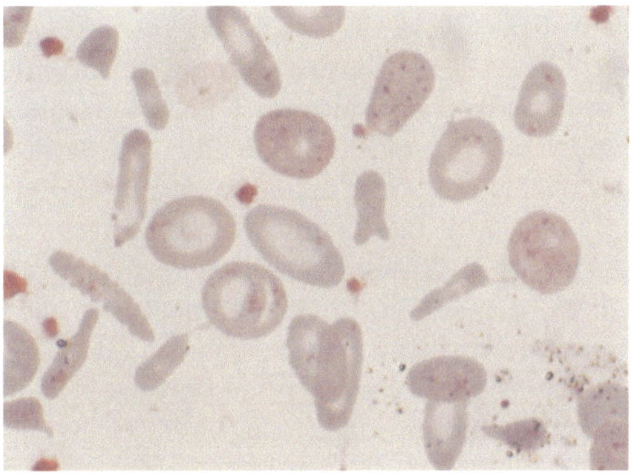

Figure 8.
Peripheral blood MGG stained examination of a newborn with hereditary pyropoikylocytosis (HPP).

lack stomatin, but mutations have not been found in the gene of affected patients and erythrocytes from stomatin knockout mice are normal. There is a variant of OHSt variant known as Cryohydrocytosis in which patient erythrocytes exhibit minimal to mild changes in cation leak at physiologic temperatures, but a marked increase in monovalent cation permeability at low temperature, typically 5°C. Erythrocytes demonstrate a sphero-stomatocytic morphology on peripheral smear. Heterozygous missense mutations in band 3, the anion exchanger (SLC4A1), have been identified in some cryohydrocytosis patients [29]. Dehydrated stomatocytosis or hereditary xerocytosis (HX) syndromes, are the most common primary disorders of erythrocyte hydration and are the most clinically heterogeneous. HX erythrocytes are dehydrated due to a cation leak, primarily of potassium, that leads to decreased potassium concentration. Because the cation leak is not accompanied by a proportional net gain of sodium and water, cellular dehydration ensues. Peripheral blood smear reveals few target cells, and occasional dessicytes (erythrocytes with haemoglobin puddled to one side), and rare stomatocytes. MCHC is increased (34–38 g/dL), and RBC osmotic fragility is decreased, both reflecting cellular dehydration [30]. Osmotic gradient ektacytometry (LoRRca Osmoscan) reflects a characteristic pattern of mixed reduced deformability index and dehydration given by a leftward shift of the minimal osmolality point (**Figure 6**).

When studied at the genetic level, in most cases of HX, mutations in PIEZO1 have been identified. PIEZO proteins are ion channels mediating mechanic sensory transduction in mammalian cells, and PIEZO1 is a large integral membrane protein

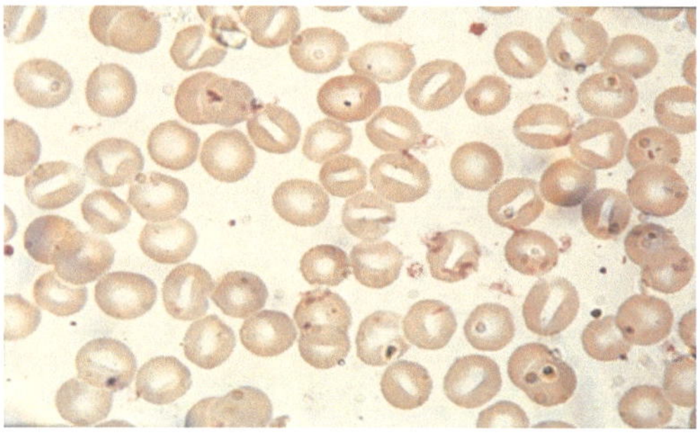

Figure 9.
Typical RBC morphology in a patient with hereditary stomatocytosis.

with numerous transmembrane domains that assemble into a homo-multimeric complex fully active as a mechanic sensitive cation channel [29]. A few HX patients do not have mutations in PIEZO1, but instead have mutations in the Gardos channel, encoded by KCNN4. The role of Gardos channel in normal erythrocytes has not yet been defined, butin HX-associated mutant KCNN4 channels demonstrate alterations in channel kinetics and trafficking. Clinically, HX patients with KCNN4 mutations experience variable degree of anaemia and RBC dehydration with typically more severe forms than in PIEZO1-mutant HX patients [29].

Treatment of HHA due to RBC membrane defects are always palliative, depending on the severity of anaemia. In HS, splenectomy allows a complete recover of haemoglobin concentration, whereas in the HE this recovery is only partial. In HS, splenectomy is not recommended because it facilitates thrombotic events due to an increased thrombophilia.

5.4 Erythroenzymopathies

Erythroenzymopathies are hereditary diseases due to a defect of RBC metabolism, in general an enzyme deficiency, that can be associated with an haemolytic crisis, a chronic haemolytic anaemia (HHA), neonatal cyanosis with metahaemoglobinemia or c) hereditary erythrocytosis. An association between enzymatic defect and HHA has been described in 14 of the 38 enzymes that make up the erythrocyte metabolism (**Table 4**). Some enzymatic defects produce haemolysis only under cellular stress produced by infections, oxidizing drugs or by the intake of fava beans. Other enzymatic deficiencies are associated with chronic non-spherocytic haemolytic anaemia (CNSHA). On some occasions, the expression of the deficiency is not restricted to the erythrocyte, but extends to other tissues, mainly the neurological, hepatic or muscular tissues, and a neuropathy, hepatopathy or myopathy, respectively, associated with anaemia appears. The RBC is especially sensible to enzymopathies because, unlike other cells, it cannot resynthesize the deficient enzymes because it lacks a nucleus and ribosomes. Enzymatic deficiencies occur when one of the enzymes of the reduced RBC metabolism is unstable and disappears very quickly, or has lost catalytic functionality and lacks activity. In the mature RBC there are two fundamental metabolic pathways: (1) the anaerobic glycolysis, by which glucose is used to generate ATP and (2) the aerobic pentose phosphate pathway (PPP), by which it eliminates any oxidative aggression to generate NADH and NADPH (**Figure 10**). ATP is used to meet energy requirements and NADH to reduce methaemoglobin. The NADPH is used to reduce the oxidized glutathione (GSH) which, in turn, is required to maintain the sulfhydryl groups of proteins in a reduced state and to detoxify hydrogen peroxide

Enzyme deficiency	Prevalence	Inheritance	Haemolysis	Comments
Hexokinase (HK)	Ultra-rare	Recessive	Yes (+++)	Low 2,3DPG level, poor tolerance of anaemia, 20 cases described.
Glucose phosphate isomerase (GPI)	Very rare	Recessive	Yes (++)	45 cases, 24 mutations re- ported; deficiency extended to leucocytes and platelets
Phosphofructokinase (PFK)	Very rare	Recessive	Variable	35 reported cases; variable degree of haemolysis and myopathy
Aldolase (ALD)	Ultra-rare	Recessive	Yes	3 cases reported
Triosephosphate isomerase (TPI)	Very rare	Recessive	Yes	Severe generalized disorder; widespread tissue involvement; neurologic, infectious and cardiac complications, 12 mutations described
Phosphoglycerate kinase (PGK)	Ultra-rare	X-linked	Yes, usually	Mental retardation and neurologic disturbances in hemizygous men; specific amino acid substitutions identified in 7 variants
Enolase (ENOL)	Ultra-rare	Dominant	Yes	3 cases described
Pyruvate kinase (PK)	The most common glycolytic defect	Recessive	Yes	First described and best studied defect, prototype for the group. 1:20,000 affected in the general population, 180 mutations described
Lactate dehydrogenase (LDH)	Ultra-rare	Recessive	No	7 cases described, myopathy with lack of M-subunit

Table 4.
Erythroenzymopathies of the glycolytic pathway.

(**Figure 11**). Enzymopathies have been described in both metabolic pathways. Glucose-6-phosphate dehydrogenase (G6PD, OMIM 300908, 134,700) is the most frequent antioxidant system, and shows hereditary transmission linked to sex. It is especially frequent in Africa, Asia and in the Mediterranean region (Greece and Italy, mainly) and, due to its polymorphic nature, it has many variants, among which the G6PD A-, predominant in black people, and the G6PD (−) Mediterranean, predominant in Caucasians. In G6PD A-forms, the enzyme is unstable but enzymatic activity is almost normal in reticulocytes, whereas in Mediterranean G6PD variants, the enzyme is even more unstable, and its activity is very low even in reticulocytes. This explains that in G6PD A-carriers, the acute haemolytic episode is self-limited and the recovery of the anaemia is faster than in the carriers of Mediterranean G6PD variants. Clinically, the G6PD deficiency occurs with haemolytic crisis sometimes associated with severe anaemia, in general triggered by the intake of oxidant substances, like fava beans (favism), or certain oxidizing drugs. Due to this, the carriers of a G6PD deficiency can remain asymptomatic for many years, until a contact occurs with the substances that may trigger the haemolytic crisis. Among the drugs that can induce haemolysis in G6PD deficiency, can be mentioned certain analgesics, sulphonamides, antimalarials, and antibiotics [31]. Favism, a severe haemolytic anaemia induced by fava beans ingestion or exposure to pollen from the plant, is the most frequent clinical manifestation in caucasians bearing the deficient G6PD Mediterranean variant, but also the G6PD A (−) variant (G66PD Betica). There are also ultra-rare forms of G6PD deficiency that do not obey to polymorphic variants but to

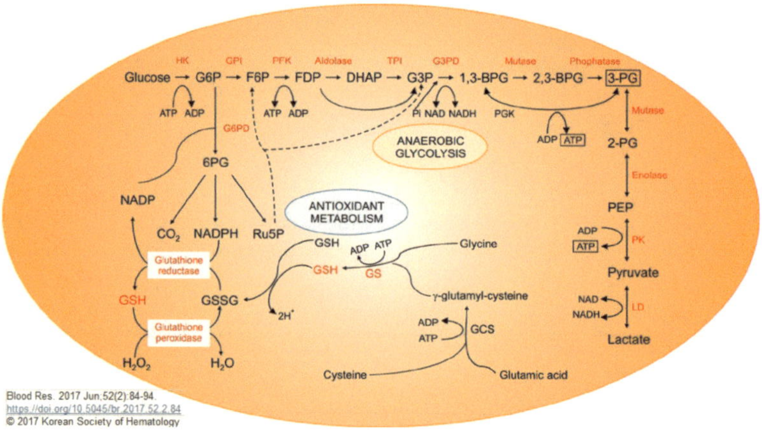

Figure 10.
Anaerobic glycolysis and antioxidant metabolic pathways of red blood cells. Abbreviations: BPG, bisphosphoglyceric acid; DHAP, dihydroxyacetone phosphate; F6P, fructose 6-phosphate; FDP, fructose-1,6-diphosphate; G3P, glycerol 3-phosphate; G3PD, glyceraldehyde 3-phosphate dehydrogenase; G6P, glucose 6-phosphate; G6PD, glucose-6-phosphate dehydrogenase; GCS, glutamylcysteine synthetase; GPI, glucose-phosphate isomerase; GS, glutathione synthetase; GSH, glutathione; GSSG, glutathione disulfide; HK, hexokinase; LD, lactate dehydrogenase; NADP, nicotinamide adenine dinucleotide phosphate; PEP, phosphoenolpyruvic acid; PFK, phosphofructokinase; PG, phosphoglyceric acid; PGK, phosphoglycerate kinase; PK, pyruvate kinase; Ru5P, ribose-5-phosphate isomerase.

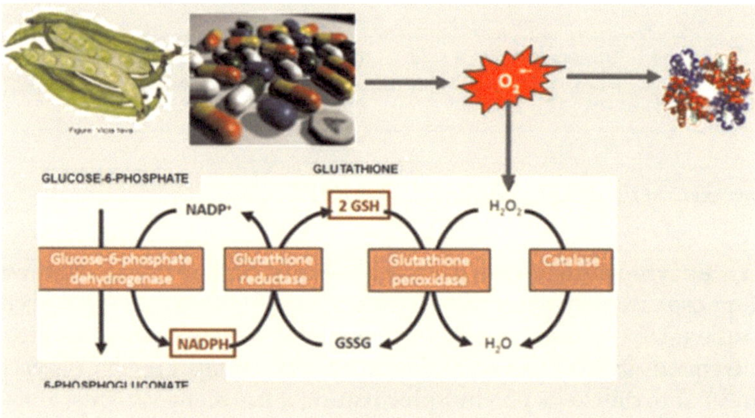

Figure 11.
Anti-oxidant system present in RBC to protect the cells against the oxidant threat generated by the ingestion of oxidant drugs of fava beans (favism).

sporadic variants that present with a chronic haemolytic syndrome (CSSHA). Other factors that can induce haemolysis in the G6PD deficiency are viral infections, especially influenza and hepatitis, diabetic ketoacidosis, and other different situations called of "stress." The diagnosis of G6PD deficiency is based on the clinical history, and the exclusion of the autoimmune mechanism through the negativity of the direct antiglobulin test (DAGT) or Coombs test. During the haemolytic crisis, the observation of the smear shows the presence of eccentrocytes or RBCs subjected to oxidative stress where haemoglobin is pushed off to one part of the cytoplasm (**Figure 12**). For screening purposes, the fluorescent spot test is used based on demonstrating the formation of NADPH (fluorescent) from NADP (non-fluorescent) in the Beutler's G6PD fluorescence spot test or the reduction of methaemoglobin in the presence of methylene blue.

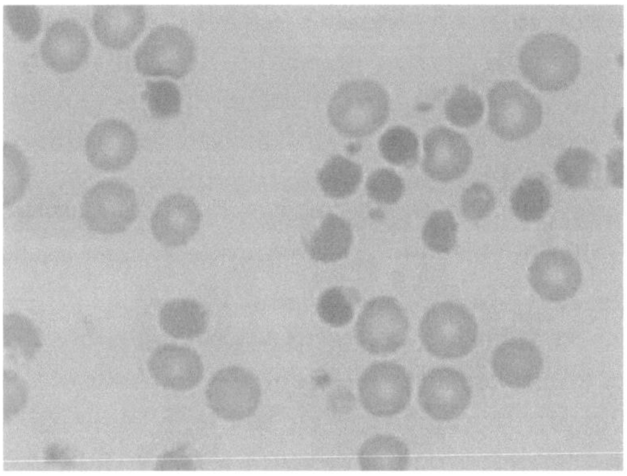

Figure 12.
Excentrocytes present in the blood of a patient with G6PD deficiency and haemolytic crisis.

The pyruvate kinase deficiency (PKD, OMIM 266200) is the most frequent enzyme of anaerobic glycolysis (Embden-Meyerhof pathway) and the most frequent cause of hereditary haemolytic anaemia (HHA), after hereditary spherocytosis [32]. It is an enzymopathy much less frequent than G6PD deficiency and its diagnosis requires the quantification of enzymatic activity in patient's haemolysates. Since haemolytic anaemia in PK deficiency is always due to mutations in the PKLR gene, leukocytes have a normal PK activity, so if they are not eliminated well when preparing the haemolysate, they can geopardise the result and mask the existence of a RBC PK deficiency (PKD). To avoid this important cause of error (false negatives), blood treated with anticoagulant must be filtered through a column of celulose-micro celulose in order to eliminate leukocytes and platelets. Also the presence of a high number of circulating reticulocytes, very frequent in newborns and children, can also give false negatives because the PK activity of the reticulocytes is much higher than that of the mature RBCs. Therefore, if in the presence of intense reticulocytosis a normal PK activity is obtained, the result should be confirmed by determining the quotient between PK activity and hexokinase (HK). HK is an enzyme whose activity also increases in the presence of reticulocytosis and, therefore, if this increase is much greater than that of PK, this enzyme deficiency is evidenced by a significant decrease in the PK / HK ratio [33].

Very recently a concise guide to PK deficiency for primary care providers, but also for haematologists, healthcare providers and medical students has been published [34]. There, the underlying PKD defect is explained in great detail together with its mode of inheritance, clinical manifestations, diagnostic procedures and an attempt for medical treatment.

6. Databases and epidemiology

Clinical epidemiology, originally confined to the global problems of infectious diseases, became, in the last 50 years, the fundament of today's evidence based medicine. No medical stakeholder is able to oversee the abundance of data describing prevalence, incidence, clinical patterns and health risks from all regions in the world. The majority of studies are concerned with common diseases, but there is still a paucity of data for rare diseases, which came in the scope of medical stakeholders in the last decade.

In RA, as in other rare and very rare disorders, only supranational networks can provide valid data. ENERCA has concentrated on data from the MS of the EU on a subset of RA. However, it is often overlooked that social-economic conditions and medical practices are different in the different MS, resulting in different recognition of the epidemiological data studied [20]. Frequency is a general term to compare differences between the occurrence of a given disease, in the case of rare anaemias between populations defined by geographic regions or populations of different origin (such as the formerly called races) in a given region. The latter became of paramount importance with the ongoing immigration of people from the Mediterranean basin to North- and Middle Europe and from Asia and Africa to all MS, as mentioned above. The frequency is a useful parameter in any first approach of disease characteristics and a useful tool to decide on the methodology to estimate more precise issues. No one would challenge the fact, that thalassemia is much more frequent in the Mediterranean area or in immigrants within the Northern European countries. However, mathematically defined parameters are needed for research and health care planning. Prevalence, or more exactly prevalence proportion, is the main indicator used for any epidemiological studies in congenital diseases, representing the vast majority of conditions considered in disease category. Paroxysmal Nocturnal Haemoglobinuria (PNH) is an exception, with prevalence being of major significance, alike for the situation of cancers. For very rare anaemias included in ENERCA, usually period prevalence is measured, using a defined number of observation years rather than an index day as used for the so called point prevalence in common diseases. Another useful measure is the number of affected children of all live births in a given observation period; in this case, the period of definition of live birth (e. g. Days after birth) should be indicated, to avoid bias due to early mortality. An effective instrument to measure true prevalence a proportion is obtained with post-natal screening programs, as described for SCD. Ideally, all cases of a given disease or disease category in a population at time should represent the "true" prevalence. However, in the case of rare anaemias, the detection rate (number of detected/number of existing cases) is often less than 1. As shown by the work of ENERCA, there are strong indicators that the detection rates in the MS vary considerably depending on socio-economic conditions, and the same is true for the proportion of misclassifications. These data are of importance for any attempt to harmonize the diagnosis of rare anaemias in the European countries.

An inherent, unsolved problem of all registries is sustainability. Time trends, so important considering the influence of scientific as well as population changes due to both demographic evolution and migration can only be ascertained if sustainability can be guaranteed by resources of much longer duration than available today. Clinical trials, even though primarily directed to progress of therapeutic measures and often dependent on industrial interests are another source of epidemiological data. We hope that final EuorBloodNet standardization will provide solutions to many of these problems.

Acknowledgements

We are indebted to the EC projects FP7 Combined Molecular Microscopy for Therapy and Personalized Medication in Rare Anaemias Treatments (CoMMiT-MenT) and H20200 Innovative Training Networks MSCA.ITN.2014 (Relevance) for their financial support. The collaboration of the J. Trujillo and J. Surrallés from the Spanish Network for Rare Diseases Investigation (CIBERER) and of J. Sevilla from the Hospital Infantil Universitario Niño Jesus (Madrid), is acknowledged. We are also grateful for the technical assistance of Mrs. Elena Krishnevskaya in the RBC ektacytometric studies and in the analysis of HHA patients mutations by Next Generation Sequencing (NGS).

Author details

Joan-Lluis Vives-Corrons[1,2,3]

1 Red Blood Cell Pathology and Haematopoietic Disorders, Rare Anaemias Expert Centre, Institute for Leukaemia Research Josep Carreras, Barcelona, Spain

2 Department of Medicine, University of Barcelona, Catalonia, Spain

3 European Network for Rare and Congenital Anaemias (ENERCA), Barcelona, Catalonia, Spain

*Address all correspondence to: jlvives@ub.edu

References

[1] World Health Organization. Worldwide Prevalence of Anaemia 1993–2005: WHO Global Database on Anaemia. Geneva, Switzerland: World Health Organization; 2008

[2] Kassebaum NJ, Jasrasaria R, Naghavi M, Wulf SK, Johns N, Lozano R, et al. A systematic analysis of global anemia burden from 1990 to 2010. Blood. 2014;**123**:615-624

[3] Vives Corrons JL, Mañú Pereira MM, Romeo-Casabona C, Nicolás P, Gulbis B, Eleftheriou A, et al. Recommendations for centres of expertise in rare anaemias. The ENERCA White Book. Proceedings of the 4th Pan-European Conference on Haemoglobinopathies and Rare Anaemias. Thalassemia Reports. 2014. Vol. 4. 4878

[4] Vives Corrons JL, Mañú Pereira MM. Enerca: The European network for patients with rare Anaemias. Journal of Rare Disorders: Diagnosis & Therapy. 2015;**1**(1):12

[5] Vives Corrons JL. EuroBloodNet: From rare anaemias to rare haematological diseases, a transitional proposal for European reference network (ERN). Journal of Rare Disorders: Diagnosis & Therapy. 2016; **2**(4):47

[6] Vives-Corrons JL, Manú Pereira MM, Romeo-Casabona C, Nicolás P, Gulbis B, Eleftheriou A, et al. Consensus Recommendations for Expert Centres in Rare Anaemias: ENERCA White Book. Madrid: Prodrug Multimedia; 2014. ISBN: 978-84-939018-8-2

[7] Gulbis B, Eleftheriou A, Angastiniotis M, Ball S, Surrallés J, Castella M, et al. Epidemiology of rare anaemias in Europe. Advances in Experimental Medicine and Biology. 2010;**686**:375-396

[8] Vives Corrons JL, Aguilar Bascompre JL. Manual de Tecnicas de Laboratorio en Hematologia. 4th ed. Elsevier Masson; 2014

[9] Bain B. Diagnosis from the blood smear. The New England Journal of Medicine. 2005;**353**:498-507

[10] Splinter K, Adams DR, Bacino CA, Bellen HJ, Bernstein JA, Cheatle-Jarvela AM, et al. Effect of genetic diagnosis on patients with previously undiagnosed disease. The New England Journal of Medicine. 2018;**379**(22):2131-2139

[11] Kasper DL, Eugene B, Anthony F, et al. Harrison's Principles of Internal Medicine. 16th ed. New York: McGraw-Hill; 2005. ISBN 978-0-07-140235-4

[12] Shimamura A, Alter BP. Pathophysiology and management of inherited bone marrow failure syndromes. Blood Reviews. 2010;**24**: 101-122

[13] Bluteau D, Masliah-Planchon J, Clairmont C, Rousseau A, Ceccaldi R, Dubois d'Enghien C, et al. Biallelic inactivation of REV7 is associated with Fanconi anemia. The Journal of Clinical Investigation. 2016;**126**:3580-3584

[14] Auerbach AD. Diagnosis of Fanconi anemia by diepoxybutane analysis. Current Protocols in Human Genetics. 2003;**37**:871-886

[15] Bogliolo M, Schuster B, Stoepker C, Derkunt B, Su Y, Raams A, et al. Mutations in ERCC4, encoding the DNA-repair endonuclease XPF, cause Fanconi Anemia. The American Journal of Human Genetics. 2013;**92**:800-806

[16] Parrella S, Aspesi A, Quarello P, Garelli E, Pavesi E, Carando A, et al. Loss of GATA-1 full length as a cause of diamond-Blackfan anemia phenotype.

Pediatric Blood & Cancer. 2014;**61**(7): 1319-1321

[17] Iolascon A, Heimpel H, Wahlin A, Tamary H. Congenital dyserythropoietic anemias: Molecular insights and diagnostic approach. Blood. 2013;**122**: 2162-2166

[18] Vives Corrons JL, Mañú Pereira MM, Trujillo JP, Surrallés J, Sevilla J. Anemias raras y fallos medulares hereditarios. Arbor. 2018; **194**(789):a463. DOI: 10.3989/arbor.2018.789n3005

[19] Angastiniotis M, Vives Corrons JL, Soteriades ES, Eleftheriou A. The impact of migrations on the health services for rare diseases in Europe: The example of haemoglobin disorders. The Scientific World Journal. 2013;**2013**:727905. DOI: 10.1155/2013/727905

[20] Aguilar Martinez P, Angastiniotis M, Eleftheriou A, Gulbis B, Mañú Pereira MM, Petrova-Benedict R, et al. Haemoglobinopathies in Europe: Health & migration policy perspectives. Orphanet Journal of Rare Diseases. 2014;**9**:97

[21] Piel FB, Steinberg MH, Rees DC. Sickle cell disease. New England Journal of Medicine. 2017;**376**:1561-1573. DOI: 10.1056/NEJMra1510865

[22] Daniel Y, Elion J, Allaf B, Badens C, Bouva MJ, Brincat I, et al. Newborn screening for sickle cell disease in Europe. International Journal of Neonatal Screening. 2019;**5**:15. DOI: 10.3390/ijns5010015

[23] Angastiniotis M, Lobitz S. Thalassemias: An overview. International Journal of Neonatal Screening. 2019;**5**:16. DOI: 10.3390/ijns5010016

[24] Thompson AA, Walters MC, Kwiatkowski J, Ribeil JJ, Hongeng S, Magrin E, et al. Gene therapy in patients with transfusion-dependent β-thalassemia. The New England Journal of Medicine. 2018;**378**:1479-1493

[25] King MJ, Zanella A. Hereditary red cell membrane disorders and laboratory diagnostic testing. International Journal of Laboratory Hematology. 2013;**35**: 237-243

[26] Christensen RD, Yaish HM, Gallagher PG. A Pediatrician's practical guide to diagnosing and treating hereditary spherocytosis in neonates. Pediatrics. 2015;**135**:1107-1114

[27] Llaudet-Planas E, Vives-Corrons JL, Rizzuto V, Gómez-Ramírez P, Sevilla Navarro J, Coll Sibina MT, et al. Osmotic gradient ektacytometry: A valuable screening test for hereditary spherocytosis and other red blood cell membrane. International Journal of Laboratory Hematology. 2018;**40**: 94-102. DOI: 10.1111/ijlh.12746 Epub 2017 Oct 10

[28] An X, Mohandas N. Disorders of red cell membrane. British Journal of Haematology. 2008;**141**:367-375. DOI: 10.1111/j.1365-2141.2008.07091.x

[29] Gallanger PG. Disorders of erythrocyte hydration. Blood. 2017;**130**: 2699-2708

[30] Vives Corrons JL, Besson I, Aymerich M, Ayala S, Alloisio M, Delaunay J, et al. Hereditary xerocytosis: A report of six unrelated Spanish families with leaky red cell syndrome and increased heat stability of the erythrocyte membrane. British Journal of Haematology. 1995;**90**:817-822

[31] Luzzatto L, Seneca E. G6PD deficiency: A classic example of pharmacogenetics with on-going clinical implications. British Journal of Haematology. 2014;**164**:469-480

[32] Zanella A, Fermo E, Bianchi P, Valentini G. Red cell pyruvate kinase

deficiency: Molecular and clinical aspects. British Journal of Haematology. 2005;**130**:11-25

[33] Montllor L, Mañú-Pereira MM, Llaudet-Planas E, Gómez Ramírez P, Sevilla Navarro J, Vives-Corrons JL. Red cell pyruvate kinase deficiency in Spain: A study of 15 cases. Medicina Clínica (Barcelona). 2017;**148**:23-27

[34] Glader B, Barcellini W, Grace R. Fast Facts: Pyruvate Kinase Deficiency. 1st ed. Oxford, UK: Karger Publishers Limited; 2018. ISBN 978-1-910797-88-4

[35] Wegman-Ostrosky T, Savage SA. The genomics of inherited bone marrow failure: From mechanism to the clinic. British Journal of Haematology. 2017; **177**:526-542

Chapter 9

Milestone Histories and Paradigmatic Genetic Discoveries of Chronic Myeloid Leukemia (CML)

Zhan He Wu

Abstract

Chronic myeloid leukemia (CML) is classified as a hematological malignant rare disease by National Organization for Rare Disease (NORD, USA) based on the estimated incidence of 1–2 cases/100,000 per year internationally. CML occurs in all ages but commonly seen in the 45–55 years group. Males are slightly more affected than females. CML is one of the oldest known diseases with new faces and one of the fastest developing diseases with many extraordinary discoveries in human history of conquering the disease. CML possesses at least Nine First findings in leukemia and cancer research and even in human medical histories: the First named as leukemia in 1845, the First of a live case of CML patient diagnosed in 1846, the First used of arsenic in CML treatment in 1865, the First defined as a myeloproliferative disorder in 1951, the First finding of Philadelphia chromosome (Ph chromosome) in 1960, the First finding of chromosome 9 and 22 translocations in 1973, the First identified as a clonal hematological malignancy derived from the stage of pluripotent bone hematopoietic stem cells in 1977, the First finding of the chromosomal fusion gene-BCR-ABL as an oncogene in 1984, and the First designed target therapy of use of tyrosine kinase inhibitor (TKI) in 1998. The footprints of the studies on CML established the milestone histories. Remarkable and fascinating genetic discoveries were made of the mysteries of human diseases, the multiway translocation of Ph chromosome, and the latest issues. The association of the combination of chronic myeloid leukemia and chronic lymphocytic leukemia will be reviewed in this chapter with the aim of increasing the understanding of CML further from laboratory bench to clinical bedside.

Keywords: rare hematological malignancy, chronic myeloid leukemia, genetic variations, Philadelphia chromosome, BCR-ABL gene

1. Introduction

Myeloproliferative neoplasm (MPN) is a rare type of hematological malignancy featured by the excessive proliferation of single or multilineages of hematopoietic cells in the bone marrow affecting fewer than six in 100,000 people. MPN mainly includes polycythemia vera (PV), essential thrombocythemia (ET), primary myelofibrosis (MF), and chronic myeloid leukemia (CML) classified by World Health Organization (WHO) [1].

Among these types of MPN, CML, with several synonyms of chronic myelogenous leukemia, chronic granulocytic leukemia, is the most common type of myeloproliferative disorder characterized by increased proliferation of the granulocytic cell line without the loss of their capacity to differentiate.

CML consists of about 20% of all leukemias affecting individuals of all ages including children and infants with chronic, accelerated, and blast crisis phases to acute leukemia resulting in life-threatening situation [2].

CML presents as easy bleeding, splenomegaly, feeling run down or tired, fever, loss of weight without trying, loss of appetite, pain or fullness below the ribs on the left side, pale skin, and excessive sweating during sleep (night sweats) [3].

CML has a very exciting history and extraordinary findings in which it has paved the way toward clinical diagnosis and treatment. It was predicted by John Gordon in 2003 that the fascinating CML could be becoming even more fascinating from now on [4].

2. Milestone histories and remarkable genetic discoveries of CML

The remarkable genetic discoveries have been translating into clinical diagnosis, effective, and specific therapies from the following so many FIRST findings.

2.1 The first named as a leukemia

CML was first named as leukemia in the nineteenth century, when it was described and recognized in 1845 from descriptions of the clinical presentations and symptoms by Bennett, Virchow, and Craigie [5–7].

Cells from blood or bone marrow morphology from patient with CML show at every stage differential cells due to partial blockage, unlike the maturation and differentiation of acute leukemia, which are blocked completely in the early cell differential stage. The chronic term of CML refers to maturation and differentiation, unlike other diseases by period of disease duration.

2.2 The first of a live case of CML patient diagnosed

The first live patient with CML was diagnosed in 1846 by Dr. Henry Fuller, a physician at St George's Hospital in London with the identification of a large proportion of abnormal, granular colorless globules under microscope [8].

2.3 The first used of arsenic in CML treatment

Fowler's solution, the compounded a potassium bicarbonate-based solution of arsenic trioxide (As_2O_3) invented by Thomas Fowler named as Fowler's solution in 1786, was first tried in CML among all leukemias in 1865 to reduce the over proliferative white cell numbers [9].

Very excitingly, the arsenic has been used to cure acute promyelocytic leukemia (APL) which it made the worst and incurable type of leukemia; APL became the best therapeutical curable type among all types of leukemias achieved by several Chinese medical researchers [10].

2.4 The first defined as a myeloproliferative disorder

CML was first introduced as a myeloproliferative disorder based on the evidence accumulated of multiple abnormalities involved in erythroblasts, granulocytes, megakaryocytes, but no fibroblasts in bone marrow by Dameshe [11].

2.5 The first finding of Ph chromosome in leukemia

Ph chromosome was first reported in 1960 by Nowell and Hungerford [12]. Originally such a finding was described as deletion of the long arm of chromosome 22, although it was thought to be chromosome 21 [13] and was even thought to be the chromosome Y due to limitation of low chromosomal resolution from the cytogenetic technique at that time [14, 15]. The smart conclusion made from this was the suggestion that such chromosome change could be associated with CML.

Since then the detection of Ph chromosome by the application of the cytogenetic (Karyotyping) and the molecular cytogenetic techniques, fluorescence in-situ hybridization (FISH) has become a very useful and practical approach in the diagnosis and monitor of CML. Cytogenetic karyotype analysis is a specific, accurate, low cost, fast technology in CML diagnosis, and disease monitoring in the detection of both classical and variant Ph translocation.

2.6 The first identified as a translocation of chromosomes 9 and 22 in leukemia

In 1973, Ph chromosome or Ph translocation was identified as balanced translocated chromosomes 9 and 22, t[q34;q11], by Rowley [16]. Such milestone finding identified and classified the Ph chromosome was not the shortening of chromosome 22 as found by Nowell and Hungerford, which it pointed out the direction and narrowed down to the discovery of CML causing gene from the initial finding of the association between Ph chromosome and CML.

2.7 The first finding of BCR-ABL gene in leukemia

Breakpoint cluster region-Abelson leukemia (BCR-ABL) virus was the first finding from CML in leukemia and oncology. BCR-ABL is a fusion oncogene, resulting in CML from the translocation at the breakpoints of the long arm of chromosome 9 and the long arm of chromosome 22 and in humans [17] and mice [18–20].

Studies found that BCR-ABL fusion gene has several types of isoform protein products from the different breakpoints of translocated. The common types are the fusion protein products (p210, p190, and p230), resulting in the enhancement of tyrosine kinase activity in CML and other types of hematological malignancies in the similar mechanism [21]. The concept from such findings obtained provided the valuable theory for the development of the target-specific therapy afterward.

The detection of BCR-ABL gene using PCR technique commonly has become a valuable/effective and sensitive approach in the diagnosis and disease monitoring of CML, which it does not require cell culture.

2.8 The first clinical therapy by using tyrosine kinase inhibitor (TKI) in leukemia

CML has a long developmental history in the trial of treatment in the past, including the first trial by using arsenic (Fowler's solution), x-irradiation, nitrogen mustard, busulfan, hydroxyurea, interferon-α, and stem cell transplantation. The tyrosine kinase inhibitor (TKI) is considered as the first and a successfully designed first-generation target therapy in cancer therapies clinically. This therapy was designed on the base of blocking and deregulating the activity of BCR-ABL fusing gene 1998 [22]. The second-generation TKI started to be used for reducing the resistance was developed in 2004. Such specific therapy significantly prolonged lifespan for patients with CML.

2.9 The first described as a clonal hematological disease in leukemia

Cells from bone marrow or peripheral blood of a patient with CML show excessive proliferation from one or multiple lineages and different maturation stages due to the partial blocking of differentiation.

CML was first identified as a clonal hematological malignancy from pluripotent bone marrow stem cells [23, 24]. Such finding increased our understanding of the stages of disease mechanism and helps in the diagnosis, differential diagnosis, and treatment.

3. Variant complex and multiway translocations of Ph chromosome

3.1 Variant complex translocation of Ph chromosome

Cytogenetically, CML is characterized by the Ph chromosome formed by the fusion gene of the reciprocal translocation t(9:22)(q34;q11), resulting in the chimeric gene breakpoint cluster region (BCR)-Abelson leukemia (ABL).

Studies demonstrated that approximately 90–95% CML patients have Ph chromosome from the classical reciprocal translocations. However, about 5–10% CML cases have variant types of the Ph chromosome. The variant Ph chromosome translocations are involving chromosomes other than 9 and 22 or multiple chromosomes involved in CML cases [25]. Some studies also suggested that the classical and variant Ph chromosome translocations in CML patient have showed different sensitivities to treatment [26].

Mysorekar et al. reported five male CML cases with variant Ph chromosome translocations. Two cases were two-way translocations, t(16;22), t(15;22), and three cases were three-way translocations, t(1;9;22), t(9;9;22), t(9;14;22), and all cases studied were with BCR-ABL fusion gene, but responded well to the tyrosine kinase inhibitors, imatinib treatment in their studied cases [27].

3.2 Three-way translocation of Ph chromosome

Three-way translocation involves three chromosomes including the Ph chromosome. Such complex translocation was found not only in adult but also in childhood.

Lee reported a 22-year-old male CML case with a three-way translocation involving in chromosomes 9, 22, and 11 at the breakpoints of q34;q11.2;q24 detected by using cytogenetic-G banding and FISH techniques, and this patient responded well to TKI treatment imatinib [28].

Asif groups reported male CML case with a three-way translocation involving chromosomes 9, 11, and 22 at the breakpoints of q34;p15;q11 in separate studies [29].

Allen-Proctor group reported a male CML case with a three-way translocation involved in chromosomes 9, 22, and 17 at the breakpoints of q34;q11.2;q12 detected by using cytogenetic analysis of G banding and FISH [30].

Most three-way translocations reported were primary abnormalities. Achkar et al. reported a male CML case with a three-way translocation involved in chromosomes 9, 10, and 22 at the breakpoints of q34;p11.2;q11.2 and also loss of Y chromosome as a secondary abnormality after the classical Ph translocation of t(9;22) followed by chemotherapy [31].

CML is very low in childhood and infant. Three-way translocation of Ph chromosome in infant is extremely rare. An 10-month-old boy infant with three-way Ph translocations involved in chromosomes 9, 22, and 14 at the breakpoints of q34;q11.2;q32 by using GTG banding and FISH techniques and confirmed the presence of BCR-ABL by

RT-PCR was reported as the first case with the accelerated phase and received favorable response with hydroxyl urea and the TKI (dasatinib) [32].

3.3 Four-way translocation of Ph chromosome

Four-way translocation involves four chromosomes including the Ph chromosome. Asif et al. reported a four-way translocation involved in chromosomes 4, 9, 19, and 22. They have reviewed and analyzed 59 cases of CML with four-way translocations reported from the literatures previously. Their analysis showed that 56% of four-way translocation was male, 39% was female, 2% was missing chromosome Y (-Y), and 3% was unidentifiable of sex [33].

Achkar group reported a four-way translocation involving chromosomes 9, 11, 20, and 22 [34]. The same group reported another case with four-way translocations involved in chromosomes 9, 11, 20, and 22. Also, BCR-ABL fusion gene was detected by reverse transcription polymerase chain reaction (RT-PCR). That patient also showed additional chromosome abnormalities involving translocations of chromosomes 7 and 8. Patient showed poor response to imatinib and died for unknown reason [35].

3.4 Five-way translocation of Ph chromosome

Five-way translocation is involved in five chromosomes including the Ph chromosome. A novel five-way translocation involved in chromosomes 7, 11, 9, 22, and 9 detected by G-banding technique and confirmed by spectral karyotyping (SKY); BCR-ABL gene was detected by fluorescence in-situ hybridization (FISH), which was reported by Yokota group in 2012, and patients showed good respond to imatinib treatment and also reviewed another nine cases of five-way translocations compared with their case reported in that article [36].

Another five-way translocations of 29-year-old male CML case involved in chromosomes 9, 11, 13, 19, and 22 by G-banding technique confirmed by SKY, and BCR-ABL gene fusion by Vaidya group reported a five-way translocation involved in chromosomes 9, 11, 13, 19, and 22, and that case responded well to imatinib treatment [37].

The mechanism of variant complex translocation is still unknown. The spatial arrangement is involved in chromosomes because they require the physical interaction of the translocation partners and the association of genomic instability could be associated with multiway translocation.

3.5 The application of next-generation sequencing (NGS) and the detection of other genes associated with CML

Currently, cytogenetics, FISH, and qRT-PCR have been using as the routine techniques in the applications of CML diagnosis. However, each of them has his/her limitation in the application. NGS technique is a powerful technique with high throughput. Lyu group identified a novel BCR-ABL1 fusion gene with breakpoints in the BCR intron 14 and the ABL1 intron 2 (with an e14a3) by using NGS [38].

Shokeen group studied CML cases by using NGS and found some variants and potential prognostic and susceptibility markers, which helped them in the prediction of TKI therapy [39].

Fu group studied BCR-ABL fusion gene variants on CML by using next-generation sequencing (NGS), and they found an e13a2-like novel form of BCR-ABL fusion, while it was negative with qRT-PCR-based test, which helped them in diagnosis and therapy. Their results suggested that NGS is a powerful technique to detect BCR-ABL fusion variants, which they could be missed by other routine techniques. In addition, other mutated genes SETBP1, PAX5, and TP53 were also detected [40]. Such findings of additional mutated genes involved in CML by NGS may increase the understanding in leukemogenesis and help in treatment for cases with CML with TKI therapy resistant.

4. Issues of the presence of Ph chromosome or BCR-ABL gene in non-CML hematological malignancies or healthy individuals

Ph chromosome, t(9;22)(q34.1;q11.2), was found in CML at 90–95% as mentioned above [41]. However, Ph chromosome has been found in other types of non-CML hematological malignancies.

Studies showed that acute myeloid leukemia (AML) about 3% of adult AML and 1% in childhood have Ph chromosome [42, 43]. Different proportions of Ph chromosome were found in patient with myelodysplasia syndrome (MDS) [44]. About 20% of adult ALL and 2–5% of children have Ph chromosome in acute lymphoblastic leukemia (ALL) [45–48]. The couple of T-ALL cases with positive Ph have been reported [49, 50]. The presence of Ph chromosome on a patient with lymphoma was detected by a study [51]. Positive Ph chromosome was reported from H929 multiple myeloma cell line [52]. Koshy group reported the presence of Ph chromosome from a case of pregnant women with unusual primary myelofibrosis [53].

Interestingly and surprisingly, BCR-ABL fusion gene was detected in healthy individuals (2/30) but without following up studies seen afterward [54]. Biernaux group studied the BCR-ABL gene of blood cells from healthy individuals and found the presence of BCR-ABL transcript (22 of 73) [55]. More evidence from a study of peripheral blood leukocytes conducted on 16 healthy individuals, and some cell lines as controls by Bose group and results showed the presence of BCR-ABL gene either p210 (27%) or p190 (69%) transcript in healthy individuals [56]. It is suggested that leukemia-associated genes in healthy individuals require the additional activations to be malignancy, although no satisfactory explanation on why BCR/ABL fusion gene detected from some healthy individuals short- and long-term following up.

5. Issues of the combination of CML and chronic lymphocytic leukemia (CLL) in the clonal association

CML and CLL are different hematological malignancies characterized by their cause of disease, their origin of hematopoietic lineages, laboratory findings and clinical presentations, and different immune phenotypes. CML and CLL require different treatment strategies. In general, there are no many problems or issues in the diagnosis and differential diagnosis on both of CML and CLL.

Recently, there were some rare cases reported in the combination of CML and CLL, which raises a question as to whether the myeloid and lymphoid malignant clones derived from the common malignant stem cells or CML and CLL are two independent simultaneous events.

A group performed a study on three-way translocations by flow cytometric sorting using monoclonal antibody anti-CD19 lacked the BCR-ABL rearrangement. Their results suggested CML and CLL were from two different clones B-cell transformation occurred in a Ph-B-cell subset [57].

Wu et al. reported a novel CML case with three-way translocations involved in chromosomes 9, 22, and 11 cytogenetically and confirmed by fluorescence in-situ hybridization (FISH). It was found the deletion of chromosome short arm (4p) confirmed by comparative genome hybridization microarray. This patient had more than 10 years indolent chronic lymphoblastic leukemia (CLL) history without progression over several years, and cytogenetic test was normal. Interestingly, both CML and CLL got remission after treatment for CML indicating the possibility of the relevant if clonal revolution [58]. These results might indicate the association of Ph chromosome in the leukemogenesis of CML and CLL.

Armarego et al. reported five CML cases in the combination of CLL history and one case with the deletion of short arm of chromosome 17(17p). All patients were treated for both CLL and CML, and a satisfactory outcome was achieved from the five cases studied separately [59].

The association of CML and CLL raises the issues that the combination of CML and CLL is the two different events or a result from a clonal evolution either from CML or CLL that needs to be classified further.

6. Conclusion

CML is a special disease with a milestone history and remarkable nonstopping genetic discoveries, which have paved the path in effective treatment of CML by translating findings into clinical settings.

It is believed that the continuing study on genetic variations will help to develop TKI therapy to minimize further therapy resistance in the future.

CML is an old disease with new face. The continuous discoveries of genetic variations and multiway translocation of Ph chromosome in CML will help in the diagnosis and monitoring of treatment.

The mystery and the associations of the combination of CML and CLL in some reported cases are still unknown.

Such fascinating stories made the best example in the process of conquering the human diseases.

Author details

Zhan He Wu
Western Sydney Genome Diagnostics, The Children's Hospital at Westmead, Affiliated to University of Sydney, Sydney, Australia

*Address all correspondence to: zhan.wu@health.nsw.gov.au

References

[1] Swerdlow SH, Campo E, Harris NL et al. WHO Classification of Tumours of Haematopoietic and Lymphoid Tissues. Revised 4th ed. Vol. 2. Lyon: International Agency for Research on Cancer; 2017. pp. 29-57

[2] Siegel RL, Miller KD, Jemal A. Cancer statistics. 2015. CA: A Cancer Journal for Clinicians. 2015;**65**(1):5-29

[3] Sawyers CL. Chronic myeloid leukemia. The New England Journal of Medicine. 1999;**340**:1330-1340

[4] Gorden J. Chronic myeloid leukemia—Past, present, and future. Seminars in Hematology. 2003;**40**(1):1-3

[5] Bennett JH. Case of hypertrophy of the spleen and liver in which death took place from suppuration of the blood. Edinburgh Medical and Surgical Journal. 1845;**64**:413-423

[6] Virchow R. Weisses Blut. Froriep's Notizen. 1845;36:151-156

[7] Craigie D. Case of disease of the spleen in which death took place from suppuration of the blood. Edinburgh Medical and Surgical Journal. 1985;**64**:400-412

[8] Fuller HW. Particulars of a case in which enormous enlargement of the spleen and liver, together with dilation of all the blood vessels of the body were found co-incident with a peculiarly altered condition of the blood. Lancet. 1846;**2**:43-44

[9] Lissauer, initials unknown. Zwei Falle von Leukamie. Berliner Klinische Wochenschrift. 1865;**2**:403-404

[10] Chen Z, Wang ZY, Chen SJ. Acute promyelocytic leukemia: Cellular and molecular basis of differentiation and apoptosis. Pharmacology and Therapeutics. 1997;**76**(1-3):141-149

[11] Dameshek W. Some speculations on the myeloproliferative syndromes. Blood. 1951;**6**(4):372-375

[12] Nowell PC, Hungerford DA. Chromosome studies on normal and leukemic human leukocytes. The Journal of the National Cancer Institute. 1960;**25**:85-109

[13] Nowell PC, Hungerford DA. A minute chromosome in human granulocytic leukemia. Science. 1960;**13**:132, 1497

[14] Tough I, Court B, Baikie WM, et al. Cytogenetic studies in chronic myeloid leukaemia and acute leukaemia associated with mongolism. Lancet. 25 Feb 1961;**1**(7174):411-417

[15] Nowell PC, Hungerford DA. Chromosome studies in human leukemia. II. Chronic granulocytic leukemia. The Journal of the National Cancer Institute. 1961;**27**:1013-1035

[16] Rowley J. A new consistent chromosomal abnormality in chronic myeloid leukemia identified by quinacrine fluorescence and Giemsa staining. Nature. 1973;**243**:290-293

[17] Groffen J, Stephenson JR, Heisterkamp N. Philadelphia chromosomal breakpoints are clustered within a limited region, bcr, on chromosome 22. Cell. 1984;**36**:93-99

[18] Groffen J, Stephenson JR, Heisterkamp N, et al. The human c-abl oncogene in the Philadelphia translocation. Journal of Cellular Physiology. Supplement. 1984;**3**:179-191

[19] Daley GQ, Van Etten RA, Baltimore D. Induction of chronic myelogenous leukemia in mice by the P210bcr/abl gene of the Philadelphia chromosome. Science. 1990;**247**:824-830

[20] Li S, Ilaria RL Jr, Million RP. The P190, P210, and P230 forms of the BCR/ABL oncogene induce a similar chronic myeloid leukemia-like syndrome in mice but have different lymphoid leukemogenic activity. The Journal of Experimental Medicine. 1999;**189**(9):1399-1412

[21] Collins SJ, Groudine MT. Rearrangement and amplification of c-abl sequences in the human chronic myelogenous leukemia cell line K-562. Proceedings of the National Academy of Sciences of the United States of America. 1983;**80**(15):4813-4817

[22] Druker BJ, Lydon NB. Lessons learned from the development of an abl tyrosine kinase inhibitor for chronic myelogenous leukemia. The Journal of Clinical Investigation. 2000;**105**(1):3-7

[23] Fialkow PJ, Jacobson RJ, Papayannopoulou T. Chronic myelocytic leukemia: Clonal origin in a stem cell common to the granulocyte, erythrocyte, platelet and monocyte/macrophage. The American Journal of Medicine. 1977;**63**(1):125-130

[24] Fialkow PJ, Jacobson RJ, Singer JW, et al. Philadelphia chromosome (Ph1)-negative chronic myelogenous leukemia (CML): A clonal disease with origin in a multipotent stem cell. Blood. 1980;**56**:70-73

[25] Melo JV. The molecular biology of chronic myeloid leukemia. Leukemia. 1996;**10**(suppl 2):S4-S9

[26] Beutler E, Lichtmann MA, Coller BS, et al. Williams Hematology. 5th ed. New York, NY: McGraw-Hill; 1995. pp. 298-330

[27] Mysorekar V, Subramanian M, Kilara N, et al. Variant Philadelphia translocations in chronic myeloid leukemia: A report of five cases. Journal of Cancer Research and Therapeutics. 2015;**11**:654

[28] Lee J, Kim DS, Lee HS, et al. A novel t(9;22;11) translocation involving 11q24 in a patient with chronic myeloid leukemia: A case report. Oncology Letters. 2017;**13**:1711-1713

[29] Asif M, Hussain A, Rasoo M. A rare case of a three way complex variant positive Philadelphia translocation involving chromosome (9;11;22)(q34;p15;q11) in chronic myeloid leukemia: A case report. Oncology Letters. 2016;**12**:1986-1988

[30] Proctor KA, Ruckdeschel E, Naous R. A novel three-way Philadelphia variant t(9;22;17)(q34;q11.2;q12) in chronic myeloid leukemia: A case report. Molecular and Clinical Oncology. 2018;**8**:300-301

[31] Achkar W, Wafa A, Ikhtiar A. Three-way Philadelphia translocation t(9;10;22)(q34;p11.2;q11.2) as a secondary abnormality in an imatinib mesylate-resistant chronic myeloid leukemia patient. Oncology Letters. 2013;**5**:1656-1658

[32] Hayek RA, Omar H, Dayel AA, et al. The first case report of an infant with three-way Philadelphia chromosome variant T(9;22;14) (Q34;Q11.2;Q32) chronic myeloid leukemia, King Fahd specialist hospital Dammam experience, Kingdom of Saudi Arabia. Cancer Therapy and Oncology International Journal. 2017;**4**(5):1-3

[33] Asif M, Jamal MS, Khan ARA. Novel four-way complex variant translocation involving chromosome 46,XY,t(4;9;19;22)(q25:q34;p13.3;q11.2) in a chronic myeloid leukemia patient. Frontiers in Oncology. 2016;**6**:124, 1-6

[34] Achkar W, Wafa A, Liehr T. A new t(9;11;20;22)(q34;p11.2;q11.21;q11) in a Philadelphia-positive chronic myeloid leukemia case. Oncology Letters. 2013;**5**:605-608

[35] Achkar W, Aljapawe A, Almedani S, et al. A novel cytogenetic abnormality t(7;8)(p11.2:q11.2) and a four-way Philadelphia translocation in an imatinib mesylate-resistant chronic myeloid leukemia patient. Oncology Letters. 2013;**5**:617-620

[36] Vaidya S, Joshi D, Ghosh K, et al. A novel five-way translocation t(9;11;13;19;22) in a case of chronic-phase chronic myeloid leukemia. Human Pathology. 2013;**44**:2365-2369

[37] Yokota S, Nakamura Y, Bessho M. A novel five-way translocation t(7;11;9;22;9)(q22; q13;q34;q11.2;q34) involving Ph chromosome in a patient of chronic myeloid leukemia: A case report. Molecular Cytogenetics. 2012;**5**(20):1-5

[38] Lyu X, Yang J, Wang X, et al. A novel BCR-ABL1 fusion gene identified by next-generation sequencing in chronic myeloid leukemia. Molecular Cytogenetics. 2016;**9**(47):1-7

[39] Shokeen Y, Sharma NR, Vats A. Identification of prognostic and susceptibility markers in chronic myeloid leukemia using next generation sequencing. Ethiopian Journal of Health Sciences. 2018;**28**(2):135-140

[40] Fu S, Hu Y, Fu Y, et al. Novel BCR-ABL1 fusion and leukemic mutations of SETBP1, PAX5, and TP53 detected by next generation sequencing in chronic myeloid leukemia. Cancer Biology and Therapy. 2016;**17**(10):1003-1009

[41] Kurzrock R, Gutterman JU, Talpaz M. The molecular genetics of Philadelphia chromosome-positive leukemias. The New England Journal of Medicine. 1988;**319**(15):990-998

[42] Whang-Peng J, Henderson ES, Knutsen T, Freireich E, Gart JJ. Cytogenetic studies in acute myelocytic leukemia with special emphasis on the occurrence of Ph chromosome. Blood. 1970;**36**(4):448-458

[43] Zhang LJ, Gan YM, Yu L. Occurrence of BCR/ABL fusion gene in a patient with acute promyelocytic leukemia. Medical Oncology. 2015;**32**(1):382

[44] Keung YK, Beaty M, Powell BL, et al. Philadelphia chromosome positive myelodysplastic syndrome and acute myeloid leukemia-retrospective study and review of literature. Leukemia Research. 2004;**28**(6):579-586

[45] Pullarkat V, Slovak ML, Kopecky KJ, et al. Impact of cytogenetics on the outcome of adult acute lymphoblastic leukemia: Results of southwest oncology group 9400 study. Blood. 2008;**111**(5):2563-2572

[46] Rafiei A, Mian AA, Doring C, et al. The functional interplay between the t(9;22)-associated fusion proteins BCR/ABL and ABL/BCR in Philadelphia chromosome-positive acute lymphatic leukemia. PLoS Genetics. 2015;**11**(4):e1005144

[47] Propp S, Lizzi FA. Philadelphia chromosome in acute lymphocytic leukemia. Blood. 1970;**36**(3):353-360

[48] Tsuchiya H, Migita M, Yamamori S, et al. A late-appearing Philadelphia chromosome in acute lymphoblastic leukemia confirmed by expression of BCR-ABL mRNA. Leukemia. 1995;**9**(10):1689-1693

[49] Tchirkov A, Bons JM, Chassagne J, et al. Molecular detection of a late-appearing BCR-ABL gene in a child with T-cell acute lymphoblastic leukemia. Annals of Hematology. 1998;**77**:55-59

[50] Verrma SP, Dutta TK, Vinod KV, et al. Philadelphia chromosome positive pre-T cell acute lymphoblastic leukemia: A rare case report and short review.

Indian Journal of Hematology and Blood Transfusion. 2014;**30**(Suppl 1):177-179

[51] Boddu P, Cameron YC, Rashmi SRK, et al. An unsuspected finding of t(9;22): A rare case of Philadelphia chromosome-positive B-lymphoblastic lymphoma. Case Reports in Hematology. 2017;**2017**:1-4

[52] Breitkopf SB, Yuana M, Pihanc GA, et al. Detection of a rare BCR–ABL tyrosine kinase fusion protein in H929 multiple myeloma cells using immunoprecipitation (IP)-tandem mass spectrometry (MS/MS). Proceedings of the National Academy of Sciences of the United States of America. 2012;**109**(40):16190-16195

[53] Koshy J, Alperin J, Jana B, et al. A case of Philadelphia chromosome positive myeloproliferative neoplasm in a pregnant woman with unusual primary myelofibrosis features. Case Reports in Hematology. 2013;**2013**:1-4

[54] Boquett JA, Alves JRP, andOliveira CEC. Analysis of BCR/ABL transcripts in healthy individuals. Genetics and Molecular Research. 2013;**12**(4):4967-4971

[55] Biernaux C, Loos M, Sels A, Huez G, et al. Detection of major bcr-abl gene expression at a very low level in blood cells of some healthy individuals. Blood. 1995;**86**:3118-3122

[56] Bose S, Deininger M, Tybor JG, et al. The presence of typical and atypical BCR-ABL fusion genes in leukocytes of normal individuals: Biologic significance and implications for the assessment of minimal residual disease. Blood. 1998;**92**(9):3362-3367

[57] Armarego M, Gottlieb D, Combined CJ. CML and CLL in four patients, including one with 17p deletion. Pathology. 2018;**50**(Suppl 1):101-102

[58] Wu ZH, Hung D, Sharma P, et al. A novel case of chronic myeloid leukaemia (CML) with a three-way t(9;22;11) translocation but with a history of indolent chronic lymphocytic leukaemia (CLL). Pathology. 2018;**50**(Suppl 1):109-110

[59] Mansat-De Mas V, Rigal-Huguet F, Cassar G, et al. Chronic myeloid leukemia associated with b cell chronic lymphocytic leukemia: Evidence of two separate clones as shown by combined cellsorting and fluorescence in situ hybridisation. Leukemia and Lymphoma. 2003;**44**(5):867-869

Chapter 10

Chronic Myeloid Leukemia

Letícia Antunes Muniz Ferreira

Abstract

Chronic myelogenous leukemia (CML) is a chronic clonal myeloproliferative disease characterized by left leukocytosis, splenomegaly, and the presence of the Philadelphia (Ph) chromosome, which results from the reciprocal and balanced translocation between the long arms of chromosomes 9q34 and 22q11, generating the hybrid protein BCR-ABL, with increased tyrosine kinase activity. The BCR-ABL protein is present in all patients with CML, and its hyperactivity triggers the release of effectors of cell proliferation and inhibitors of apoptosis, and its activity is responsible for the initial oncogenesis of CML. This chapter will review CML from its discovery, molecular and epigenetic mechanisms of disease progression to current treatments.

Keywords: chronic myeloid leukemia, hematologic malignancy, hematopoietic neoplasm, myeloproliferative disorder, Philadelphia chromosome

1. Introduction

Chronic myeloid leukemia (CML) is a neoplasm characterized by clonal expansion of hematopoietic stem cells, resulting in increase of peripheral blood myeloid, erythroid, and platelet cells, with bone marrow (BM) myeloid hyperplasia [1, 2]. Typical symptoms of CML include fatigue, anorexia, and weight loss. However, about 40% of patients are asymptomatic, and in these patients the diagnosis is based on an abnormal blood count [1].

CML is categorized into three phases: chronic, accelerated, and blast crisis. At the beginning of the chronic phase (CP), some patients are asymptomatic, but others have fatigue, weakness, headaches, irritability, fever, night sweats, and weight loss. The accelerated phase (AP) comes after a variable period of diagnosis from a few months to several years, and it is characterized by increased bone marrow and peripheral blood blasts, peripheral blood leukocytosis and basophilia, anemia and thrombocytopenia unrelated to treatment, or the development of cytogenetic evolution. Subsequently, the disease progresses to the blast phase (BP), defined hematologically by the increase of leukemic blasts in the peripheral blood and/or bone marrow (more than 20%). At this stage of the disease, many patients die within 3–6 months. The progression to AP and BP seems to be associated mainly with genomic instability, which predisposes to the appearance of other molecular abnormalities [3].

The average diagnosis of CML is 64 years. However, all age groups, including children, are affected. About 15% of all leukemias are CML. It is estimated for the USA that 1 out of 526 people will have CML in their lifetime. The American Cancer Society estimates for CML in the USA by 2019: about 8990 new cases will be diagnosed with CML (5250 in men and 3740 in women) and about 1140 CML deaths (660 men and 480 women) [4].

1.1 Discovery of leukemias

The first case of leukemia was described in 1827 by Alfred Velpeau. Velpeau observed in a 63-year-old patient an enlarged spleen and liver associated with fever, weakness, and the presence of blood pus [5]. Later, Alfred Donné described the autopsy of a patient who had an enlarged spleen and semi-purulent blood under a microscope [6].

However, the first description of leukemia was credited to John Hughes Bennett in 1845. Bennett gave a more complete and scientific description of a 28-year-old patient who had postmortem examination with massive enlargement of the liver, spleen, and lymph nodes, in addition to the presence of purulent blood [7]. In the same year, Rudolf Virchow described the autopsy of a 50-year-old female patient with splenomegaly and pus in her blood vessels [8].

In 1852, Bennett described 37 cases of leucocythemia [9]. Later, in 1856, Virchow noted that cases of splenomegaly leukemia had some granular blood cells with irregular or divided nuclei, while patients with lymphadenopathy already had smooth nucleus cells [10]. Virchow proposed two main varieties of chronic leukemia, splenic and lymphatic, which today are identified as leukemia and lymphoma, respectively [11].

The introduction of blood cell staining techniques in 1878 by Paul Ehrlich revolutionized hematology, allowing a differentiation of different types of leukocytes [12]. With this, Ehrlich distinguished lymphoid and myeloid leukemias [13].

1.2 Discovery of Philadelphia chromosome

The improvement of cytogenetic techniques allowed the study of chromosomal arrangements in various pathological conditions. Thus, specific human disorders were found to be associated with specific chromosomal abnormalities (e.g., Down syndrome, associated with an extra copy of chromosome 21) [14].

In 1960, Peter Nowell and David Hungerford identified a small chromosome in two CML patients. This chromosome was called the Philadelphia (Ph) chromosome, according to the chromosome standardization committee, which suggested that abnormal chromosomes be designated by the name of the city in which they were discovered [11, 14, 15]. The discovery of this chromosome was a very important step in understanding the pathophysiology of CML.

Chromosome banding techniques revolutionized the cytogenetic approach. Thanks to this advance in 1973, Janet Rowley demonstrated that the Ph chromosome was not a simple deletion but a reciprocal and balanced translocation between the long arms of chromosomes 9 and 22 [16]. Still in the 1970s, Herbert Abelson and Louise Rabstein identified the *ABL* gene, located on chromosome 9, position 9q34 [11]. Protein tyrosine kinase *ABL* is related to the processes of regulation of cell proliferation, survival, cell adhesion, and migration [17].

In 1984, Groffen et al., through the cloning of genomic DNA from CML patients, identified chromosome breaks within a limited region on chromosome 22, which they called the breakpoint cluster region (BCR) [18, 19]. Thus, the highly specific presence of the BCR chromosome breakpoint in patients with Ph-positive CML strongly suggested the involvement of this gene in leukemia.

In the formation of the Ph chromosome, the *ABL1* proto-oncogene (Abelson leukemia 1) is translocated from chromosome 9 to the *BCR* gene on chromosome 22 at position 22q11. This process gives rise to the chimeric *BCR-ABL1* gene, which encodes a constitutively active protein tyrosine kinase, considered central in the mechanism involved in chronic phase-chronic myeloid leukemia (CP-CML) [20–22]. Identification of this anomaly is extremely important for the diagnosis of the disease and for treatment purposes.

1.3 Variants of Ph chromosome

The Ph is detected by G-band karyotyping in around 90% of CML patients among whom 5–10% may have variant chromosome types [23–25]. Variants of Ph chromosome are characterized by the involvement of another chromosome in addition to chromosomes 9 and 22. Variant rearrangements can be simple or complex. Simple-type variants involve another chromosome, for example, t (9; 22; 6). Complex variants participate in the translocation of two or more chromosomes, besides chromosomes 9 and 22 [26, 27].

Variant Ph breakpoints occur in hotspots across the genome, usually in the G-light bands, within the cytosine and guanine (CG) richest parts of the genome [28]. CG content correlates with chromatin condensation and transcription activity; that is, open chromatin is transcriptionally active and relatively likely to undergo breakage and repair with a consequent tendency to illegitimate recombination and translocation [24].

Variant Ph chromosomes are distinguished from additional chromosomal abnormalities or clonal evolution that drives disease progression. The clonal evolution is a reflection of a genetic instability that characterizes the transition to advanced phase [29]. However, the mechanism of variant Ph generation and the molecular bases of biological differences between classic Ph and variant Ph chromosomes are not fully understood [30].

In atypical CML (aCML), patients are Ph-negative. This leukemia presents initial characteristics and clinical course similar to those of Ph-positive patients. However, Ph-negative patients have more heterogeneous characteristics, often more aggressive disease progresses with worse prognosis [31].

2. Molecular characterization of CML

The *BCR-ABL* fusion protein with strong tyrosine kinase activity is one of the molecular biological bases of leukemia [32]. The Ph chromosome is generated by the translocation t (9; 22) (q34; q11). The normal *c-ABL* gene is located on chromosome 9 and has 11 exons (1b, 1a, a2–a11). During chromosomal translocation, *c-ABL* gene breakdown can occur at three points: upstream of 1b, between 1b and 1a, and between 1a and a2. Regardless of the breakpoint, the first two alternative exons (1b and 1a) are always separated [21].

The normal *BCR* gene is located on chromosome 22 and consists of 23 exons (e1–e23). In generation of the *BCR-ABL* fusion gene, there are three breakpoints that can occur in the *BCR* gene: major (*M-BCR*), minor (*m-BCR*), and micro (*μ-BCR*). The M-*BCR* break can generate junctions e14a2, e13a2, e14a3, and e13a3; m-BCR breakdown can induce junctions e1a2 and e1a3; and the breakdown in μ-BCR can give rise to e19a2 junction [21].

Despite the many junctions that exist, in Ph-positive hematological neoplasms, the junctions e14a2 and e13a2 are the most frequent. These two junctions generate the same transcript encoding the p210 BCR-ABL protein. The junction e19a2 produces a transcript encoding the p230 BCR-ABL protein. And junction e1a2 creates a transcript that encodes p190 BCR-ABL [21, 29].

All domains of c-ABL protein—SRC-homology-2 (SH2) domain, SH3 domain, tyrosine kinase domain, nuclear localization signal (NLS), nuclear export signal (NES), DNA-binding domain (DBD), and actin-binding domain (ABD)—are present in the three BCR-ABL proteins. However, the three BCR-ABL proteins have different BCR domains [33].

The SH2 and SH3 regulatory domains mediate protein-protein interactions and control activation of transduction signals. The SH3 domain is known as a negative regulator of kinase activity, acting as a counterpoint to the SH2 domain, inactivating its tyrosine kinase-activating and receptor potential [34]. In BCR-ABL products, a partial or complete deletion of the SH3 domain occurs, losing negative control. In contrast, the SH2 domain is eventually activated by the presence of a tyrosine kinase-activating component [35].

The BCR-ABL fusion protein acts as an oncoprotein by activating several signaling pathways that lead to transformation. Myc, Ras, c-Rafn MAP/ERK, SAPK/JNK, STAT, NFKB, PI-3kinase, and c-Jun are included as signal cascade molecules. Many signaling proteins have been shown to interact with BCR-ABL through various functional domains and/or to become phosphorylated in BCR-ABL-expressing cells. In brief, BCR-ABL activates the main signal pathways, such as RAS/MAPK, PI-3kinase, c-ABL pathways and CRKL pathways, and JAK-STAT, and the Src pathway to play a major role in transformation and proliferation. Inhibition of apoptosis is thought to result from activation of the PI-3 kinase and RAS pathways with induction through AKT of Myc and BCL-2 [36].

Activation of these signaling pathways leads to deregulation of cellular processes such as proliferation, differentiation, DNA repair, decreased adhesion of leukemic cells to bone marrow stroma, and reduced apoptotic response to mutagenic stimulation, leading to uncontrolled clonal proliferation [37].

3. Diagnostic of CML

Approximately 40% of patients are asymptomatic, and the diagnosis is made with a blood count [1], performed by any clinical situation, preoperatively or even at a checkup. Several methodologies may be employed for the diagnosis of CML patients, including microscopic examination of peripheral blood and bone marrow, cytogenetics, and molecular biology.

3.1 Blood count

In peripheral blood of patients with CML, there is a leukocytosis of approximately 225,000/mm^3 ranging from 20,000 to 600,000/mm^3 and an intense increase in circulation granulocytes. Granulocytosis is characterized by a small proportion of leukemic blasts and promyelocytes and predominance of intermediate forms (such as myelocytes and metamyelocytes), in addition to maturing and fully mature neutrophils (rods and segmented). Differential leukocyte count shows staggered left shift from mature neutrophils to myeloblasts. Fifteen to 20% proportions of basophils may be found [1, 37].

The presence of mild anemia and thrombocytosis are also common in CML. There is a small correlation between hemoglobin concentration and the total number of white blood cells (hemoglobin values range from 9.7 g/dL ranging from 5.4 to 14.4 g/dL). Depending on the stage of the disease, the number of platelets ranges from 485,000/mm^3, ranging from 25,000 to 1,400,000/mm^3. Basophilia and eosinophilia are common findings. Leukocyte alkaline phosphatase is generally low and can be used to distinguish CML from other myeloproliferative diseases [1, 37, 38].

3.2 Myelogram

Analysis of bone marrow (BM) through myelogram reveals granulocytic hyperplasia, leading to a leukoerythroblastic ratio of 20:1. The differentiation sequence is maintained, however with a predominance of younger cells such as promyelocytes and myelocytes. The number of megakaryocytes is increased. Other nonspecific biopsy findings include reticulin fibrosis and vascularization [1, 37].

3.3 Cytogenetics

The cytogenetic picture of CML provides unique and crucial information for diagnosis. Cytogenetic analysis of bone marrow or peripheral blood cells allows the identification of the Ph translocation and other chromosome changes that are associated with the leukemic process. Diagnostic assays at baseline for CML patients are based on the standard banding cytogenetics (chromosome banding analysis or CBA) and fluorescence in situ hybridization (FISH) [39].

Cytogenetic examination is preferably performed on bone marrow cells. The t (9; 22) (q34; q11) is easily recognized when the cell cycle of leukemic cells is disrupted in the metaphase. Identification of translocation 9; 22 requires analysis of at least 20 metaphases [40].

The FISH technique is used when the result is urgent. Fast and specific, this technique allows detection of *BCR-ABL* rearrangement through the use of molecular probes [37].

3.4 Molecular biology

The most modern and effective methods for detecting BCR-ABL transcripts are based on molecular biology techniques. Polymerase chain reaction (PCR) testing of peripheral blood RNA is highly sensitive: it can detect 1 Ph-positive cell expressing the BCR-ABL fusion transcript in 10^5–10^6 normal cells [1].

Real-time PCR is a great ally of clinical oncologist seeking better therapeutic outcomes because it helps in defining treatment, which can be more or less aggressive according to each patient's response [41]. Importantly, molecular methods, although extremely sensitive, do not allow observation of concomitant gene or chromosomal alterations.

4. Treatment of CML

Therapy for treatment of CML developed very slowly. Heinrich Lissauer, in 1865, described the use of arsenic in two leukemia patients [42], nothing new in view of the fact that the use of arsenic for cancer therapy had been described in the Indian Ramayana more than 2000 years earlier [43].

In the 1920s, radiotherapy entered clinical practice, and it was soon used for the treatment of CML, and for over 50 years, radiotherapy was considered the standard treatment. Radiation was usually directed to the spleen for symptomatic relief [43–45].

After the Second World War, there was the rapid development of alkylating agents. Thus, busulfan largely replaced radiotherapy in the 1960s. Later, hydroxyurea (hydroxycarbamide) was introduced in the USA (United States of America). Prospective studies showed that patients treated with hydroxyurea survived longer than those treated with busulfan. However, it was not clear whether this was due to the beneficial effect of hydroxyurea or a mitogenic effect of busulfan [44].

In the early 1980s, interferon-α (IFN-α) was introduced for the treatment of CP-CML. Few patients achieved any level of Ph-negative hematopoiesis, and others achieved a complete and lasting Ph-negative hematopoiesis. In rare cases, IFN-α may be discontinued without subsequent relapse. Thus, IFN-α replaced busulfan and hydroxyurea in the treatment of CP-CML if the patient was not eligible for allogeneic BM transplantation [46].

In 1979, Fefer and colleagues treated four CP-CML patients with high doses of chemoradiotherapy, followed by transfusion of stem cells from their genetically identical twins [47]. At follow-up intervals of 22–31 months, these patients remained well absent of Ph-positive metaphases in their marrow. The previously fatal leukemia brought the possibility of treatment and cure through BM transplantation [45].

Researchers began to treat CP-CML patients with allogeneic BM transplantation between identical HLA siblings. In the beginning, conditioning consisted of the use of cyclophosphamide and full body irradiation. However, years later, it was decided to use busulfan with cyclophosphamide [48]. According to the Center for International Blood & Marrow Transplant Research, allograft-associated transplant-related mortality for CP-CML patients is about 10–20% at 1 year, and the survival at 5 years is about 60% [49]. Most survivors have no evidence of leukemia, but occasional patients relapse early after transplantation [44].

Thus, from the 1990s, the treatment of choice for all relatively young CP-CML patients (under 50 years old) was an allogeneic stem cell transplant (SCT). In France, patients with CML who were not eligible for allograft were treated with IFN-α plus cytarabine [50], although more recent data from Italy cast doubt on this conclusion [51].

4.1 Tyrosine kinase inhibitors

Accumulated knowledge of action mechanism of BCR-ABL was sufficient to initiate experiments with target molecule designs to be used in the treatment of CML. From the knowledge that tyrosine kinase is the effective portion of oncoprotein, it was evident that its inhibition would be the most attractive target as a therapeutic strategy. The goal was to design a small chemical compound that would compete with ATP binding at the kinase domain site. Thus, with this site occupied by an “ATP-like” molecule, it would not be possible to provide any phosphate group for substrate transfer. With this, the tyrosine residues would remain in the “non-phosphorylated” form, and the protein substrate would not be able to change its conformation so that it could be associated with the effectors described above, resulting in the interruption of oncogenetic signals to the nucleus of cell.

This “ATP-like” molecule, known as imatinib, revolutionized the treatment in oncology and specifically of CML, opening the “era of targeted specific therapy.” One of the first studies on the effectiveness of imabinib treatment (the International Randomized Study of Interferon and STI571 [IRIS] trial) estimated the rate of complete cytogenetic response (CCyR) at 12 months in the imatinib arm was 69%. Such responses are in relation to the standard treatment of the time (IFN-α and cytarabine) [52].

One of the last IRIS updates showed an estimated overall survival (OS) rate of 83% at 10 years (20.1% of patients had unknown survival status when data was analyzed). It should be mentioned that, despite these excellent results, 31 and 52% of patients assigned to imatinib discontinued treatment by 5 and 10 years of follow-up, respectively. The main cause of treatment discontinuation was the unsatisfactory therapeutic effect (11%), while only 4% of patients discontinued treatment due to side effects [53].

Treatment with imatinib induces a hematological response in 90% of patients diagnosed in the CP and a cytogenetic response in 80% of them, which made bone marrow transplantation, the only curative treatment for CML, to be indicated only in those patients who develop imatinib resistance, observed in 20–25% of cases [52].

Known mechanisms of imatinib resistance include the presence of mutation point in the BCR-ABL tyrosine kinase domain, amplification of the BCR-ABL gene, overexpression of the multidrug resistance gene known as P-glycoprotein, and low expression of pickup transporters such as SLC22A1 (hOCT1) [54].

The second generation TKIs (2GTKIs), dasatinib, nilotinib, and bosutinib, were initially approved in CML patients who were resistant or intolerant to imatinib. Due to a more potent in vitro inhibition of the unmutated BCR-ABL kinase with a good safety profile, these second generation TKIs were later evaluated and approved in the first-line setting [55].

Dasatinib is an oral, second generation TKI that is 350 times more potent than imatinib in vitro. It also inhibits the Src family of kinases, which may be important in blunting critical cell signaling pathways [56]. Compared to the structure analog of imatinib, nilotinib's affinity for the ATP-binding site on BCR-ABL1 is 30–50 times more potent in vitro [57]. Like dasatinib, nilotinib initially demonstrated the ability to induce hematologic and cytogenetic responses in patients who had failed imatinib [56]. Bosutinib appeared to retain activity across most known mutations that confer imatinib resistance, except for T315I. Responses were independent of whether patients had resistance to or intolerance of imatinib [56].

A subset of patients with CML exhibited either primary or secondary resistance to imatinib. Primary resistance refers to patients never responding to imatinib, whereas secondary resistance occurs when a patient who had an initial response to imatinib eventually loses the response [36]. Although a significant proportion of patients respond to 2GTKI therapy after imatinib failure, most of them (70%, approximately) will eventually discontinue such treatment in the short term due to loss of response or toxicity [55].

There are many treatment mechanisms of resistance, and several of them, mostly in vitro or in selected patient samples, have been reported. However, their individual contribution to this phenomenon has not been completely defined. The most frequently identified mechanism of resistance is the development of mutations in the ABL tyrosine kinase domain [55].

A third generation TKI, ponatinib, is approved in CML patients with refractory CML or Ph-positive acute lymphoblastic leukemia (Ph + ALL) and those harboring the BCR-ABL1T315I mutant [58]. Clinical trials using the approved dose of 45 mg/day of ponatinib show the main concern with this drug is the increased incidence of cardiovascular complications [55]. **Table 1** shows the target recommendations for CML, according to the American Cancer Society.

First generation TKI	CML patients newly diagnosed
Second generation TKI	CML patients resistant or intolerant to imatinib
Third generation TKI	CML patients with refractory CML or Ph-positive acute lymphoblastic leukemia and those harboring the BCR-ABL1T315I mutant
Interferon or chemotherapy	CML patients who cannot take TKI or those who are not responding to treatment
Allogeneic stem cell transplantation	CML who have failed at least two TKIs and for all patients in advanced phase disease

Table 1.
Target recommendations for CML [4].

4.1.1 Definition of therapeutic response

The quality of response to TKI treatment is categorized according to the laboratory method used. Patients are monitored by hematological, cytogenetic, and molecular response, and their terminology has been standardized by the European Leukemia Net [59].

Hematologic response is defined by the presence of platelets <450 × 10^9L, without differential immature granulocytes and <5% basophils, and a non-palpable spleen. Cytogenetic response (CyR) is defined according to the proportion of positive Philadelphia chromosome (Ph +) in bone marrow cells. The association between CyR and improved survival made the cytogenetic response the gold standard of CML therapy [36]. **Table 2** shows the cytogenetic response definition.

The IRIS study, conducted in 2003, defined two types of molecular response assessed by real-time PCR: major molecular remission (MMR) and complete molecular remission (CMR). Major molecular remission is defined as a three-log drop of the initial load of BCR-ABL at the time of diagnosis; this value is equal to or less than 0.1%. Complete molecular remission is defined when the BCR-ABL transcript is undetectable [60].

Response to treatment is monitored during the first 3 months through clinical evaluation, blood count, and biochemical exams every 2 weeks. After the third month, cytogenetics is recommended every 6 months until complete CCyR is achieved. From the moment the patient reaches CCyR (Ph + 0%), monitoring is performed through real-time PCR quarterly to detect minimal residual disease [61].

4.2 Allogeneic stem cell transplantation

For patients who fail frontline therapy, the second-line options include second and third generation TKIs. Even though second and third generation TKIs are potent and selective TKIs, some patients still do not respond to treatment. Allogeneic stem cell transplantation (allo-SCT) remains an important therapeutic option for patients with CML-CP who have failed at least two TKIs and for all patients in advanced phase disease [56].

Patients exposed primarily to TKI treatment do not respond negatively to allo-SCT. Conversely, if patients referred for transplant have the lower CML burden, they may respond better to allo-SCT [62].

Allo-SCT is the only treatment with healing potential. However, it remains associated with substantial risks of morbidity and mortality. For appropriate counselling of patients, a rapid and simple way to assess risk is needed [63]. Pre-allo-SCT risk factors for CML are donor type, disease stage, recipient age, recipient-donor gender combination, and, lastly, time between diagnosis and allo-SCT. **Table 3** presents the risk factors for allo-STC [63–67].

Complete cytogenetic response (CCyR)	0% Ph-positive metaphases
Partial cytogenetic response (PCyR)	1–35% Ph-positive metaphases
Minor cytogenetic response (mCyR)	36–65% Ph-positive metaphases
Minimal cytogenetic response (min CyR)	66–95% Ph-positive metaphases
No response (NR)	>95% Ph-positive metaphases

Table 2.
Cytogenetic response definition [59].

Prognostic factors	Score
Donor type	0—related identical human leukocyte antigen (HLA)
	1—unrelated identical HLA
Disease stage	0—chronic phase (CP)
	1—accelerated phase (AP)
	2—blast phase (BP)
Receiver age	0—< 20 age
	1—20–40 age
	2—> 40 age
Gender donor/receiver	1—female/male
	0—male/female
Time from diagnosis to transplant	0—< 12 months
	1—> 12 months

Table 3.
Risk factors for allo-STC [63–67].

In the era of TKIs, there is no doubt for the first-line treatment for CML patients. But when allo-SCT is indicated, this scoring system is still of great value in estimating overall disease-free survival and procedure-related mortality.

When considering allo-SCT for CML patients, it is important to know that a poor response to one or more TKIs does not predict a negative transplant response. TKIs pharmacologically block BCR-ABL activity, while allo-SCT depends on graft-versus-leukemia (GVL) effect [68].

The challenge of allo-SCT for treatment of leukemia and other malignancies of the hematopoietic system is the prevention of graft-versus-host disease (GVHD) without losing the GVL effect. Depletion of T cells abrogates GVHD and GVL effects. Delayed transfusion of donor lymphocytes into chimeras after T-cell-depleted stem cell transplantation produces a GVL effect without necessarily producing GVHD [69].

Allo-SCT should not be seen as a last resort but as a treatment strategy to be considered viable at the beginning of treatment for patients who have suboptimal responses to TKIs. The key issues for HSCT in CML are those of patient selection, risk stratification, and outcome optimization by means of regimen selection and improved supportive care [68].

5. Conclusions

CML is a myeloproliferative disease, resulting from clonal expansion of hematopoietic progenitor stem cells, characterized by *BCR-ABL* fusion gene, resulting from reciprocal translocation t (9; 22) (q34; q11) that gives rise to Ph chromosome. All the accumulated knowledge about action mechanisms of BCR-ABL1 has enabled the development of very efficient target-specific drugs, as well as molecular methods for disease monitoring.

Allo-SCT is a possible cure for CML; however, it is associated with mortality and morbidity increased due to complications in the pre- and posttransplantation periods, such as GVHD, immunosuppression, and multiple organ toxicity.

Although great progress has been made for the improvement in clinical treatment during the past decades, it is common for patients to develop resistance to treatments. Therefore, further exploring the novel therapeutic strategies is still crucial for improving disease outcome.

Author details

Letícia Antunes Muniz Ferreira
University Center of Jales—UNIJALES, Jales, SP, Brazil

*Address all correspondence to: leticiaamferreira@gmail.com

References

[1] Sawyers CL. Chronic myeloid leukemia. The New England Journal of Medicine. 1999;**340**(17):1330-1340. DOI: 10.1056/NEJM199904293401706

[2] Ayala M, Ávila E, Domínguez J, Aquino X, Vela J. Diagnosis and treatment of chronic myeloid leukemia in the imatinib mesylate era: Report of the experience at "La Raza" Medical Center in Mexico. Clinical Lymphoma, Myeloma & Leukemia. 2016;**16**(2): 57-62. DOI: 10.1016/j.clml.2015.10.006

[3] Chen R, Chen B. The role of dasatinib in the management of chronic myeloid leukemia. Drug Design, Development and Therapy. 2015;**9**:773-779. DOI: 10.2147/DDDT.S80207

[4] American Cancer Society [Internet]. 2019. Available from: https://www.cancer.org/cancer/chronic-myeloid-leukemia.html [Accessed: 20 July 2019]

[5] Velpeau A. Sur la résorption du pus et sur l'altération du sang dans les maladies. Revue Médicale Suisse. 1827;**2**:216-240

[6] Donné A. Cours de microscopie complémentaire des études médicales. Paris: Ballière; 1844. p. 550

[7] Bennett J. Case of hypertrophy of the spleen and liver in which death took place from suppuration of the blood. Edinburgh Medical and Surgical Journal. 1845;**165**:1-11

[8] Virchow R. Weisses Blut. Froiep's Notizen. 1845;**36**:151-156

[9] Bennett J. Leucocythaemia, or White Cell Blood in Relation to the Physiology and Pathology of the Lymphatic Glandular System. Sutherland and Knox: Edinburg; 1852

[10] Virchow R. Die Leukämie. Gesammelte Abhandlungen Zur Wissenschaftlichen Medizin. Meidinger: Frankfurt; 1856

[11] Gonon-Demoulian R, Goldman JM, Nicolini FE. History of chronic myeloid leukemia: A paradigm in the treatment of cancer. Bulletin du Cancer. 2014;**101**(1):56-67. DOI: 10.1684/bdc.2013.1876

[12] Ehrlich P. Über die specifischen granulationen des blutes. Archiv für Anatomie, Physiologie und Wissenschaftliche Medicin. 1879:571-579

[13] Ehrlich P. Farbenanalytische Untersuchungen Zur Histologie und Klinik Des Blutes. Berlin: Hirschwald; 1891

[14] Nowell PC. Discovery of the Philadelphia chromosome: A personal perspective. The Journal of Clinical Investigation. 2007;**117**(8):2033-2035. DOI: 10.1172/JCI31771

[15] Nowell P, Hungerford D. A minute chromosome in human chronic granulocytic leukemia. Science. 1960;**142**:1497

[16] Rowley JD. Letter: A new consistent chromosomal abnormality in chronic myelogenous leukaemia identified by quinacrine fluorescence and Giemsa staining. Nature. 1973;**243**(5405):290-293. DOI: 10.1038/243290a0

[17] Pendergast AM. The Abl family kinases: Mechanisms of regulation and signaling. Advances in Cancer Research. 2002;**85**:51-100. DOI: 10.1016/S0065-230X(02)85003-5

[18] Groffen J, Stephenson JR, Heisterkamp N, de Klein A, Bartram CR, Grosveld G. Philadelphia chromosomal breakpoints are clustered within a limited region, bcr, on chromosome 22. Cell. 1984;**36**(1):93-99. DOI: 10.1016/0092-8674(84)90077-1

[19] Chandra HS, Heisterkamp NC, Hungerford A, Morrissette JJ, Nowell PC, Rowley JD, et al. Philadelphia Chromosome Symposium: Commemoration of the 50th anniversary of the discovery of the Ph chromosome. Cancer Genetics. 2011;**204**(4):171-179. DOI: 10.1016/j.cancergen.2011.03.002

[20] Melo JV, Gordon DE, Cross NC, Goldman JM. The ABL-BCR fusion gene is expressed in chronic myeloid leukemia. Blood. 1993;**81**(1):158-165

[21] Melo JV. The diversity of BCR-ABL fusion proteins and their relationship to leukemia phenotype. Blood. 1996;**88**(7):2375-2384

[22] Chauffaille MLLF, Bandeira ACA, Silva ASG. Diversity of breakpoints of variants Philadelphia chromosomes in chronic myeloid leukemia in Brazilian patients. Revista Brasileira de Hematologia e Hemoterapia. 2015;**37**:17-20. DOI: 10.1016/j.bjhh.2014.07.006

[23] Ishihara T, Minamihisamatsu M. The Philadelphia chromosome. Considerations based on studies of variant Ph translocations. Cancer Genetics and Cytogenetics. 1988;**32**(1):75-92. DOI: 10.1016/0165-4608(88)90026-x

[24] Fisher AM, Strike P, Scott C, Moorman AV. Breakpoints of variant 9;22 translocations in chronic myeloid leukemia locate preferentially in the CG-richest regions of the genome. Genes, Chromosomes & Cancer. 2005;**43**(4):383-389. DOI: 10.1002/gcc.20196

[25] Marzocchi G, Castagnetti F, Luatti S, Baldazzi C, Stacchini M, Gugliotta G, et al. Variant Philadelphia translocations: Molecular-cytogenetic characterization and prognostic influence on frontline imatinib therapy, a GIMEMA Working Party on CML analysis. Blood. 2011;**117**(25):6793-6800. DOI: 10.1182/blood-2011-01-328294

[26] Sandberg AA. Chromosomes and causation of human cancer and leukemia: XL. The Ph1 and other translocations in CML. Cancer. 1980;**46**(10):2221-2226. DOI: 10.1002/1097-0142(19801115)46:10<2221::aid-cncr2820461019>3.0.co;2-8

[27] Heim S, Mittelman F. Cancer Cytogenetics: Chromosomal and Molecular Genetic Aberrations of Tumor Cells. 2nd ed. New York: Wiley Liss; 1995

[28] Jeffs AR, Benjes SM, Smith TL, Sowerby SJ, Morris CM. The BCR gene recombines preferentially with Alu elements in complex BCR-ABL translocations of chronic myeloid leukaemia. Human Molecular Genetics. 1998;**7**(5):767-776. DOI: 10.1093/hmg/7.5.767

[29] Quintás-Cardama A, Cortes J. Molecular biology of bcr-abl1-positive chronic myeloid leukemia. Blood. 2009;**113**(8):1619-1630. DOI: 10.1182/blood-2008-03-144790

[30] Chauffaille MLLF. Cytogenetics and FISH monitoring CML during tyrosine kinase inhibitors treatment. Revista Brasileira de Hematologia e Hemoterapia. 2008;**30**(1):13-139. DOI: 10.1590/S1516-84842008000700005

[31] Koldehoff M, Beelen DW, Trenschel R, Steckel NK, Peceny R, Ditschkowski M, et al. Outcome of hematopoietic stem cell transplantation in patients with atypical chronic myeloid leukemia. Bone Marrow Transplantation. 2004;**34**(12):1047-1050. DOI: 10.1038/sj.bmt.1704686

[32] Zhu HQ, Gao FH. Regulatory molecules and corresponding processes of BCR-ABL protein degradation. Journal of Cancer. 2019;**10**(11):2488-2500. DOI: 10.7150/jca.29528

[33] Zhou T, Medeiros LJ, Hu S. Chronic myeloid leukemia: Beyond BCR-ABL1. Current Hematologic Malignancy Reports. 2018;**13**(6):435-445. DOI: 10.1007/s11899-018-0474-6

[34] Marcucci G, Perrotti D, Caligiuri MA. Understanding the molecular basis of imatinib mesylate therapy in chronic myelogenous leukemia and the related mechanisms of resistance. Commentary re: A. N. Mohamed et al. The effect of imatinib mesylate on patients with Philadelphia chromosome-positive chronic myeloid leukemia with secondary chromosomal aberrations. Clin. Cancer Res., 9: 1333-1337, 2003. Clinical Cancer Research. 2003;**9**(4):1248-1252

[35] Di Bacco A, Keeshan K, McKenna SL, Cotter TG. Molecular abnormalities in chronic myeloid leukemia: Deregulation of cell growth and apoptosis. The Oncologist. 2000;**5**(5):405-415. DOI: 10.1634/theoncologist.5-5-405

[36] Bennour A, Saad A, Sennana H. Chronic myeloid leukemia: Relevance of cytogenetic and molecular assays. Critical Reviews in Oncology/Hematology. 2016;**97**:263-274. DOI: 10.1016/j.critrevonc.2015.08.020

[37] Dulley F, Hamerschlack N. Leucemia mielóide crônica. Associação Brasileira de Linfoma e Leucemia. 2004;**25**:11-12

[38] Jamur VR. Estudo citogenético de pacientes com Leucemia Mielóide Crônica tratados com o Mesilato de Imatinibe [dissertation]. Curitiba: Universidade Federal do Paraná; 2005

[39] Molica M, Massaro F, Breccia M. Diagnostic and prognostic cytogenetics of chronic myeloid leukaemia: An update. Expert Review of Molecular Diagnostics. 2017;**17**(11):1001-1008. DOI: 10.1080/14737159.2017.1383156

[40] Webber LM, Garson OM. Fluorodeoxyuridine synchronization of bone marrow cultures. Cancer Genetics and Cytogenetics. 1983;**8**(2):123-132. DOI: 10.1016/0165-4608(83)90044-4

[41] Anunciação SF, Elias LFQ, Guimarães DC, Neto Filho JL, Sadi VA. Aspectos diagnósticos da leucemia mieloide crônica e detecção de doença residual mínima. Estudos. 2008;**35**(11/12):1069-1083

[42] Lissauer H. Zwei Falle von Leucaemie. Berliner Klinische Wochenschrift. 1865;**2**:403-404

[43] Deininger MW. Chronic myeloid leukemia: An historical perspective. Hematology. American Society of Hematology. Education Program. 2008:418. DOI: 10.1182/asheducation-2008.1.418

[44] Goldman JM, Majhail NS, Klein JP, Wang Z, Sobocinski KA, Arora M, et al. Relapse and late mortality in 5-year survivors of myeloablative allogeneic hematopoietic cell transplantation for chronic myeloid leukemia in first chronic phase. Journal of Clinical Oncology. 2010;**28**(11):1888-1895. DOI: 10.1200/JCO.2009.26.7757

[45] Goldman JM. Chronic myeloid leukemia: A historical perspective. Seminars in Hematology. 2010;**47**(4):302-311. DOI: 10.1053/j.seminhematol.2010.07.001

[46] Talpaz M, Kantarjian HM, McCredie K, Trujillo JM, Keating MJ, Gutterman JU. Hematologic remission and cytogenetic improvement induced by recombinant human interferon alpha A in chronic myelogenous leukemia. The New England Journal of Medicine. 1986;**314**(17):1065-1069. DOI: 10.1056/NEJM198604243141701

[47] Fefer A, Cheever MA, Thomas ED, Boyd C, Ramberg R, Glucksberg H, et al. Disappearance of Ph1-positive

cells in four patients with chronic granulocytic leukemia after chemotherapy, irradiation and marrow transplantation from an identical twin. The New England Journal of Medicine. 1979;**300**(7):333-337. DOI: 10.1056/NEJM197902153000702

[48] Goldman JM, Baughan AS, McCarthy DM, Worsley AM, Hows JM, Gordon-Smith EC, et al. Marrow transplantation for patients in the chronic phase of chronic granulocytic leukaemia. Lancet. 1982;**2**(8299):623-625. DOI: 10.1016/s0140-6736(82)92736-2

[49] Horowitz MM, Rowlings PA, Passweg JR. Allogeneic bone marrow transplantation for CML: A report from the International Bone Marrow Transplant Registry. Bone Marrow Transplantation. 1996;**17**(Suppl 3):S5-S6

[50] Guilhot F, Chastang C, Michallet M, Guerci A, Harousseau JL, Maloisel F, et al. Interferon alfa-2b combined with cytarabine versus interferon alone in chronic myelogenous leukemia. French Chronic Myeloid Leukemia Study Group. The New England Journal of Medicine. 1997;**337**(4):223-229. DOI: 10.1056/NEJM199707243370402

[51] Baccarani M, Rosti G, de Vivo A, Bonifazi F, Russo D, Martinelli G, et al. A randomized study of interferon-alpha versus interferon-alpha and low-dose arabinosyl cytosine in chronic myeloid leukemia. Blood. 2002;**99**(5):1527-1535. DOI: 10.1182/blood.v99.5.1527

[52] O'Brien SG, Guilhot F, Larson RA, Gathmann I, Baccarani M, Cervantes F, et al. Imatinib compared with interferon and low-dose cytarabine for newly diagnosed chronic-phase chronic myeloid leukemia. The New England Journal of Medicine. 2003;**348**(11):994-1004. DOI: 10.1056/NEJMoa022457

[53] Gugliotta G, Castagnetti F, Breccia M, Levato L, D'Adda M, Stagno F, et al. Long-term outcome of a phase 2 trial with nilotinib 400 mg twice daily in first-line treatment of chronic myeloid leukemia. Haematologica. 2015;**100**(9):1146-1150. DOI: 10.3324/haematol.2015.129221

[54] Branford S, Rudzki Z, Walsh S, Parkinson I, Grigg A, Szer J, et al. Detection of BCR-ABL mutations in patients with CML treated with imatinib is virtually always accompanied by clinical resistance, and mutations in the ATP phosphate-binding loop (P-loop) are associated with a poor prognosis. Blood. 2003;**102**(1):276-283. DOI: 10.1182/blood-2002-09-2896

[55] García-Gutiérrez V, Hernández-Boluda JC. Tyrosine kinase inhibitors available for chronic myeloid leukemia: Efficacy and safety. Frontiers in Oncology. 2019;**9**:603. DOI: 10.3389/fonc.2019.00603

[56] Jabbour E, Kantarjian H. Chronic myeloid leukemia: 2016 update on diagnosis, therapy, and monitoring. American Journal of Hematology. 2016;**91**(2):252-265. DOI: 10.1002/ajh.24275

[57] Weisberg E, Manley PW, Breitenstein W, Brüggen J, Cowan-Jacob SW, Ray A, et al. Characterization of AMN107, a selective inhibitor of native and mutant Bcr-Abl. Cancer Cell. 2005;7(2):129-141. DOI: 10.1016/j.ccr.2005.01.007

[58] O'Hare T, Shakespeare WC, Zhu X, Eide CA, Rivera VM, Wang F, et al. AP24534, a pan-BCR-ABL inhibitor for chronic myeloid leukemia, potently inhibits the T315I mutant and overcomes mutation-based resistance. Cancer Cell. 2009;**16**(5):401-412. DOI: 10.1016/j.ccr.2009.09.028

[59] Baccarani M, Cortes J, Pane F, Niederwieser D, Saglio G, Apperley J, et al. Chronic myeloid leukemia: An update of concepts and management

recommendations of European LeukemiaNet. Journal of Clinical Oncology. 2009;**27**(35):6041-6051. DOI: 10.1200/JCO.2009.25.0779

[60] Hughes TP, Kaeda J, Branford S, Rudzki Z, Hochhaus A, Hensley ML, et al. Frequency of major molecular responses to imatinib or interferon alfa plus cytarabine in newly diagnosed chronic myeloid leukemia. The New England Journal of Medicine. 2003;**349**(15):1423-1432. DOI: 10.1056/NEJMoa030513

[61] Baccarani M, Saglio G, Goldman J, Hochhaus A, Simonsson B, Appelbaum F, et al. Evolving concepts in the management of chronic myeloid leukemia: Recommendations from an expert panel on behalf of the European LeukemiaNet. Blood. 2006;**108**(6):1809-1820. DOI: 10.1182/blood-2006-02-005686

[62] Lee SJ, Kukreja M, Wang T, Giralt SA, Szer J, Arora M, et al. Impact of prior imatinib mesylate on the outcome of hematopoietic cell transplantation for chronic myeloid leukemia. Blood. 2008;**112**(8):3500-3507. DOI: 10.1182/blood-2008-02-141689

[63] Gratwohl A, Hermans J, Goldman JM, Arcese W, Carreras E, Devergie A, et al. Risk assessment for patients with chronic myeloid leukaemia before allogeneic blood or marrow transplantation. Chronic Leukemia Working Party of the European Group for Blood and Marrow Transplantation. Lancet. 1998;**352**(9134):1087-1092. DOI: 10.1016/s0140-6736(98)03030-x

[64] Bittencourt H, Funke V, Fogliatto L, Magalhães S, Setubal D, Paz A, et al. Imatinib mesylate versus allogeneic BMT for patients with chronic myeloid leukemia in first chronic phase. Bone Marrow Transplantation. 2008;**42**(9):597-600. DOI: 10.1038/bmt.2008.218

[65] Gratwohl A, Brand R, Apperley J, Crawley C, Ruutu T, Corradini P, et al. Allogeneic hematopoietic stem cell transplantation for chronic myeloid leukemia in Europe 2006: Transplant activity, long-term data and current results. An analysis by the Chronic Leukemia Working Party of the European Group for Blood and Marrow Transplantation (EBMT). Haematologica. 2006;**91**(4):513-521

[66] van Rhee F, Szydlo RM, Hermans J, Devergie A, Frassoni F, Arcese W, et al. Long-term results after allogeneic bone marrow transplantation for chronic myelogenous leukemia in chronic phase: A report from the Chronic Leukemia Working Party of the European Group for Blood and Marrow Transplantation. Bone Marrow Transplantation. 1997;**20**(7):553-560. DOI: 10.1038/sj.bmt.1700933

[67] Devergie A, Apperley JF, Labopin M, Madrigal A, Jacobsen N, Carreras E, et al. European results of matched unrelated donor bone marrow transplantation for chronic myeloid leukemia. Impact of HLA class II matching. Chronic Leukemia Working Party of the European Group for Blood and Marrow Transplantation. Bone Marrow Transplantation. 1997;**20**(1):11-19. DOI: 10.1038/sj.bmt.1700844

[68] Innes AJ, Milojkovic D, Apperley JF. Allogeneic transplantation for CML in the TKI era: Striking the right balance. Nature Reviews. Clinical Oncology. 2016;**13**(2):79-91. DOI: 10.1038/nrclinonc.2015.193

[69] Kolb HJ. Graft-versus-leukemia effects of transplantation and donor lymphocytes. Blood. 2008;**112**(12):4371-4383. DOI: 10.1182/blood-2008-03-077974

Section 4

Diagnosis, Management/ Treatment Prevention and Advocacy of Rare Diseases

Chapter 11

Rare Disease Advocacy Groups and Their Significance in Diagnosis, Management, Treatment, and Prevention of Rare Diseases

Yashodhara Bhattacharya, Gayatri Iyer, Aruna Priya Kamireddy, Subhadra Poornima, Keerthi Konda Juturu and Qurratulain Hasan

Abstract

Rare diseases are those diseases that are not seen frequently in a population. There are about 7000 rare diseases that have been identified worldwide, and 80% of them are caused by genetic changes. Since a small number of individuals are affected with rare diseases, most clinicians are not aware of such diseases, and thus, they remain undiagnosed and untreated. Awareness regarding such diseases is essential to train clinicians to diagnose individuals affected with these disorders and to develop National/International Registries, which will serve to give information about the disease prevalence, its natural course, treatment, and management options available, to the medical fraternity. Patient advocacy groups play a remarkable and unique role in forming the collective voice of individuals living with rare diseases. They help in the identification, diagnosis, management, treatment, and prevention of such diseases. Advocacy Groups form collaborative partnerships with scientists studying such rare diseases, clinicians managing these diseases, pharmaceutical companies developing drugs, and Government officials overseeing and policy makers implementing medical regulatory processes. Thus, advocacy groups play a key role in helping patients and families with rare diseases.

Keywords: rare disease, patient advocacy group, rare disease registry, diagnosis, management, treatment

1. Introduction

A rare disease is so called because its frequency in any given population is very low [1]. There are about 7000 rare diseases that have been discovered, and more are being described in medical literature. Rare diseases have different causes, and about 80% of them have a genetic basis that could be chromosomal or genomic [2]. Rare diseases also include certain rare infections, cancers, and even autoimmune disorders. A rare disease is defined differently in individual countries and is based on the following parameters:

- The total number of people affected by the disease in that country
- Prevalence of the disease in that country
- Non-availability of treatment for the disease in that country

The USA defines a rare disease as a condition that affects less than 200,000 people. The definition of rare diseases as is defined in the USA was coined in the Congress during the Orphan Drug Act of 1983. Such diseases also came to be known as Orphan Diseases as drug companies were indifferent to adopting the research and manufacture of novel drugs for their treatment [2, 3]. The World Health Organization defines a rare disease as a disease with a frequency of less than 6.5–10 per 10,000 people. In Europe, it is defined as a disease seen in less than 5 of every 10,000 people, while in Australia, it is taken as one in 10,000 individuals, and in India, it is taken as one in 5000 individuals [4, 5].

A rare disease in isolation may affect a small population because of which clinicians are not aware of the disease and their symptoms, hence such individuals remain undiagnosed and untreated [1, 6, 7]. Although individually these disorders are rare, when taken together the people affected with rare diseases constitute a large population of the country. Such diseases are debilitating and without a proper diagnosis may cause gross morbidity and mortality, thereby posing a challenge to the healthcare system of the country [8]. A rare disease has an adverse impact on the everyday lives of the whole family and their care givers [9–12]. The cost of treatment/management is high and causes considerable financial burden to the individuals and their families [8, 11, 12], as there is a lack of Government policies regarding this aspect, hindering their treatment.

2. Advocacy groups

Since several rare diseases are being diagnosed and brought into light, it is required that more time and effort should go into research for understanding and preventing such diseases. A remarkable and unique aspect of rare disease treatment and management is the evolving role of advocacy groups and their collaborative partnerships with scientists studying such diseases, pharmaceutical companies developing drugs, and Government officials and policy makers overseeing medical research and health care [3, 6]. Rare disease advocacy groups have played a vital role over the years in the adoption of public policies, relocation of available research funding, and other factors affecting the research for rare diseases [1, 7]. In most settings, the rare disease advocacy groups are created by the family members of the affected individuals. They are the ones who look into the formation of public policies, help fast-track treatment approvals by regulatory bodies, and facilitate the welfare of individuals and their care givers.

The National Organization for Rare Disorders (NORD) in the USA was one of the first advocacy groups to be formed, followed by Rare Diseases International, which is a global alliance of patients with rare diseases across various nationalities and is dedicated for supporting treatment and formulating policies for rare disorders. Apart from these, patient advocacy groups have been formed all over the world, which individually or in alliance help to alleviate the various problems faced by individuals with rare diseases and to pressurize companies and countries to provide life-saving drugs and at a reasonable cost.

3. Patient advocacy groups in India

There are many patient advocacy groups currently active in India. The Pompe Foundation started by Mr. Prasanna Shirol in 2008 and caters to individuals and families affected with Lysosomal Storage Disorders. The Metabolic Errors and Rare Diseases Organization of India (MERD), founded by Mr. Vikas Bhat, promotes awareness regarding Inborn Errors of Metabolism and newborn screening. Both these organizations have been founded by parents having an affected child. There are a few other advocacy groups for Spinal Muscular Atrophy (SMA), Spino-Cerebellar Ataxia (SCA), Duchenne Muscular Dystrophy (DMD), and Osteogenesis Imperfecta. Twenty-five such organizations together joined hands to form the Organization for Rare Diseases India (ORDI), which is actively involved in helping patients and their families through the involvement of NGOs. These advocacy groups, however, need to be better organized, so that they can obtain and disseminate information about diseases, diagnostics, and treatment avenues to the affected families.

India has a huge diversity in the kind of rare diseases seen in different states, which can be attributed to certain cultural practices such as consanguinity in South India and endogamy in the North [13]. Based on the data from these organizations, a Rare Disease Registry has been initiated. This has helped in re-classifying rare diseases based on their prevalence in different states. Diseases like β-thalassemia are more prevalent in Punjab, Gujarat, West Bengal, Odisha, and Andhra Pradesh but are rare in other states [14, 15]; hence, they cannot be classified under rare diseases in these states. Similarly, house-to-house survey carried out by Molecular Diagnostics, Counseling, Care and Research Center (MDCRC) Coimbatore estimates that the prevalence of Duchenne Muscular Dystrophy in Tamil Nadu is high and cannot come under a rare disorder in that state [16]. Gradually, such data need to be combined, so that advocacy groups can focus their efforts on rare diseases and would help in developing a comprehensive and factual National registry, which would further aid in framing the National Policy for Rare Diseases [17, 18].

4. Multi-specialty hospital-based advocacy group

In this chapter, we would like to highlight our study that was to evaluate the feasibility of initiating an advocacy group for rare diseases in a multi-specialty hospital setting with the support of the Department of Genetics and Molecular Medicine. The genetic counselors were instrumental in liaising between different departments such as pediatrics, nephrology, neurology, orthopedics, and oncology for the identification of patients with suspected rare disease. Around 200 such patients were identified during the period of April 2016 to April 2019. The patient families were encouraged to register with the advocacy group, which would support and follow-up the patient and their families and provide the necessary management and treatment options as required.

Patients evaluated were identified and categorized based on age into the pediatric and the adult age group. About 63% of the patients were in the pediatric age group, and the remaining 37% were in the adult age group.

4.1 Rare disease advocacy group at Kamineni Hospital

To cater to patients affected with such diverse diseases, the first hospital-based advocacy group was created at Kamineni Hospital, a multi-specialty hospital located in the cosmopolitan city of Hyderabad in South India. It was named Maitri, which originates from the Sanskrit word meaning "friendship." Maitri looks into the collective interests of individuals with rare diseases. The rare disease community is often denied the most basic of rights. Society is ill-equipped to understand the cause and gravity of the diseases. This often leads to a number of psychological problems. A diagnosis is important to understand a disease, its progression, symptoms, possible treatment options, and also for its prevention in future generations. Most individuals can lead a normal life. However, due to the lack of awareness, such individuals are not allowed to do so. People in general lack the sensitivity to accept and work alongside individuals suffering from such diseases. Maitri aims to change this scenario by raising awareness among clinicians, the general public, in schools, and colleges. It also looks into extended family screening and counseling for making informed reproductive decisions.

4.1.1 MAITRI (bond of friendship) – Kamineni Hospital's rare disease advocacy group

The Department of Genetics and Molecular Medicine along with its team of genetic counselors created Maitri to collectively address the various problems faced by individuals suffering from rare diseases.

Objectives of Maitri:

- To raise awareness about rare diseases among healthcare professionals, general public, and policy makers
- To evaluate and diagnose an individual with a suspected rare disease
- To identify individuals with rare diseases at Kamineni Hospital and include them in the Kamineni Rare Disease Registry
- To counsel the patient, parents, and family about the disease and its prognosis, management, and treatment options (if any)
- To identify individuals in the extended family at risk of having the disease
- To create self-help groups of individuals with similar symptoms/problems for discussion and possible management options
- To help cope with psychosocial issues
- To conduct parental/family group sessions about the different rare diseases and on the various psychosocial problems faced by them
- To involve teachers from the pre-school level, school, special schools, and college level in the advocacy group. To create awareness among them and other teaching staff about dealing with an individual affected with rare diseases to integrate individuals into the mainstream schools/colleges and allow them to lead a normal life.

4.2 General workflow of Maitri

Every patient visiting the Department of Genetics and Molecular Medicine was evaluated in two or more sessions as a part of primary evaluation (**Figure 1**).

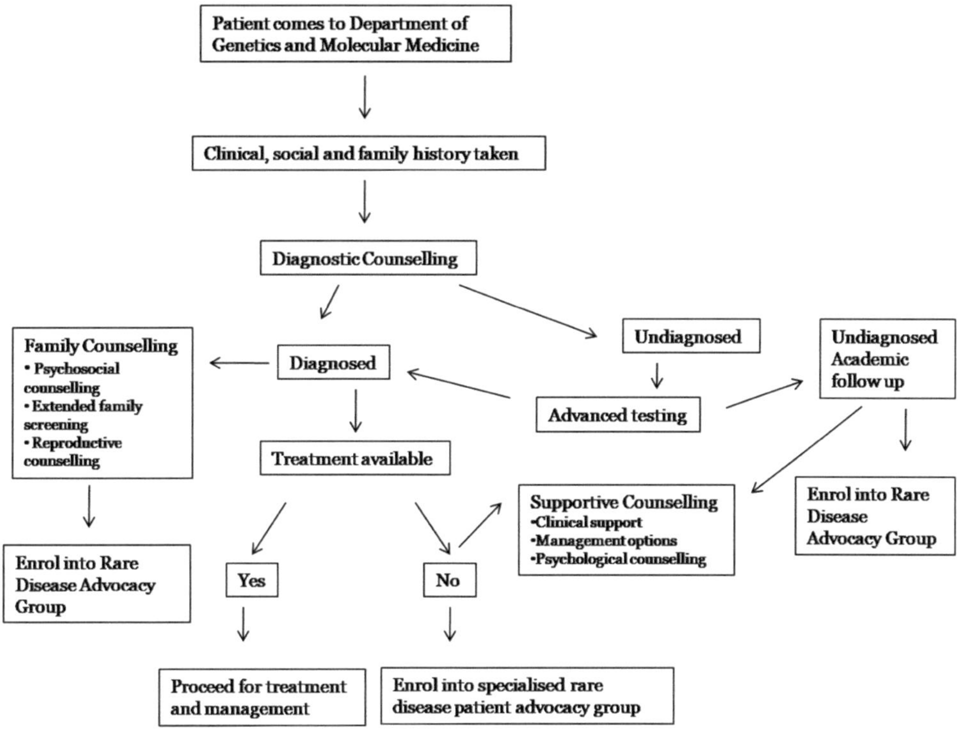

Figure 1.
Flowchart for the working of Maitri.

Patients were segregated based on the following age groups and advised accordingly.

a. Pediatric age group:

Age 0–5 years: Parental discussions on symptom management, addressing various needs of the child. Refer for clinical follow-up and psychological evaluation of the child prior to school admission.

Age 6–15 years: Addressing psychological needs of the patient. Group discussion programs with teachers, parents, and other healthcare professionals. Address issues faced at school and mitigate it.

b. Adult age group:

Age 16–22 years: Patient and parental psychological consultation to address various psychosocial issues. One-on-one patient meetings with geneticist and psychologist to address puberty-related problems. Reproductive counseling is also given.

Age 23–40 years: Pre-marital, pre-pregnancy genetic counseling, group sessions with other patients and their family to address common issues. Refer for clinical follow-up if needed.

Age > 40 years: Group sessions for patient and families for discussion of symptoms, their management, possible treatment options, and psychosocial problems faced due to the condition. Pre-symptomatic genetic testing and subsequent advice for children of individuals affected with rare diseases.

- Individual patients requiring vocational, behavioral, or occupational therapy are referred for the same

The importance of a rare disease advocacy group at the National and International level has been established by many esteemed clinicians, geneticists, and social workers. However, such groups at a hospital setting are important in a country like India, where there are limited electronic medical records, and there is huge literary and financial disparity in the population, such advocacy groups may contribute to maintaining crucial information for providing better healthcare and support to patient families.

5. Conclusion

Hospital-based Rare Disease Advocacy Groups like Maitri are crucial in a number of ways they help in establishing prevalence of rare disorders through the hospital-based registries. They promote awareness, so that every affected individual may be tested for a diagnosis. Such advocacy groups help bring together families with same, similar, or even different rare diseases, so that they can help and support each other. Groups like Maitri also perform a very important role in extended family screening, wherein they identify individuals at risk of developing the disorder and are counseled regarding appropriate testing and preventive measures. It also encourages reproductive genetic counseling for the families with an affected individual, which would help prevent the disorder in the future generations.

Advocacy groups along with policy makers are instrumental in creating public awareness about such diseases. Increase in awareness would make their prevention a public health concern, thus making it mandatory to have definitive screening and preventive strategies in the country. Not only advocacy groups are important for the support of individual families, but they also play a role in mass awareness and prevention of rare diseases.

Acknowledgements

We would like to thank Kamineni Hospitals Ltd. for the support they have extended to us for this project. We would also like to thank all the clinicians and other healthcare providers who have referred patients to the Department of Genetics and Molecular Medicine. They have been instrumental in the identification and diagnosis. We would also like to thank our patients for the support and cooperation.

Conflict of Interest

There was no conflict of interest for the given project.

Author details

Yashodhara Bhattacharya, Gayatri Iyer, Aruna Priya Kamireddy, Subhadra Poornima, Keerthi Konda Juturu and Qurratulain Hasan*
Department of Genetics and Molecular Medicine, Kamineni Hospitals, Hyderabad, India

*Address all correspondence to: qhasan2000@yahoo.com

References

[1] Choudhury MC, Saberwal G. The role of patient organizations in the rare disease ecosystem in India: An interview based study. Orphanet Journal of Rare Diseases. 2019;**14**(1):117. DOI: 10.1186/s13023-019-1093-6

[2] Melnikova I. Rare diseases and orphan drugs. Nature Reviews Drug Discovery. 2012;**11**(4):267-268. DOI: 10.1038/nrd3654

[3] Merkel PA, Manion M, Gopal-Srivastava R, Groft S, Jinnah HA, Robertson D, et al. The partnership of patient advocacy groups and clinical investigators in the rare diseases clinical research network. Orphanet Journal of Rare Diseases. 2016;**11**:66. DOI: 10.1186/s13023-016-0445-8

[4] Gammie T, Lu CY, Babar Z. Access to orphan drugs: A comprehensive review of legislations, regulations and policies in 35 countries. PLoS One. 9 Oct 2015;**10**(10):e0140002. DOI: 10.1371/journal.pone.0140002

[5] Rajasimha HK, Shirol PB, Ramamoorthy P, Hegde M, Barde S, Chandru V, et al. Organization for rare diseases India (ORDI) - addressing the challenges and opportunities for the Indian rare diseases' community. Genetical Research. 2014;**96**:e009

[6] Dunkle M, Pines W, Saltonstall PL. Advocacy groups and their role in rare diseases research. Advances in Experimental Medicine and Biology. 2010;**686**:515-525. DOI: 10.1007/978-90-481-9485-8_28

[7] Song P, Gao J, Inagaki Y, Kokudo N, Tang W. Rare diseases, orphan drugs and their regulation in Asia: Current status and future perspectives. Intractable & Rare Diseases Research. 2012;**1**(1):3-9. DOI: 10.5582/irdr.2012.v1.1.3. PMID: 25343064

[8] Valdez R, Ouyang L, Bolen J. Public health and rare diseases: Oxymoron no more. Preventing Chronic Disease. 2016;**13**:150491. DOI: 10.5888/pcd13.150491

[9] Shapiro E et al. Analysis of the caregiver burden associated with Sanfilippo syndrome type B: Panel recommendations based on qualitative and quantitative data. Orphanet Journal of Rare Diseases. 2019;**14**:168. DOI: 10.1186/s13023-019-1150-1

[10] Somanadhan S, Larkin PJ. Parents' experiences of living with, and caring for children, adolescents and young adults with mucopolysaccharidosis (MPS). Orphanet Journal of Rare Diseases. Dec 2016;**11**(1):138. DOI: 10.1186/s13023-016-0521-0

[11] Rofail D, Maguire L, Kissner M, Colligs A, Abetz-Webb L. A review of the social, psychological, and economic burdens experienced by people with spina bifida and their caregivers. Neurology and Theory. 2013;**2**(1-2):1-12

[12] Ouyang L, Grosse SD, Riley C, Bolen J, Bishop E, Raspa M, et al. A comparison of family financial and employment impacts of fragile X syndrome, autism spectrum disorders, and intellectual disability. Research in Developmental Disabilities. 2014;**35**(7):1518-1527

[13] Tamang R, Singh L, Thangaraj K. Complex genetic origin of Indian populations and its implications. Journal of Biosciences. 2012;**37**:911-919

[14] Mohanty D, Colah RB, Gorakshakar AC, Patel RZ, Master DC, Mahanta J, et al. Prevalence of β-thalassemia and other haemoglobinopathies in six cities in India: A multicentre study. Journal of Community Genetics. 2013;**4**:33-42. DOI: 10.1007/s12687-012-0114-0

[15] Colah R, Italia K, Gorakshakar A. Burden of thalassemia in India: The road map for control. Pediatric Hematology Oncology Journal. 2017;**2**:79-84

[16] Murugan S, Chandramohan A, Lakshmi BR. Use of multiplex ligation-dependent probe amplification (MLPA) for Duchenne muscular dystrophy (DMD) gene mutation analysis. The Indian Journal of Medical Research. 2010;**132**:303-311

[17] van der Weide J et al. Rare disease registries: Potential applications towards impact on development of new drug treatments. Orphanet Journal of Rare Diseases. 2018;**13**:154. DOI: 10.1186/s13023-018-0836-0

[18] Khosla N, Valdez R. A compilation of national plans, policies and government actions for rare diseases in 23 countries. Intractable & Rare Diseases Research. 2018;**7**(4):213-222

Section 5

Therapies and Monitoring of Rare Diseases

Chapter 12

Pharmacotherapy of Rare Diseases in Serbia: The Current State of Art

Branislava Medić Brkić, Bojan Stopić, Katarina Savić Vujović, Nevena Divac, Sonja Vučković, Radan Stojanović, Dragana Srebro, Miloš Basailović and Milica Prostran

Abstract

Rare diseases affect less than 1 in 2000 or 5 in 10,000 people by definition. Most of those diseases have genetic basis (80% of cases) and first symptoms appear in early childhood (50% of cases). Most of these diseases are chronic and degenerative and pharmacotherapy is not available for many of them. Until today, there are more than 7000 rare diseases. In Serbia, the problem of diagnosis and pharmacotherapy of rare diseases is currently under public scrutiny. Patients who suffer from rare diseases in Serbia face many challenges in terms of awareness, timely diagnosis, and adequate treatment. These people are often misdiagnosed or the diagnosis is delayed due to several problems: lack of awareness among medical professionals, lack of expertise, unavailability and/or high costs of diagnostic tests, etc. According to the National Organization of Patients with Rare Diseases in Serbia (NORBS), many diagnostic procedures have to be conducted abroad and the process comprises many difficulties: high costs, travel expenses, or transportation of biological material. Although national legislation ensures the availability of drugs for those diseases, pharmacotherapy is faced with many problems. In this work, we aim to show that improvement of the knowledge regarding rare diseases among both professionals and patients represents a crucial step for enhancement of perspectives for those patients in our community.

Keywords: rare diseases, pharmacotherapy, physicians, patients, knowledge, attitudes

1. Introduction

A rare disease or an orphan disease represents any disease that affects a small percentage of the population. According to data from Europe, a disease or disorder is defined as rare when it affects less than 1 in 2000 citizens (there are so rare diseases that affect 1 person in 100,000 or even less) [1].

The most significant matters concerning rare diseases (RDs) are as follows: (1) these diseases are often chronic, progressive, degenerative, and life-threatening; (2) most of them (80%) have identified genetic base; (3) in the majority of cases (75%), the first symptoms appear in early childhood (30% of rare disease patients die before the age of 5); (4) RDs represent disabling conditions: they have tremendous social and socio-economic impact on one country, because they affect not only the patients but also their families and the whole society.

It is estimated that more than 7000 rare diseases have been detected and described so far. European Organization for Rare Diseases (EURORDIS) represents a unique, non-profit alliance of rare disease patient organizations from 72 European countries. According to this organization, 30 million people in Europe suffer from some of the numerous rare diseases. A similar organization exists in Serbia (NORBS), which estimates that such patients are about half a million in our community [2].

Patients suffering from RDs are faced with numerous complications: deficit of public and scientific education of the diseases, delay in diagnosis (or lack of access to correct diagnosis), heavy social consequences (stigmatization, isolation, discrimination, reducing professional opportunities, etc.), lack of appropriate quality healthcare, high prices of these drugs and complicated procedures for their procurement, etc. [3]. Also, people affected with RDs may require other medicinal devices (diapers, special nutritional preparations, wheelchairs, etc.). The fact that these expenses are not reimbursed by the national health insurance represents additional problem in everyday life of these patients and their family. All these obstacles have led to many charitable actions aimed at collecting donations in order to improve treatment solutions as well as to involve media in raising public awareness of this topic [2, 3].

Although national legislation ensures the availability of drugs for those diseases, ("orphan drugs"), the National Register of RDs still does not exist in Serbia. It is important to know that there are hospital registries for some rare diseases but a systemic and universal approach is still missing. Additionally, most of these conditions are not coded in the ICD-10, which only has codes for 500 of the rare diseases [4].

Beside this, pharmacotherapy of rare diseases in our country is also challenged with many difficulties, not just due to legislative obstacles. Although there are not enough registered orphan drugs, many of them can be found on the "black" market, in private pharmacies at very high prices and without adequate supervision [5].

Serbia has made certain progress in the area, but numerous unresolved issues remain. It should be point out that the importance of this topic was recognized in our country for the first time few years ago, in 2014. At that moment, certain amendments displayed the need for the development of centers for rare diseases and also declared this group of patients as a special category with the right to use free health insurance. In addition, a special budget from the Ministry of Health was assigned to finance treatment with orphan drugs [6, 7].

In addition to the above, National Organization for Rare Diseases in Serbia (NORBS) represents a non-governmental, non-profit organization that was founded in 2010 with an aim to improve the quality of life for people affected with RDs in Serbia.

2. Rare diseases patients as vulnerable subjects in clinical trials: bioethical challenges

The particular question that arises here is related to bioethical aspects of pharmacotherapy of these diseases and all obstacles along the way of examination of special kind of drugs intended to treat small number of patients (the so-called orphan drugs).

The issue of ethical and bioethical aspects of experiments including humans (which was the forerunner of clinical trials) was almost completely ignored by medical ethics of the late nineteenth and early twentieth century. It is relevant to mention that the sensitivity toward medical research subjects belonging to vulnerable groups was first expressed clearly in the Declaration of Helsinki (it was adopted by the 18th World Medical Association General Assembly in Helsinki in 1964, and revised several times (most recently in 2013) [8].

Generally, patients suffering from rare diseases could be considered as the members of vulnerable groups. As we already mentioned, most of these conditions are chronic, degenerative, and life-threatening, of unknown or genetic origin, and mainly affect children [2, 3]. Some of these diseases have a devastating impact on all aspects of the patients' lives and their careers. Additionally, the development and availability of drugs for RDs could challenge basic bioethical principles. Four commonly accepted principles of health care ethics, excerpted from *Beauchamp and Childress*, include the: (1) principle of respect for autonomy, (2) principle of non-maleficence, (3) principle of beneficence, and (4) principle of justice [9].

The first bioethical principle—respect for the autonomy of the patient—means that the patient has the capacity to act intentionally, with understanding, and without controlling influences that would mitigate against a free and voluntary act. This principle is the basis for the practice of "informed consent" in the physician/patient transaction regarding health care, which represents one of postulates of modern clinical trial. The principle of non-maleficence requires us, as medical professionals, to not intentionally create harm or injury to the patient, either through acts of commission or omission. The meaning of the Principle of Beneficence is that health care providers have a duty to be of benefit to the patient, as well as to take positive steps to prevent and to remove harm from the patient. Finally, justice in health care is usually defined as a form of fairness, or as Aristotle once said, "giving to each that which is his due." [9].

In addition to the above, the utilitarian concept of bioethics could not be fully applied in this matter since it favors development of drugs for common disorders instead of the rare ones. One could argue that diseases are rare but there are a lot of patients suffering from them [5, 6]. These diseases represent a challenge not only for the individual and the family of the patient but also for the medical professionals, the entire health care system, and the complete society.

By considering the patients suffering from rare diseases as the members of vulnerable groups, we want to stress the presence of individualized medicine trend in contemporary medicine. Ethical declarations, codices, bioethical documents, and the function of the ethical committees were the indicators of individualizing medicine trend. Regarding the rare diseases issue, the indicators of individualizing medicine trend are certain documents: (1) EU Regulation on Orphan Medicinal Products (1999); (2) EU Regulation on Pediatric Drugs (2006); (3) Programme of Community Action in the Field of Public Health (2007–2013); and (4) EU 7th Framework Programme for Research (2007–2013) [8].

It can be concluded that above-mentioned case of "moving" from a random sample of hospitalized patients to specific group of patients, members of vulnerable groups, is the indicator of individualizing medicine trend and it continues to develop. One of its goals is certainly, we consider, the rare disease issue and the specific patient-physician encounter that includes the rare disease patient, namely, the patient *sui generis* as the subject of specific therapeutic research [8].

3. The aim of our study

Our research group deals with different aspects of rare diseases in our community: pharmacotherapy, bioethical issues, social significance, importance of education among medical students, patients, and professionals, etc.

In the first part of this work, we will briefly present the main results of the pilot study regarding pharmacotherapy of rare diseases conducted among physicians and clinical pharmacists who deal with these kinds of patients in Serbia.

In the next part of examination, we will present the main results of the survey conducted among patients suffering from rare diseases in our country.

4. The knowledge and attitudes of physicians and clinical pharmacists regarding pharmacotherapy of rare diseases in Serbia: a pilot study

In Serbia, clinical trials in the field of rare diseases are extremely rare and mainly relate to rare oncological diseases.

We considered that it would be important to examine the attitudes and knowledge of physicians and clinical pharmacists regarding the pharmacotherapy of rare diseases in Serbia. An anonymous pilot survey entitled "Attitudes of Physicians and Pharmacists Regarding Pharmacotherapy of rare diseases in Serbia" was designed and conducted by employees of the Department of Pharmacology, Clinical Pharmacology and Toxicology in a selected sample of subjects (N = 11, Internal Medicine Clinic and Central Pharmacy, KBC "Bezanijska Kosa" in Belgrade). The survey consisted of both open- and closed-ended questions. The attitudes of medical professionals were assessed by the 10-point Likert scale. The total response rate was 97.2%.

4.1 Physicians' and pharmacists' knowledge and attitudes concerning rare diseases: results

Our respondents found that the greatest problems of patients suffering from rare diseases in our environment are: lack of scientific knowledge (23%), complicated procedures for the procurement of drugs (21%), the lack of a sufficient number of registered medicines for these diseases (14%), etc. Although our examinees considered this issue as highly important in our country (on a scale of 0–10, our respondents gave an average score of 9), the majority of them (64%) assessed they were not sufficiently familiar with the existing legislation. According to our respondents, the treatment of patients with rare diseases in our environment can be improved: by forming a National Strategy for RDs (23%), raising general and professional awareness (20%), by creating a register of patients with rare diseases (20%), etc.

5. The knowledge and attitudes of patients suffering from rare diseases in Serbia

In the next part of our investigation, we performed a cross-sectional study for 5 weeks on outpatients and inpatients (Neurology Clinic, Department for Neuromuscular Disorders, Clinical Center of Serbia) who suffered from rare neurological diseases.

The anonymous questionnaire concerning the knowledge and attitudes of rare diseases and its pharmacotherapy was completed by a total of 60 patients (39 were male and 21 were female). The questionnaire consisted of both open- and closed-ended questions, and patients' attitudes were assessed by the 10-point Likert scale.

All of our respondents suffered from different neurological diseases (myasthenia gravis, myotonic dystrophy, polyneuropathy, multiple sclerosis, syringomyelia, amyotrophic lateral sclerosis, etc.). The total response rate was 95.83%.

5.1 Patients' knowledge and attitudes concerning rare diseases: results

This part of our survey showed that slightly more than a third of participants knew the exact prevalence and definition of rare diseases in Europe. Although more than 70% of patients answered they knew what kind of disease is defined as "rare," only half of the participants believed that they suffered from rare disease.

Our respondents found that dealing with this issue in our community is very important (median value: 9; interquartile range: 8–10), while availability of "orphan drugs" is still poor (median value: 2; interquartile range: 1–6).

The most important problems faced by patients suffering from rare diseases in Serbia include: lack of public and scientific knowledge (21.83% and 14.78%), insufficient number and cost of orphan drugs (14.08%), legislative obstacles (12.67%), delay in diagnosis and misdiagnosis (12.67%), etc.

It should be pointed out that only 16.6% of examined patients were part of some rare diseases patients' organizations and just a quarter of our respondents (26.6%) agreed to participate in clinical trials concerning orphan drugs.

According to our participants, the availability of drugs for RDs could be enhanced by the efforts of: the state (55%), medical doctors (30%), pharmaceutical companies and pharmacies (10%), rare diseases patients' organizations (3.33%), etc.

Finally, in order to improve the pharmacotherapy of RDs in our country, the examined participants suggested the following: well-timed diagnostics (25.78%), progress of the general awareness regarding this topic (22.64%), clarified orphan drug approval processes (16.9%), registration of more RDs drugs (11.3%), creating a RDs patients' register (7.6%), forming a National Strategy for RDs (6.2%), full implementation of legislation (4.7%), adequate control of orphan drugs available in private pharmacies in Serbia (4.25%), etc.

6. Discussion

In general, our questionnaires showed that the examined physicians and clinical pharmacists, as well as patients, were very interested in expressing their attitudes regarding the issue of rare diseases and their treatment in our country. This is confirmed by the high percentage of provided answers (the total response rate was 97.2% and 95.83%, respectively).

The first thing to notice here is that both the patients and medical professionals did not show sufficient knowledge regarding this topic. It is important to emphasize that both groups of our participants were directly involved in this issue (for survey, medical professionals who were in daily practice in contact with RDs patients and patients who belonged to the RDs patients' group by definition were selected).

Our respondents estimated the importance of rare diseases in our society as a problem of crucial importance. Here, we noticed a significant difference in attitudes between RDs patients and third- and sixth-year medical students that we have examined in previous research ($P < 0.01$). In opposite, the observed patients and examined students showed a similar opinion regarding the overall quality of health care of RDs patients, rated it as insufficient ($P < 0.05$) [10].

We need to reveal that the issue of pharmacotherapy of rare diseases involves different kind of ethical dilemmas and controversies. That is why we strongly believe that understanding and analyzing such a sensitive topic must also implement knowledge of basic principles of biomedical ethics [11–14].

In our survey, respondents found that the state was most responsible for the improvement of availability of orphan drugs. However, we need to be aware that national policies and activities of the state start from the initiative of those who participate in the health system of one country (policy-makers, members of the regulatory bodies, medical doctors, pharmacists, patients, etc.). Our research has shown that patients do not participate sufficiently in these activities and do not take an active role in the fight to improve their position in society. Related to these findings, *Baker* and *Trisnadi* in their works emphasized the importance of understanding personal responsibility to address a bioethically vulnerable issue in one community [15, 16].

In the last three decades, the concept of "medicalization" of society ("a pill for every ill") has been increasingly present in numerous bioethical debates [17]. In contrast to this phenomenon, there is a real need to develop novel drugs for rare diseases and their inaccessibility in many societies, on the one hand, and the lack of concern of the pharmaceutical industry regarding this topic, on the other [18, 19].

A controversial and substantive question would be is it reasonably and ethically justified to invest large amounts of money to treat a small number of patients? In a previous study performed on third- and sixth-year medical students, we received an affirmative answer to this question in both groups ($P < 0.05$) [10].

The most important results of survey conducted among third- and sixth-year medical students are shown in **Table 1**.

Finally, in order to improve the pharmacotherapy of rare diseases in Serbia, medical professionals and patients similarly suggested: improvement of general and scientific knowledge, well-timed diagnostics, simplified procedures for drug provision, registration of more appropriate drugs, etc. (see **Tables 2** and **3**).

The first comprehensive study was recently published by Joldic et al. related to the needs of patients with rare diseases in Serbia. According to this paper, four different groups of needs are identified: needs for health care, needs for social care, psychological needs, and other needs. The most important problems of RDs patients and their families arise first from the insufficient information and knowledge on this topic and second from the non-recognition of rare diseases in the legislation of health care system [7, 20–24].

The most important problems of patients (%)	**Third year**	**Sixth year**	**P value**
Lack of information in general public	67.71	56.61	**<0.01**
Lack of scientific knowledge	31.42	37.19	>0.05
Lack of access to correct diagnosis	46.28	42.56	>0.05
Lack of appropriate quality health care	49.71	40.08	**<0.05**
Lack of a sufficient number of registered drugs	41.43	70.24	**<0.0001**
Complicated procedures of drug provision	60.00	63. 22	>0.05
High prices of drugs	86.29	80.58	>0.05
Other causes	2.00	1.65	>0.05
How to improve pharmacotherapy of rare diseases (%)			
Raise general awareness and expertise	30.57	60.00	**<0.0001**
Well-timed diagnostics	44.86	63.22	**<0.0001**
Simplified procedures for drug provision	50.00	70.66	**<0.0001**
Registration of more appropriate drugs	55.43	69.01	**<0.01**
The establishment of the National Plan for Rare Diseases	64.57	74.38	**<0.05**
Create the registry of rare diseases	54.58	53.72	>0.05

Bold values are represented statistically significant difference between groups.

Table 1.
Medical students' knowledge and attitudes concerning rare diseases.

The most important problems of patients (%)	
1. Lack of scientific knowledge	23
2. Complicated procedures for the procurement of drugs	21
3. Lack of a sufficient number of registered drugs for these diseases	14
4. Lack of access to correct diagnosis	12
5. Complicated procedures of drug provision	11
6. High prices of drugs	11
7. Other	8
How to improve pharmacotherapy of rare diseases (%)	
1. The establishment of the National Strategy for Rare Diseases	23
2. Raise general and professional awareness	20
3. Create registries of rare diseases	20
4. Well-timed diagnostics	18
5. Registration of more appropriate drugs	13
6. Other	6

Table 2.
Physicians' and pharmacists' knowledge and attitudes concerning rare diseases.

The most important problems of patients %	
1. Lack of public knowledge	21.83
2. Lack of scientific knowledge	14.78
3. Lack of a sufficient number of registered drugs	14.08
4. Lack of access to correct diagnosis	12.67
5. Complicated procedures of drug provision	11.75
6. High prices of drugs	11.30
7. Unavailability of these drugs in private pharmacies	8.40
8. Other	5.19
How to improve pharmacotherapy of rare diseases %	
1. Well-timed diagnostics	25.78
2. Raise general awareness	22.64
3. Simplified procedures for drug provision	16.90
4. Registration of more appropriate drugs	11.30
5. Create registries of rare diseases	7.60
6. The establishment of the National Strategy for Rare Diseases	6.20
7. Full implementation of legislation	4.7
8. Other	4.88

Table 3.
The knowledge and attitudes of patients suffering from rare diseases

7. Conclusions

We can conclude that our participants showed will to express their attitudes regarding this important medical, societal, and bioethical concern in our community. Patients, as well as medical doctors and pharmacists, are aware of the most significant challenges concerning this topic in Serbia.

However, we need to improve both knowledge and attitudes of all participants in the health care system. Patients should be encouraged to more actively advocate for their rights through the formation of associations, and medical professionals to make greater efforts in the field of education on this subject.

Additionally, we believe that education is very important among medical students as future physicians, as our previous research has proven.

Finally, we would like to point out that at this moment our country has already conducted different kind of activities in order to create national strategy and registries of RDs, to form centers of expertise, to improve accessibility of orphan drugs, etc. Concerning this, we consider this is the critical point for conducting public discussion regarding this issue. An initiative like this should involve not just medical professionals and regulatory bodies, but the RDs patients and the general public as well. We strongly believe this is the unique way to significantly improve the position of these patients in our community in future.

Acknowledgements

This work was supported by the Ministry of Education, Science and Technological Development of Serbia (Grant no. 175023).

Conflict of interest

The authors declare no conflict of interest.

Author details

Branislava Medić Brkić[1]*, Bojan Stopić[2], Katarina Savić Vujović[1], Nevena Divac[1], Sonja Vučković[1], Radan Stojanović[1], Dragana Srebro[1], Miloš Basailović[1] and Milica Prostran[1]

1 Department of Pharmacology, Clinical Pharmacology and Toxicology, Faculty of Medicine, University of Belgrade, Serbia

2 Department of Nephrology, University Medical Center Zvezdara, Belgrade, Serbia

*Address all correspondence to: brankicamedic@gmail.com

References

[1] Rare Diseases Europe (EURORDIS): About Rare Diseases [Online]. Available from: http://www.eurordis.rs/about-rare-diseases [Accessed: November 2019]

[2] Serbian National Organization for Rare Diseases (NORBS): About Rare Diseases [Online] (Serbian). Available from: http://www.norbs.rs/norbs-o-retkim-bolestima.php [Accessed: November 2019]

[3] 14th Sitting of the Health and Family Committee. 2017. Available from: http://www.parlament.gov.rs/14th_Sitting_of_the_Health_and_Family_Committee.34262.537.html [Accessed: November 2019]

[4] Društveni i pravni položaj osoba sa retkim bolestima i njihovih porodica u Srbiji. 2016. pp. 66-81. Available from: http://www.idn.org.rs/biblioteka/Polozaj%20osoba%20sa%20retkim%20bolestima.pdf [Accessed: November 2019] (Serbian)

[5] Ten Years of Orphan Medicines Legislation in Europe—European Medicines Agency Reviews Success and Looks Ahead. Available from: http://www.ema.europa.eu/pdfs/general/direct/pr/29156010en.pdf [Accessed: November 2019]

[6] Amandments to the Law on Health Care. Official Gazette Republic of Serbia 2011, no. 57/2011. Belgrade: Official Gazzete of the Republic of Serbia

[7] Joldic M, Todorovic J, Terzic-Supic Z. The needs of patients with rare disease in Serbia. Why do we need National Strategy for rare disease? Health & Social Care in the Community. 2019;**00**:1-10. DOI: 10.1111/hsc.12813

[8] Radenović S. Bioetika i medicina—Odnos lekar-pacijent u paradigmi integrativne bioetike (in Serbian) Novi Sad: Akademska knjiga; 2012. pp. 161-163

[9] Beauchamp T, Childress J. Principles of Biomedical Ethics. 7th ed. New York: Oxford University Press; 2013. pp. 10-17

[10] Medić B, Divac N, Stopić B, Savić Vujović K, Glišić A, Cerovac N, et al. The attitudes of medical students towards rare diseases: A cross-sectional study. Vojnosanitetski Pregled. 2015;**73**:94

[11] Macklin R. Applying the four principles. Journal of Medical Ethics. 2009;**29**(5):275-280

[12] Todorović Z, Prostran M, Medić B, Vučinić M. Bioehics and pharmacology. In: Todorović Z, Prostran M, Turza K, editors. Bioethics and Pharmacology: Ethics in Preclinical and Clinical Drug Development. Kerala, India: Transworld Research Network; 2012. pp. 7-13

[13] Beauchamp TL, Childress JF. Principles of Biomedical Ethics. 6th ed. Oxford: Oxford University Press; 2008. pp. 23-27

[14] Prostran M, Todorović Z, Stojanović R, Potpara T, Nešić Z, Lazić J, et al. Bioethics in clinical trials: Vulnerable subjects. In: Todorović Z, Prostran M, Turza K, editors. Bioethics and Pharmacology: Ethics in Preclinical and Clinical Drug Development. Kerala, India: Transworld Research Network; 2012. pp. 87-100

[15] Baker I. To what extent can we overcome the "bystander effects" of collective responsibility in matters of global injuctice? Emergent Australasian Philosophers. 2001;**1**(4):1-11

[16] Trisnadi S. The legal protection of Indonesian physicians the medical dispute settlement based on principle standard norms and rules of physician profession in doctor patient relationship. International Journal of Humanities Social Sciences and Education (IJHSSE). 2016;**3**(1):146-155

[17] Hawkins C. For every ill a pill. Annals of the Rheumatic Diseases. 1980;**39**:198-199

[18] Gericke CA, Riesberg A, Busse R. Ethical issues in funding orphan drug research and development. Journal of Medical Ethics. 2005;**31**:164-168

[19] Jezela-Stanek A, Karczmarewicz D, Chrzanowska KH, Krajewska-Walasek M, Aktualny O, et al. Polish activity within Orphanet Europe—State of art of database and services. Developmental Period Medicine. 2015;**19**(4):536-541

[20] Pavan S, Rommel K, Marquina MEM, Höhn S, Lanneau V, Rath A. Clinical practice guidelines for rare diseases: The orphaned database. PLoS One. 2017;**12**(1):1-14. DOI: 10.1371/journal.pone.0170365

[21] Government of Serbia Earmarks RSD 2 bn for Treatment of Patients with Rare Diseases. 2019. Available from: https://www.srbija.gov.rs/vest/en/136760/government-earmarks-rsd-2-bn-for-treatment-of-patients-with-rare-diseases.php

[22] Ministry of Health of Serbia. 2017. Available from: http://www.zdravlje.gov.rs/showelement.php?xml:id=12287

[23] Official Gazzete of the Republic of Serbia. Rulebook on Forming the Prices of Medication Used in Humane Medicine. 2019. Available from: https://www.paragraf.rs/propisi_download/uredba_o_kriterijumima_za_formiranje_cena_lekova_za_upotrebu_u_humanoj_medicini_ciji_je_ezim_izdavanja_na_recept.pd

[24] The Law on Social Protection. Belgrade: Official Gazette Republic of Serbia 2011: no. 24; 2011

Chapter 13

Suitable Molecular Genetic Methods for the Monitoring of Cell Chimerism

Hana Cechova, Lucie Pavlatova, Monika Leontovycova and Milena Vrana

Abstract

The molecular analysis of individual hematopoietic chimerism at a defined time after allogeneic hematopoietic stem cell transplantation represents an important non-specific marker of posttransplant course. The monitoring of its dynamic allows the identification of patients at a high risk of relapse. A variety of methods are used for the monitoring of cell chimerism. It is necessary to use sensitive molecular genetic methods for early detection of the autologous hematopoiesis. Quantitative multiplex real-time polymerase chain reaction (PCR) analysis can serve as a very sensitive (0.01–0.1%), relatively quick, and inexpensive method to detect <1% of minor genotype. With an increasing ratio of minor genotype (>1%), it is more suitable to use short tandem repeats (STRs) for its analysis. Based on the differences in recipient/donor pair genotypes, at least two suitable informative polymorphisms located at different chromosomes can be selected. The combination of methods is appropriate, and the choice of the used method depends on the patient's actual chimerism status. The cohort of 207 patients monitored at the Institute of Hematology and Blood Transfusion was divided into three subgroups according to their chimerism status (complete chimerism (CC), microchimerism, mixed chimerism (MC)) 3 years after allogeneic hematopoietic stem cell transplantation (allo-HSCT). A significant difference in the 3-year survival and 3-year relapse rates in all three subgroups was found.

Keywords: chimerism, hematopoietic stem cell transplantation, real-time polymerase chain reaction, short tandem repeats

1. Introduction

The term chimerism comes from Greek mythology. A chimera is a creature with a lion's head, a goat's body, and a snake's tail. In biology, it is a unique state where cells from genetically different individuals coexist within one body [1].

A chimerism can spontaneously occur in several situations; probably the most common is the persistence of fetal progenitor cells in maternal blood [2]. On rare occasions, a chimerism can be developed in the uterus through the fusion of two genetically different zygotes (so-called tetragametic chimerism) or from a stem cell transfusion between dissimilar fraternal twins that share a placenta [3].

The latter possibility is an engraftment of maternal hematopoietic stem cells, especially in children with severe combined immunodeficiency.

Artificial cell chimerism can arise after transplantation of an organ, tissue, or hematopoietic stem cells (HSCT). The allogeneic HSCT (allo-HSCT) is one of the most used curative options for the treatment of hematological malignant and nonmalignant diseases, and for some diagnoses, it is currently the only available therapy. The long-term success of allo-HSCT depends on many factors such as an appropriate condition regimen (which destroys all leukemic cells), the state of patient in the time of HSCT (active disease vs. disease remission), the donor's age (T lymphocytes of younger donors are more willing to activate and destroy leukemic cells), the modification of the graft (T-cell-depleted graft vs. unmanipulated graft), and engraftment dynamic of HSC (it was proved that early achievement of full donor chimerism predicts lower relapse risk in acute lymphoblastic leukemia (ALL) patients) [4].

The analysis of cell chimerism is an integral part of the posttransplant monitoring of patients. In the immediate posttransplant period, this determination enables the identification of engraftment dynamics or graft failure, and it allows the early detection of a patient's increasing hematopoiesis which indicates a disease relapse.

The principle of the examination is based on the fact that each person has a unique DNA structure that comprises a set of highly variable polymorphisms; most polymorphisms are found in the noncoding regions of the genome [5, 6]. Thus, a comparison of the variable DNA polymorphisms of a patient and a donor provides information about the origin of the cells in almost every case.

2. Methods for the monitoring of cell chimerism

There are a number of molecular methods (e.g., sex-specific markers, fluorescence in situ hybridization (FISH), cytogenetic methods, erythrocyte phenotyping) that have been used for some time for the monitoring of cell chimerism; however, all of these techniques have their own limitations. They are laborious or time-consuming as well as have low informativity and sensitivity, (for a review, see [7, 8]).

2.1 History of molecular genetic methods

The first method of DNA analysis to take advantage of sequence polymorphisms was the method of restriction fragment length polymorphism (RFLP) where genomic DNA is digested with restriction endonucleases (restrictases) [9]. The size of the generated fragments is individually specific and depends on the various numbers of repetitive units in different individuals. All restriction fragments can be subsequently separated by gel electrophoresis. Southern blotting is used to transfer DNA from gel to filter membrane. The fragments are then detected by probe hybridization. For RFLP analyses it is necessary to extract high molecular weight undegraded genomic DNA.

The revolution in the monitoring cell of chimerism arose with the introduction of polymerase chain reaction (PCR) [10]. The first historical method based on PCR is amplified fragment length polymorphism (AFLP) [11]. Genomic DNA is digested by restriction enzymes, and the adaptors are subsequently ligated to the restriction fragments followed by selective PCR amplification with primers compatible to the adaptor's sequence. The amplicons are then separated by gel electrophoresis.

In laboratory practice, the most common current methods for long-term monitoring of cell chimerism are summarized in **Table 1**. They are based on the

	VNTR	STR	InDel	SNP
Type of polymorphisms	Length	Length	Insertion and deletion	Point
Sequence motif size	10–100 bp	2–6 bp	1–10,000 bp	1 bp
Analysis	PCR-specific repetitive sequence and subsequent to the fragment separation on agarose gel by electrophoresis	PCR-specific repetitive sequence and subsequent to the fragment separation on polymer by capillary electrophoresis	Quantitative real-time PCR	Quantitative real-time PCR
Sensitivity	1–5%	0.4–1%	0.01–0.1%	0.01–0.1%
Advantages	High informativity, unlimited quantitative determination	High informativity, unlimited quantitative determination	Highest sensitivity, rapid	Highest sensitivity, rapid
Disadvantages	Low sensitivity, time-consuming	Moderate sensitivity	Lower informative, lower accuracy in the majority of genotype quantification	Lower informative, lower accuracy in the majority of genotype quantification

VNTR, variable number of tandem repeats; STR, short tandem repeats; InDels, short insertions and deletions; SNP, single-nucleotide polymorphism; PCR, polymerase chain reaction.

Table 1.
Current possibilities of polymorphism analysis.

genotyping and quantification of different polymorphisms using PCR which provides an unlimited number of copies of a specific DNA segment based on a single copy.

2.2 Types of polymorphism

Length polymorphisms (loci) are repetitive tandem sequences and individual alleles (gene forms) that differ in the number of repeats of a sequence motif. These loci are widespread throughout the human genome and show sufficient variability among individuals in a population. They have become important in several fields including genetic mapping; linkage analysis; and human identity testing. These tandemly repeated regions of DNA are typically classified into several groups depending on the size of the repeat region such as variable number of tandem repeats (VNTRs) and short tandem repeats (STRs). The other types of polymorphisms are short insertions and deletions (InDels) or single-nucleotide polymorphisms (SNPs).

2.2.1 VNTR

VNTR polymorphisms are minisatellite DNAs with a total sequence length of up to 1000 base pairs and with a repetitive sequence motif of more than 6 base pairs. The benefit of VNTR analyses by PCR is a high degree of discrimination and unlimited quantitative determination, but, on the other hand, the disadvantage is the low sensitivity of the method (ranges from 1 to 5% depending on the analyzed VNTR locus and the combination of recipient-donor allele pair). The PCR products

(VNTR alleles) are visualized by fragment analysis via agarose gel electrophoresis, and when the donor's and the recipient's genotypes are detected in the sample together, the level of chimerism is determined densitometrically.

2.2.2 STR

STR polymorphisms are the repetitive sequences of microsatellite DNAs composed of up to one to six base pairs [12]. However, the most common STRs can reach, in their final range, from 100 to 500 base pairs [13]. The number of STR repetitive units may vary widely in populations. There are literally hundreds of STR systems which have been mapped throughout the human genome [14]. These STR loci are found on almost every chromosome. Since 1997, the National Institute of Standards and Technology (NIST) has compiled and maintained a Short Tandem Repeat DNA Internet Database [15] commonly referred to as STRBase. This STRBase includes used resources and the summary of human STR polymorphisms, their basic information, chromosomal location, overview of alleles, population studies, or available commercial kits. Observed alleles and annotated sequences for each STR locus are described along with a review of STR analysis technologies [16]. STR markers show a high level of polymorphism and consequently provide a significant degree of dissimilarity between individuals [17]. At present, they are considered to be the most informative genetic markers in the characterization of biological material. STR analysis is a very robust method with a sensitivity of 0.4–1% of minor genotype. Compared to VNTR, this method uses smaller quantities of DNA, including degraded DNA. STR polymorphisms may be amplified using a variety of PCR primers. Nowadays, a lot of multiplex kits are available on the market for human genotyping. The method is based on selective PCR of DNA segments with examined polymorphisms. PCR primers are fluorescently labeled. Separation of the fragments takes place subsequently in the genetic analyzer by capillary electrophoresis, as the carrier medium is used a polymer. In the genetic analyzer, fluorophores are excited by a laser ray to label DNA fragments. Fluorophores absorb laser light and emit light at a longer wavelength. Using an optical system, the emitted light is detected and recorded on a charge-coupled device (CCD) chip. STR alleles are visualized by specific software-like peaks. The area or height of peaks is used for quantification.

2.2.3 InDel and SNP

InDels are biallelic polymorphisms classified among small genetic variations, measuring from 1 to 10,000 base pairs in length [18, 19].

SNP is the smallest possible change in DNA sequence in individuals of a given population. SNPs are most often formed by a point mutation mechanism that is substitution-like, less often by deleting or inserting at a particular DNA site. The distribution of SNPs in the genome is not homogeneous. More often, they occur in noncoding regions, on average 1 of 1000 bp in any selected region of the genome.

SNP and InDel analysis are performed by real-time quantitative polymerase chain reaction (RQ-PCR) with specific primers designed to contain appropriate insertions or deletions or point-to-point substitutions. Real-time PCR allows accurate quantification of amplified products by detection of fluorescence released during the exponential phase of the reaction. This method can use the non-specific intercalating fluorescent DNA-binding dye SYBR Green that binds all double-stranded DNA [20]. More often TaqMan technology is used [21], which utilizes a fluorescent-labeled target-specific probe resulting in an increased specificity and sensitivity compared to the SYBR Green method. Additionally, a variety of fluorescent dyes are available so that multiplex PCR can be used to simultaneously amplify and detect many sequences. The TaqMan probe consists of a fluorophore covalently attached to the 5′ end of the oligonucleotide and the quencher at the 3′ end. If the probe is in an intact state, even when the probe is hybridized to the target sequence, the emitted fluorescence is suppressed by the quencher. Only during the elongation phase, when the Taq polymerase with its 5′ exonuclease activity degrades the specifically bound TaqMan probe complex and releases the fluorophore from the quencher, can fluorescence occur and then be measured. The fluorescence intensity is directly proportional to the amount of PCR product. The calculation of the relative amount of target DNA in a sample is done by comparing the Ct values (the threshold cycle, at which the emitted fluorescent signal exceeds the statistical significance level). The resulting portion of the gene of interest (GOI) is calculated by the ΔΔCT method [22]. Data are normalized with the reference (housekeeping) gene, and the amplification and detection of the GOI and the reference gene can be analyzed as a singleplex or multiplex reaction. The multiplex RQ-PCR assay is a quick, sensitive, reproducible, and cost-effective method for an accurate assessment [23]. Multiplex RQ-PCR in a routine practice enables an increase in throughput and reliability, with a reduction in pipetting errors. The sensitivity of this method is about 0.01% of the minor genotype. Due to the influence of the so-called Monte Carlo effect (a greater degree of random effect on very low percentages), it is appropriate to define the lowest significant detection limit of the method. On the other hand, the RQ-PCR is suitable to use for the quantification of up to about 10% of the minor genotype, since it has a lower accuracy at higher percentages.

3. Standard procedures for the monitoring of cell chimerism at the Institute of Hematology and Blood Transfusion

3.1 Informativity determination

The informativity determination always precedes the monitoring of cell chimerism. Recipient and donor DNAs are tested by a panel of highly polymorphic STRs and InDels by multiplex kits. VNTRs and SNPs are not used in our laboratory. Currently, the PowerPlex 16HS System (Promega, Madison, WI, USA) kit is used routinely for STR analysis; the kit contains 13 basic Combined DNA Index System (CODIS) core STR loci [24], sex-specific locus amelogenin, and 2 other pentanucleotide repeat polymorphisms Penta D and Penta E. For the genotyping of deletion–insertion polymorphisms (DIP), a Mentype DIPscreen (Biotype, Dresden, DE) kit is used that amplifies 33 DIP loci and amelogenin. A comparison of the donor's and the recipient's DNA profiles allows to select the specific informative markers suitable for the monitoring of cell chimerism during the posttransplantation course. We choose at least two informative polymorphisms located at different chromosomes specific for the recipient. It is necessary to take into account the potential cytogenetic changes that are associated with different types of cancer (such as genome instability, loss of heterozygosity, and chromosomal changes) [25, 26]. Only informative recipient alleles by at least $n \pm 2$ repeats outside stutter region (preferably by 2–4 longer) are used for calculation. An artifact of PCR, the so-called DNA stutter, is a result of strand slippage during DNA synthesis, showing up primarily one repeat before and, less frequently, one repeat after the true allele. The result of quantification is that such an allele would lead to an incorrect interpretation. It is always appropriate to quantify the minor genotype; therefore, in the case of graft rejection or graft failure (the donor's cells are present in <50%), we choose two informative polymorphisms specific for donor in the same way as the recipient.

3.2 Interpretation of chimerism status

Chimerism is a dynamic process, so the proportion of autologous cells after allo-HSCT can change during monitoring. It is therefore necessary to approach each patient individually and to select appropriate methods for quantification.

An overview and definition of the chimerism status are given in **Table 2**. Under optimal conditions, we can detect only the donor's genotype after allo-HSCT; thus, the recipient's hematopoiesis is completely replaced with the donor's graft. We interpret this as a complete chimerism (CC). In our laboratory the CC is detected by RQ-PCR, and, based on clinical validation, the significant detection limit was defined as ≤0.035% of the recipient's genotype (due to Monte Carlo effect as mentioned in point 2.2.3). The detection of recipient's genotype of less than 1% is interpreted as a microchimerism (range from ≥0.036 to <1%), and the presence of more than or equal 1% is interpreted as mixed chimerism (MC). The percentages of the individual alleles are then quantified by STR analysis. If we detect only the recipient's genotype or the donor's genotype less than 0.035%, transplant rejection and a complete recovery of the original hematopoiesis have occurred. Split chimerism can be seen in the analysis of cell fractions. This means that MC is detected in a certain leukocyte line, but in another cell line, it is CC. The analysis of cell subpopulations makes it possible to distinguish between residual malignant cells and nonmalignant hematopoiesis. More often, the fraction of monocytes, granulocytes, natural killer (NK) cells, T lymphocytes, and B lymphocytes is examined. The analysis of chimerism of T lymphocytes and NK cells can help, especially, as a guide to additional therapy in order to avoid graft rejection. The analysis of chimerism in cell fractions is particularly important for patients with a reduced intensity regimen before allo-HSCT or patients with autoimmune disease.

The interpretation of bone marrow samples is more difficult. Microchimerism is often detected as a result of the contamination of the primary sample by bone marrow stromal cells of the recipient. Therefore, microchimerism below 0.5% of the recipient's genotype is considered to be insignificant. The proportion of autologous hematopoiesis in the bone marrow can fluctuate over time, especially in the early period after allo-HSCT. In making a clinical decision, it is more important to watch the dynamics of chimerism and take into account the patient's diagnosis rather than the individual values of microchimerism or MC.

Chimerism status	Definition
Complete chimerism (CC)	Detection of donor's genotype only or ≤0.035% recipient's genotype
Microchimerism	Detection of donor/recipient ratio ≥0.036 to <1%
Mixed chimerism (MC)	Detection of donor/recipient ratio ≥1%
Split chimerism	Mixed chimerism is detected in a certain leukocyte line, but in another cell line, it is complete chimerism
Autologous hematopoiesis	Detection of recipient's genotype only or ≤0.035% donor's genotype

Table 2.
Interpretation of chimerism status.

3.3 Posttransplant monitoring

The monitoring of cell chimerism consists of analyzing 2–3 selected informative polymorphisms. The frequency of monitoring after graft transfer is performed under our standard days (D) +14, +21, and +28 after allo-HSCT in both adult and pediatric patients. Subsequently, in pediatric patients, the intervals of examination are every 2–3 weeks up to D + 180, once a month to the first year after allo-HSCT, later every 2–4 months up to 3 years after allo-HSCT, and every 6–12 months up to 5 years after allo-HSCT according to the dates of outpatient's controls. In adult patients, examinations from the second month after allo-HSCT are carried out in monthly intervals up to 2 years and, throughout the next period, at least every 6 months. The frequency of examinations depends on the patient's medical condition, diagnosis, the dynamics of their chimerism status, and especially the physician's decision. In cases of increasing microchimerism or MC detection after the previous period of CC, an intensive investigation scheme is recommended due to the risk of graft rejection or relapse of the primary disease.

In the first samples after allo-HSCT, the detection of MC can be expected. If the recipient's genotype fraction falls below 50%, we can interpret this as the so-called engraftment of the donor's cells. The MC gradually decreases until the patient reaches CC. The median achievement of CC is most often D + 21 or D + 28 after allo-HSCT and depends on the patient's diagnosis and many other factors such as the regimen of allo-HSCT or the quality of the graft.

The choice of method used depends on the patient's actual chimerism status. Due to the high sensitivity of the RQ-PCR method, in combination with STR analysis, it is advisable to use RQ-PCR for the monitoring of patients in cases where CC, microchimerism, or MC up to 10% has been detected. On the other hand, with a rising trend of MC, it is better to use only STR analysis for quantification. For more accurate determination, it is always necessary to analyze the informative polymorphisms that detect a minority genotype. This means that in cases where the MC increases over 50% of the recipient's genotype, it is preferable to select donor-specific polymorphisms for quantification.

3.4 The importance of microchimerism

The introduction of the RQ-PCR method for the monitoring of cell chimerism as a part of routine examination has improved significantly the sensitivity of the assessment. Its high sensitivity of 0.035% allows for a much earlier detection of relapses than conventional methods (VNTR and STR). The importance of microchimerism detection was confirmed by us and many other studies [27–30], and we would like to present our retrospective data below.

3.4.1 Patients and methods

A group of 224 patients, from HLA-identical-related and HLA-identical-unrelated donors, who underwent allo-HSCT between 2011 and 2015 at the Institute of Hematology and Blood Transfusion, were enrolled in this study. Patients with early HSCT-associated mortality (less than 14 days), another allo-HSCT before the third year, with no RQ-PCR analyses or with a loss of follow-up were excluded. In total, 207 patients were eligible for analysis of cell chimerism dynamics. The test group was divided into 3 subgroups according to chimerism status 3 years after allo-HSCT: patients with CC (137), patients with microchimerism (38), and patients with MC (32). The patients' characteristics are listed in **Table 3**.

	Number	%
Patient characteristic	207	100
Age		
Median: 53 years (range 20–67 years)		
Sex		
Male	130	63
Female	77	57
Diagnostic group		
AML	91	44.0
CML	9	4.3
MDS	22	9.6
ALL and LBL	20	9.7
Myeloproliferative disease and MDS/MPS	18	8.7
B-cell non-Hodgkin's lymphoma	10	4..8
CLL, SLL, PLL	17	8.2
Mature T-cell and NK-cell lymphomas	11	5.3
Hodgkin's lymphoma	2	1.0
Other diseases	7	3.4
Transplant characteristic		
Donor		
HLA match	207	100
Match family donor	64	31
Match unrelated donor	143	69
Conditioning regimen		
Myeloablative	126	61
Nonmyeloablative	81	39
Stem cell source		
PBPC	180	87
BM	27	13

Abbreviations: AML, acute myeloid leukemia; CML, chronic myeloid leukemia; MDS, myelodysplastic syndrome; ALL and LBL, acute lymphoblastic leukemia and lymphoblastic lymphoma; MDS/MPS, myelodysplastic/myeloproliferative neoplasms; CLL, SLL, PLL, chronic lymphoblastic leukemia, small lymphocytic lymphoma, prolymphocytic leukemia; PBPC, peripheral blood progenitor cells; BM, bone marrow.

Table 3.
Patient characteristics.

DNA from whole peripheral blood samples was isolated by means of a salting-out procedure [31] and diluted to a final concentration of 50 ng/μL. The combination of InDels by RQ-PCR, in conjunction with STR analysis by fragment analysis, was used to determine the chimerism status. Fragment analysis of the resulting PCR products was performed on an automated 3500 Series Genetic Analyzer (Thermo Fisher Scientific, Waltham, MA, USA), and data were processed by GeneMapper v5 software (Thermo Fisher Scientific). Quantification of MC was determined using the peak areas representing specific alleles. InDel analysis was performed by means of TaqMan technology. Rotor-Gene machine (Corbett Life Science, Sydney, New

South Wales) and Rotor-Gene 6 software were used for evaluation. The percentage of microchimerism was calculated by the ΔΔCT method. Data were normalized with the glyceraldehyde-3-phosphate dehydrogenase as a reference gene.

The impact of chimerism status on the 3-year overall survival of allo-HSCT patients and 3-year relapse rates was evaluated using GraphPad Prism 7 software (La Jolla, CA, USA). The logrank (Mantel-Cox) test was used for comparison of survival curves.

3.4.2 Results

The 3-year overall survival probability (**Figure 1**) in our cohort was 59%, and a significant difference was found in all three subgroups: CC vs. MC ($p < 0.0001$); CC vs. microchimerism ($p < 0.0001$); and MC vs. microchimerism ($p = 0.0485$). Overall 85 patients died: the main cause of death was a relapse of the primary disease (24%); in the second it was pneumonia (20%); and in the third it was multiple organ failure (15%). Infections, acute GvHD, cerebrovascular accident, other pulmonary complications, and heart attack occurred less frequently. However, if we take into account the distribution of patients in the three subgroups according to their chimerism status, the main cause of death in the CC subgroup was pneumonia (24%), other infections (16%), and multiple organ failure (16%); the relapse was only 5% (two patients). In these patients, the last available sample was taken 2–3 months prior to the relapse date. In the microchimerism subgroup, the main cause of death was relapse (36%), the second most often was multiple organ failure (18%), and in the third, it was pneumonia (14%). In the MC subgroup, most patients died of a relapse (38%), followed by pneumonia (19%), and multiple organ failure (12%).

Overall, the relapse mortality was 67%. In a correlation of 3-year overall relapse rates (**Figure 2**), there was a significant difference between all subgroups: CC vs. MC patients ($p < 0.0001$), CC vs. microchimerism patients ($p = 0.0073$), and MC vs. microchimerism patients ($p = 0.0007$). Patients with MC relapsed in 72% of cases, and the subsequent mortality was 87%. The detection of MC, especially in the early period after allo-HSCT, is thus an important high-risk factor for a relapse of the disease. In the microchimerism subgroup, patients relapsed in 34% of cases with a mortality rate of 69%. The patients with microchimerism are considered to be potentially at risk. In the CC subgroup, patients relapsed in 15% of cases with a mortality rate of 29%.

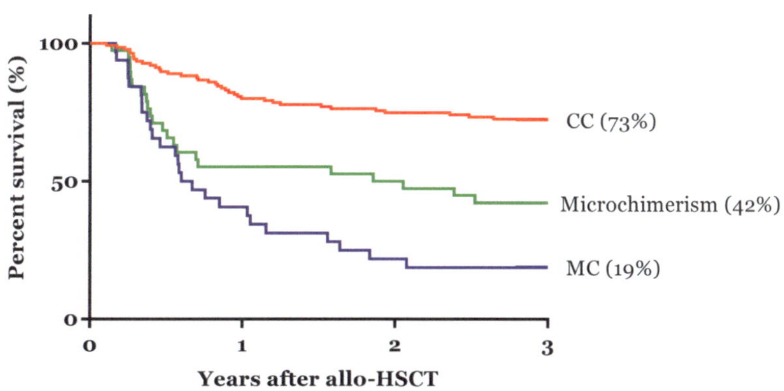

Figure 1.
Three-year overall survival probability according to chimerism status.

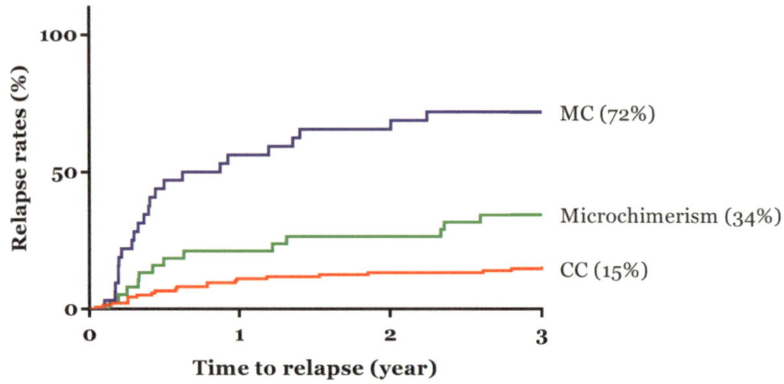

Figure 2.
Three-year overall relapse rates according to chimerism status.

4. Discussion

During the last decades, the effect of MC on the occurrence of imminent relapse has been investigated. At the beginning of the monitoring of cell chimerism by RFLP, red cell phenotyping, cytogenetic analysis, or VNTR analysis, there was no correlation found between the presence of MC and a relapse of the primary disease [32, 33]. Following the advances in methodology and the introduction of more sensitive methods for the monitoring of cell chimerism, scientists are increasingly convinced that there is a connection between the presence of MC and the incidence of relapse [34, 35]. These observations also support findings that studied the correlation of MC, minimal residual disease, and the presence of a relapse [36, 37]. Our results support this notion since we found a statistical significant difference between 3-year relapse rates and 3-year survival probability between all three subgroups based on their chimerism status. In addition, there were differences in the main causes of death: patients with MC and microchimerism died most often with a relapse, whereas CC patients died mostly of pneumonia.

In the group of patients with MC, it is also advisable to consider the issue of persisting MC (PMC). In the case of PMC, it depends on the diagnoses. In some diagnoses, PMC is typical and, usually, does not lead to a relapse (e.g., in nonmalignant diseases). In another diagnosis, PMC could be a problem; for instance, in MC patients who have a high percent of autologous cells immediately after the transplantation, it can often lead to a relapse, and the patients are often retransplanted. In our cohort of MC patients, there were eight patients without relapse. One of them relapsed shortly after 3 years, six patients died within first year after allo-HSCT from other causes, and one patient with primary myelofibrosis has never reached CC, and he is still around 1% of autologous hematopoiesis without recurrence of the disease 7 years after allo-HSCT.

The introduction of the RQ-PCR method for cell chimerism level monitoring as a part of routine examination has improved significantly the detection of microchimerism. The early identification of patients at risk is now possible, and, due to the early therapeutic intervention, we can avoid the progression to a high-risk category of MC. Thus, early detection of autologous hematopoiesis is essential for survival. In the case of MC or microchimerism detection, it is necessary to accurately quantify the proportion of recipient genotype and monitor its dynamics over time.

Recently, other studies have also begun to focus on the monitoring of cell chimerism using the latest technologies such as digital PCR [38] or next-generation sequencing [39]. The incorporation of these techniques into routine investigations depends on subsequent validations that will reveal their advantages or disadvantages.

5. Conclusion

Molecular analysis of hematopoietic chimerism at a defined period after allo-HSCT represents a valuable non-specific marker of posttransplant course for all diagnoses. For some diagnoses this is the only available marker for monitoring. The aim of cell chimerism analysis is to provide a conclusive base for informed, clinical decision-making. The establishment of an adequate monitoring schedule, as well as the selection of appropriate markers and interpretation criteria, will improve the clinical value of this analysis. The use of sensitive methods, like RQ-PCR for the monitoring of cell chimerism, is important for the early detection of relapse and allows the early initiation of medical treatment.

Acknowledgements

The authors are indebted to their colleagues Bara Cizkova, Pavla Hrabakova, and Renata Prerovska for expert routine analysis and Martina Stankova and Dagmar Brezinova for technical support. This work was supported by the Ministry of Health, Czech Republic—conceptual development of research organization (00023736, UHKT).

Conflict of interest

The authors declare no competing financial interests.

Author details

Hana Cechova*, Lucie Pavlatova, Monika Leontovycova and Milena Vrana
Institute of Hematology and Blood Transfusion, Prague, Czech Republic

*Address all correspondence to: hana.cechova@uhkt.cz

References

[1] Anderson D, Billingham RE, Lampkin GH, Medawar PB. The use of skin grafting to distinguish between monozygotic and dizygotic twins in cattle. Heredity. 1951;5:379-397

[2] Bianchi DW, Zickwolf GK, Weil GJ, Sylvester S, DeMaria MA. Male fetal progenitor cells persist in maternal blood for as long as 27 years postpartum. Proceedings of the National Academy of Sciences of the United States of America. 1996;**93**(2):705-708. DOI: 10.1073/pnas.93.2.705. PubMed PMID: 8570620; PubMed Central PMCID: PMC40117

[3] Yunis EJ, Zuniga J, Romero V, Yunis EJ. Chimerism and tetragametic chimerism in humans: Implications in autoimmunity, allorecognition and tolerance. Immunologic Research. 2007; **38**(1–3):213-236. Review. PubMed PMID: 17917028

[4] Chen CT, Gau JP, Liu JH, Chiou TJ, Hsiao LT, Liu YC. Early achievement of full donor chimerism after allogeneic hematopoietic stem cell transplantation predicts lower relapse risk in patients with acute lymphoblastic leukemia. Journal of the Chinese Medical Association. 2018;**81**(12):1038-1043. DOI: 10.1016/j.jcma.2018.06.005. Epub 2018 Aug 9. PubMed PMID: 30100353

[5] Shastry BS. SNP alleles in human disease and evolution. Journal of Human Genetics. 2002;**47**(11):561-566. Review. PubMed PMID: 12436191

[6] Harris H. Polymorphism and protein evolution. The neutral mutation-random drift hypothesis. Journal of Medical Genetics. 1971;**8**(4):444-452. Review. PubMed PMID: 4948373; PubMed Central PMCID: PMC1469095

[7] Bader P, Niethammer D, Willasch A, Kreyenberg H, Klingebiel T. How and when should we monitor chimerism after allogeneic stem cell transplantation? Bone Marrow Transplantation. 2005;**35**(2):107-119. Review. PubMed PMID: 15502849

[8] Khan F, Agarwal A, Agrawal S. Significance of chimerism in hematopoietic stem cell transplantation: New variations on an old theme. Bone Marrow Transplantation. 2004; **34**(1):1-12. Review. PubMed PMID: 15156163

[9] Botstein D, White RL, Skolnick M, Davis RW. Construction of a genetic linkage map in man using restriction fragment length polymorphisms. American Journal of Human Genetics. 1980;**32**(3):314-331. Review. PubMed PMID: 6247908; PubMed Central PMCID: PMC1686077

[10] Lawler M, McCann SR, Conneally E, Humphries P. Chimaerism following allogeneic bone marrow transplantation: Detection of residual host cells using the polymerase chain reaction. British Journal of Haematology. 1989;**73**(2): 205-210. PubMed PMID: 2818939

[11] Schreiner T, Prochnow-Calzia H, Maccari B, Erne E, Kinzler I, Wölpl A, et al. Chimerism analysis after allogeneic bone marrow transplantation with nonradioactive RFLP and PCR-AFLP using the same DNA. Journal of Immunological Methods. 1996;**196**(1): 93-96. PubMed PMID: 8841447

[12] Tautz D. Notes on the definition and nomenclature of tandemly repetitive DNA sequences. EXS. 1993;**67**:21-28. Review. PubMed PMID: 8400689

[13] Edwards A, Civitello A, Hammond HA, Caskey CT. DNA typing and genetic mapping with trimeric and tetrameric tandem repeats. American Journal of Human Genetics. 1991;**49**(4): 746-756. PubMed PMID: 1897522; PubMed Central PMCID: PMC1683171

[14] The Utah Marker Development Group. A collection of ordered tetranucleotide-repeat markers from the human genome. American Journal of Human Genetics. 1995;**57**:619-628

[15] STRBase, National Institute of Standards and Technology. 2019. Available from: https://strbase.nist.gov/index.htm

[16] Ruitberg CM, Reeder DJ, Butler JM. STRBase: A short tandem repeat DNA database for the human identity testing community. Nucleic Acids Research. 2001;**29**(1):320-322. PubMed PMID: 11125125; PubMed Central PMCID: PMC29767

[17] Kayser M, de Knijff P, Dieltjes P, Krawczak M, Nagy M, Zerjal T, et al. Applications of microsatellite-based Y chromosome haplotyping. Electrophoresis. 1997;**18**(9):1602-1607. PubMed PMID: 9378129

[18] Weber JL, David D, Heil J, Fan Y, Zhao C, Marth G. Human diallelic insertion/deletion polymorphisms. American Journal of Human Genetics. 2002;**71**:854-862

[19] Mills RE. An initial map of insertion and deletion (INDEL) variation in the human genome. Genome Research. 2006;**16**(9):1182-1190. DOI: 10.1101/gr.4565806. PMC 1557762

[20] van der Velden VH, Hochhaus A, Cazzaniga G, Szczepanski T, Gabert J, van Dongen JJ. Detection of minimal residual disease in hematologic malignancies by real-time quantitative PCR: Principles, approaches, and laboratory aspects. Leukemia. 2003; **17**(6):1013-1034. DOI: 10.1038/sj.leu.2402922. Review. PubMed PMID: 12764363

[21] Alizadeh M, Bernard M, Danic B, Dauriac C, Birebent B, Lapart C, et al. Quantitative assessment of hematopoietic chimerism after bone marrow transplantation by real-time quantitative polymerase chain reaction. Blood. 2002;**99**(12):4618-4625. PubMed PMID: 12036896

[22] Livak KJ, Schmittgen TD. Analysis of relative gene expression data using real-time quantitative PCR and the 2(-Delta Delta C(T)) method. Methods. 2001;**25**(4):402-408. DOI: 10.1006/meth.2001.1262. PubMed PMID: 11846609

[23] Nadvornikova S, Leontovycova M, Pegova K, Hrabakova P, Prerovska R, Cechova H. Multiplex real-time quantitative polymerase chain reaction assay for rapid and sensitive detection of hematopoietic chimerism. HLA. 2018;**92**(4):215-223. DOI: 10.1111/tan.13383. PubMed PMID: 30129247

[24] Butler JM. Genetics and genomics of core STR loci used in human identity testing. Journal of Forensic Sciences. 2006;**51**(2):253-265

[25] Fröhling S, Döhner H. Chromosomal abnormalities in cancer. The New England Journal of Medicine. 2008;**359**:722-734

[26] Bernheim A. Cytogenomics of cancers: From chromosome to sequence. Molecular Oncology. 2010;**4**(4): 309-322. DOI: 10.1016/j.molonc.2010.06.003. Epub 2010 Jun 11. Review. PubMed PMID: 20599448; PubMed Central PMCID: PMC5527907

[27] Koldehoff M, Steckel NK, Hlinka M, Beelen DW, Elmaagacli AH. Quantitative analysis of chimerism after allogeneic stem cell transplantation by real-time polymerase chain reaction with single nucleotide polymorphisms, standard tandem repeats, and Y-chromosome-specific sequences. American Journal of Hematology. 2006; **81**(10):735-746. DOI: 10.1002/ajh.20693. PubMed PMID: 16838323

[28] Horky O, Mayer J, Kablaskova L, Razga F, Krejci M, Kissova J, et al. Increasing hematopoietic microchimerism is a reliable indicator of incipient AML relapse. International Journal of Laboratory Hematology. 2011;**33**(1):57-66. DOI: 10.1111/j.1751-553X.2010.01249.x. PubMed PMID: 20681999

[29] Jacque N, Nguyen S, Golmard JL, Uzunov M, Garnier A, Leblond V, et al. Chimerism analysis in peripheral blood using indel quantitative real-time PCR is a useful tool to predict post-transplant relapse in acute leukemia. Bone Marrow Transplantation. 2015;**50**(2):259-265. DOI: 10.1038/bmt.2014.254. Epub 2014 Nov 10. PubMed PMID: 25387089

[30] Ahci M, Stempelmann K, Buttkereit U, Crivello P, Trilling M, Heinold A, et al. Clinical utility of quantitative PCR for chimerism and engraftment monitoring after allogeneic stem cell transplantation for hematologic malignancies. Biology of Blood and Marrow Transplantation. 2017;**23**(10):1658-1668. DOI: 10.1016/j.bbmt.2017.05.031. Epub 2017 Jun 8. PubMed PMID: 28603070

[31] Miller SA, Dykes DD, Polesky HF. A simple salting out procedure for extracting DNA from human nucleated cells. Nucleic Acids Research. 1988;**16**(3):1215

[32] Schattenberg A, De Witte T, Salden M, Vet J, Van Dijk B, Smeets D, et al. Mixed hematopoietic chimerism after allogeneic transplantation with lymphocyte-depleted bone marrow is not associated with a higher incidence of relapse. Blood. 1989;**73**(5):1367-1372. PubMed PMID: 2564791

[33] van Leeuwen JE, van Tol MJ, Joosten AM, Wijnen JT, Khan PM, Vossen JM. Mixed T-lymphoid chimerism after allogeneic bone marrow transplantation for hematologic malignancies of children is not correlated with relapse. Blood 1993;**82**(6):1921–1928. PubMed PMID: 8400242

[34] Lamba R, Abella E, Kukuruga D, Klein J, Savasan S, Abidi MH, et al. Mixed hematopoietic chimerism at day 90 following allogenic myeloablative stem cell transplantation is a predictor of relapse and survival. Leukemia. 2004;**18**(10):1681-1686. DOI: 10.1038/sj.leu.2403468. PubMed PMID: 15318247

[35] Cechova H, Leontovycova M, Pavlatova L. Chimerism as an important marker in post-transplant monitoring chimerism monitoring. HLA. 2018;**92** (Suppl 2):60-63. DOI: 10.1111/tan.13407. PubMed PMID: 30362266

[36] Formánková R, Honzátková L, Moravcová J, Sieglová Z, Dvořáková R, Nádvorníková S, et al. Prediction and reversion of post-transplant relapse in patients with chronic myeloid leukemia using mixed chimerism and residual disease detection and adoptive immunotherapy. Leukemia Research. 2000;**24**(4):339-347. PubMed PMID: 10713331

[37] Terwey TH, Hemmati PG, Nagy M, Pfeifer H, Gökbuget N, Brüggemann M, et al. Comparison of chimerism and minimal residual disease monitoring for relapse prediction after allogeneic stem cell transplantation for adult acute lymphoblastic leukemia. Biology of Blood and Marrow Transplantation. 2014;**20**(10):1522-1529. DOI: 10.1016/j.bbmt.2014.05.026. Epub 2014 Jun 4

[38] Valero-Garcia J, González-Espinosa MC, Barrios M, Carmona-Antoñanzas G, García-Planells J, Ruiz-Lafora C, et al. Earlier relapse detection after allogeneic hematopoietic stem cell transplantation by chimerism assays: Digital PCR versus quantitative real-time PCR of insertion/deletion polymorphisms. PLoS One. 2019;**14**(3):e0213966. DOI: 10.1371/journal.pone.0212708

[39] Kim J, Hwang IS, Kim HS, Joo DJ, Hong KR, Choi JR. Bone marrow chimerism detection using next generation sequencing based on single nucleotide polymorphisms following liver transplantation: Comparison with short tandem repeat-PCR. Annals of Laboratory Medicine. 2016;**36**(1):82-84. DOI: 10.3343/alm.2016.36.1.82. PubMed PMID: 26522768; PubMed Central PMCID: PMC4697352

Chapter 14

Monitoring of Chimerism in Rare Haematological Malignant Diseases after Allogeneic Haematopoietic Stem Cell Transplantation

Eva Hanusovska and Sabina Sufliarska

Abstract

Allogeneic haematopoietic stem cell transplantation (allo-hSCT) is one of the most important therapeutic options for patients with both malignant and non-malignant life-threatening rare disorders. Assessment of chimerism following allo-hSCT has been established as an indispensable tool for the clinical management of transplant recipients. The number of allo-hSCT among *CML* patients is decreasing due to tyrosine-kinase-inhibitor treatment. However, allo-hSCT in adult and paediatric patients with AML, ALL, and different non-malignant diseases is still increasing. For sex-independent patient chimerism monitoring, PCR-based short tandem repeat (PCR-STR) DNA markers with subsequent fragment analysis ('FA') and SYBR Green-based real-time PCR (SNPs or NPs markers of DNA) ('RQ PCR') were used. Specific features of chimerism assessment in non-malignant (n = 74) and malignant (n = 169) diseases were monitored by 'FA'. Complete and mixed chimerism was monitored also by SYBR Green-based real-time PCR method ('RQ PCR') (n = 188). By comparing the results of two chimerism monitoring methods ('FA' and 'RQ PCR') (n = 65), the higher sensitivity for the detection of the autologous DNA markers was observed by 'RQ PCR' (<1%) than 'FA' (1–5%). The lower detection limit of mixed chimerism could reveal an eventual relapse earlier. But the quantification of donor's DNA markers is more precise estimated by the FA.

Keywords: allo-hSCT, chimerism monitoring, diallelic indel polymorphisms, PCR-STR, rare diseases

1. Introduction

Bone marrow transplantation is widely used for many different kinds of haematological malignancies such as leukaemias/lymphomas and immunodeficiency which are rare diseases. Over the past decades, allogeneic haematopoietic stem cell transplantation (allo-hSCT) has gained increasing importance as a treatment option for patients with both malignant and non-malignant life-threatening disorders in adult as well as paediatric patients. High risk leukaemias that are indicated for allo-hSCT are acute myeloid leukaemia (AML) [1], acute lymphoblastic leukaemia (ALL) and chronic myeloid leukaemia (CML) resistant to tyrosine-kinase inhibitor targeted treatment [2]. Also, myelodysplastic syndrome (MDS) and many other non-malignant disorders (bone marrow failure syndromes, haemoglobinopathies, immunodeficiencies and osteopetrosis) can profit from allo-hSCT [3].

Considerable progress has been made in the analysis of haematopoietic chimerism afterwards, and the molecular monitoring of the genotypic origin of engrafted cells has become a routine diagnostic tool to document engraftment and to detect graft rejection or impending relapse, at most centres performing allogeneic hSCT [4]. The term 'chimerism' was introduced in the field of medicine by Anderson et al. [5] to describe organisms whose cells derive from two or more zygote lineages. Close surveillance of chimerism within total peripheral blood leukocytes after an allogeneic hSCT seems an indispensable tool for the clinical management of transplant recipients [6]. In order to identify donor cells and even small amounts of residual host cells, many genetic methods have been established for this purpose. Cytogenetics and fluorescence in situ hybridization (FISH) analysis are the older ones and are applicable only in sex-mismatched transplantations where the proportion of X and Y chromosomes are detected [7]. The variability between individuals can be found both on the phenotype and on the genotype levels, especially in non-coding areas of the DNA. The later can be used not only in the population genetics, evolutionary studies and forensic and paternity proofs but also in the medicine as appropriate DNA informative markers to identify the donor and the recipient (host; patient) on the molecular level and monitor chimerism after allo-hSCT. For sex-independent patient chimerism monitoring, the PCR-based analyses of highly polymorphic short tandem repeats (STR; PCR-STR) DNA markers with subsequent fragment analysis ('FA') on Genetic Analyser are frequently used [8, 9]. Single-nucleotide polymorphism (SNP) or nucleotide polymorphisms (NPs) assessment by relative quantification SYBR Green-based real-time PCR, ('RQ PCR') Real-time PCR and semi-nested real-time PCR are used less [10–12], but due to increased interest in diallelic insertion/deletion polymorphisms 'DIPs' [13, 14], many new commercially kits for chimerism monitoring are available. In spite of the different analytical approaches to detect post-transplant chimerism, it seems to be useful to explain some common features. The term 'complete chimerism' (CC) expresses the status, where only the donor genotype is detected in the patient blood sample after allo-hSCT by the certain method. The term 'mixed chimerism' (MC) expresses the status, where both donor and recipient (host) genotypes are detected in the patient blood sample after allo-hSCT by the certain method. However, the post-transplant chimerism is a dynamic process. Several days, weeks, or months after allo-hSCT, the mixed chimerism is usually slowly changed to complete donor chimerism named 'decreasing mixed chimerism'. Vice versa in the case of a relapse when autologous haematopoiesis is appeared often the complete chimerism becomes to the status of mixed chimerism named 'increasing chimerism'. The coexistence of donor and recipient haematopoiesis for months or a longer period (especially in non-malignant disorders) is named 'stable mixed chimerism' [3].

In following chapters, we would like to describe not only two different DNA molecular methods ('FA' and 'RQ PCR'), which have been used in chimerism monitoring after allo-hSCT in our laboratories, but also its comparison from our results.

2. PCR-STR DNA markers in chimerism monitoring by 'FA'

2.1 Introduction

Quantitative monitoring of chimerism after allo-hSCT based on PCR amplification of microsatellite STR markers has become an important component of post-transplant surveillance of patients. Each STR marker is a system of many alleles, all sharing the basic structure of a repeat (2–8 bp in length), (4–5 bp in our study) but differing in the number of tandem repeats of this sequence. They can be applied for follow-up of virtually all patients and only small amounts of DNA are required for the test to estimate to donor/recipient chimerism after allo-hSCT [15–17]. Quantitative chimerism monitoring can document engraftment, predict graft failure or rejection, identify those patients who are at the highest risk to develop relapse and clarify the origin of the cells after relapse [18–23].

2.2 Methods

The PCR-based STR (PCR-STR) DNA markers were amplified using fluorescently labelled allele-specific primers, and different amplicons were separated by capillary electrophoresis on Genetic analyser. The direct quantification of donor and recipient PCR-STR DNA markers was provided by fragment analysis (FA) of GeneMapper software (Applied Biosystems) [20, 24–28].

2.3 Sample collection

Whole peripheral blood samples were collected for DNA extraction from both the donor and recipient before transplantation in order to determine an informative STR marker. The samples were collected at weekly or monthly intervals during the first 100 days, and monthly or every 2–3 months thereafter during the first year according to the transplantation centre. During the second year, the frequency was reduced to twice a year, only if the clinical situation warranted, more frequent chimerism analyses were performed.

2.4 DNA extraction

Genomic DNA was extracted from 200 μl of fresh or frozen peripheral blood using a column-based DNA isolation technique (Qiagene DNA Blood mini kit, QIAGEN, Hilden, Germany) according to the manufacturer's instructions. DNA quantification was performed using standard UV absorption at 260 nm, and DNA samples were stored until use at −80°C. To obtain an informative STR system for chimerism analysis, we performed a donor/recipient genotyping using a commercially available STR multiplex amplification kit PowerPlex 16 (Promega, Madison, WI, USA) that contains tetranucleotide STR markers, e.g. D18S51, D21S11, TH01 and D3S1358, as well as pentanucleotide STRs Penta E and Penta D and the primers specific for the Amelogenin locus [27, 28].

2.5 PCR amplification

About 10–50 ng of genomic DNA and BioThermStar DNA polymerase (GeneCraft, Lüdinghausen, Germany) instead of AmpliTaq Gold DNA polymerase (Applied Biosystems, Foster City, CA, USA) in some reactions. The denaturation, annealing and extension cycles were programmed in Techgene thermal cycler (Techne Inc., Burlington, NJ, USA) as follows: preincubation 95°C for 10 min, 96°C for 1 min, 10 cycles with 96°C/30 s, 60°C/30 s, 70°C/45 s and 14 and 18 cycles with 96°C/30 s, 60°C/30 s, 70°C/45 s for monoplex and multiplex kits, respectively, and final elongation step performed at 60°C for 30 min.

2.6 Fragment analysis

For fragment analysis, a mixture of 1 μl of the PCR product with 8.5 μl deionised formamide and 0.5 μl of the size standard ILS 600 (Promega, Madison, WI, USA) was prepared and was subjected to capillary electrophoresis in an ABI Prism 3100-Avant Genetic Analyser (Applied Biosystems, Foster City, CA, USA). The injection times varied between 4 and 36 s. Fragment length and fluorescence intensity were analysed using GeneMapper Software (Applied Biosystems, Foster City, CA, USA), and the detection threshold was set for 50 RFU. The selection of informative STR loci was based on previously described experiences [29, 30], where in such loci donor and recipient alleles should be individually distinguishable [15, 18].

2.7 Chimerism in adult malignant disease following hSCT monitored by 'FA'

2.7.1 Cohort

The cohort consisted of 169 adult and paediatric malignant patients from three Slovak bone marrow transplantation centres who underwent allo-hSCT between the years 1993 and 2010, and chimerism analysis of polymorphic STR markers was performed by 'FA'. A prospective evaluation of chimerism was performed in 171 patients transplanted after the year 2003 also by 'FA' from fresh or frozen DNA samples which were available.

2.7.2 Methods

The method included PCR-based analysis (with fluorescent allele specific primers) of short tandem repeats (PCR-STR) markers by fragment analysis ('FA') following capillary electrophoresis in Genetic analyser.

2.7.3 Results

The chimerism analysis of transplant patients was done for the first time no later than 1 month after allo-hSCT and further on 1–4 weekly intervals up to day +200 after transplantation and then according to the chimerism result and the timing of clinical controls. Patients who showed no evidence of autologous (recipient) DNA at any time in the post-transplantation follow-up were considered to have complete chimerism (CC). Patients with both donor and recipient DNA in any of the samples analysed were defined as having mixed chimerism (MC). An example of patient's mixed chimerism is presented in **Figure 1**. The average quantity of donor alleles 30.2 and 31.2 is 77%. The average quantity of recipient's alleles 16 and 25.2 is 23%, which means patient's mixed chimerism is 23% (MC = 23%). Patients who showed an increase (5% or more) in the proportion of recipient DNA or who changed from CC to any level of MC between two consecutive assessments were referred as having increasing MC. Those patients with decreasing recipient DNA content (5% or more) or transforming from MC to CC in two successive samples were categorised

DOI: http://dx.doi.org/10.5772/intechopen.89845

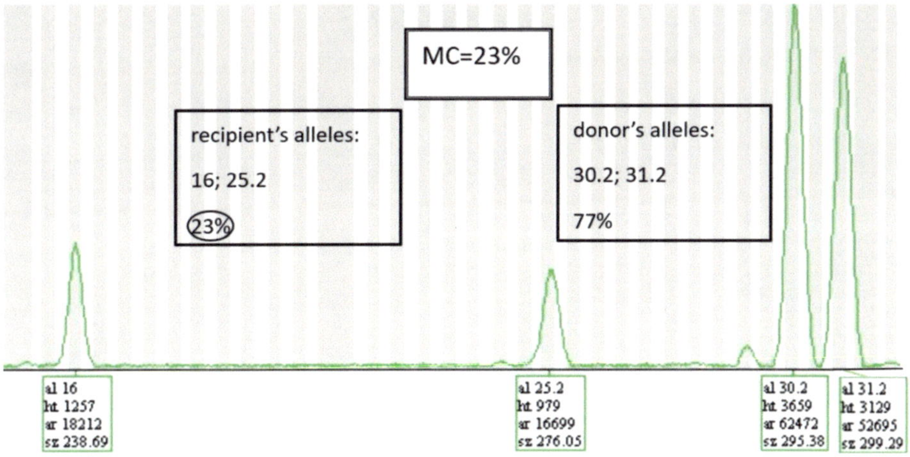

Figure 1.
Mixed chimerism (MC) in a patient after allo-hSCT

as having decreasing MC [26, 31]. Patients from our cohort with CC, stable MC, and decreasing MC showed a significantly better (p = 0.005) overall survival rate (OSR = 0.83) after allo-hSCT (**Figure 2**), compared to those with increasing MC (OSR = 0.25) after allo-hSCT (**Figure 3**) detected at any time after allo-hSCT.

2.7.4 Conclusion

Our observation shows that chimerism analysis gives clear information about engraftment, its failure, or graft rejection but is not a sufficiently sensitive method to detect an imminent relapse in acute lymphoblastic leukaemia patients. According to the changes in chimerism status after transplantation, early implementation of immunotherapeutic measures such as rapid cessation of immunosuppression and donor lymphocyte infusion (DLI) with or without cytokine coadministration can be delivered as prophylaxis and seems to be highly efficacious in restoring CC and decreasing autologous cell contents [18, 27, 32].

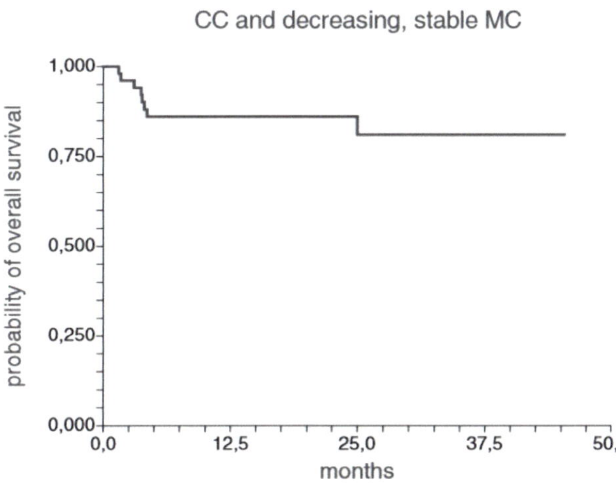

Figure 2.
Kaplan-Meier analysis of overall survival in patients with complete chimerism (CC), decreasing, stable mixed chimerism (MC) after allo-hSCT.

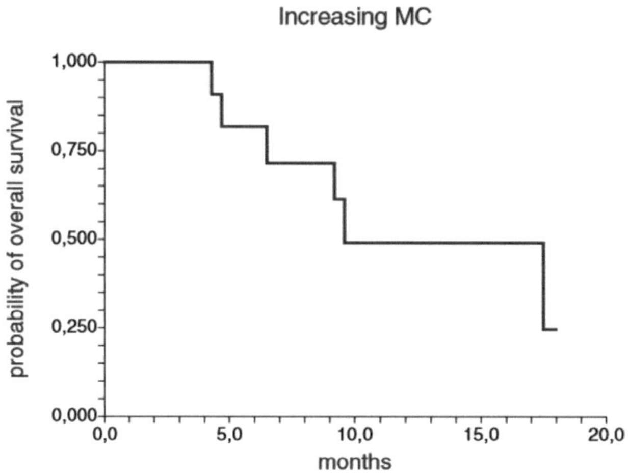

Figure 3.
Kaplan-Meier analysis of overall survival in patients with increasing mixed chimerism (MC) after allo-hSCT

2.8 Specific features of chimerism assessment in non-malignant diseases monitored by 'FA'

2.8.1 Introduction

Allo-hSCT is a well-established treatment not only for high risk leukaemias and myelodysplastic syndrome (MDS) but also for several non-malignant diseases, including acquired and inherited bone marrow failure (BMF) syndromes like aplastic anaemia (AA) and Fanconi anaemia (FA), immunodeficiencies like severe combined immunodeficiency (SCID), Wiskott–Aldrich syndrome (WAS), chronic granulomatous disease (CGD), haemoglobinopathies and metabolic disorders, mostly transplanted in childhood. The aim of transplantation in these diseases is to achieve sustained engraftment of donor stem cells to improve haematopoietic function, provide immune competence and increase or normalise enzyme deficiency. It can completely transform the lives of children for whom life expectancy or quality of life would otherwise be very poor. Although complete donor haematopoiesis is a desirable outcome of SCT in malignant disorders, complete replacement of recipient's haematopoietic system is not considered necessary to improve the underlying disease state in patients with non-malignant disorders [33, 34].

2.8.2 Cohort

The cohort consisted of 74 different adult and paediatric non-malignant patients from three Slovak bone marrow transplantation centres who underwent allo-hSCT.

2.8.3 Methods

The method included PCR-based analysis (with fluorescent allele specific primers) of short tandem repeats (PCR-STR) markers by fragment analysis ('FA') following capillary electrophoresis in Genetic analyser. Surveillance of chimerism was done within total peripheral blood leukocytes or as lineage-specific chimerism in selected T cells, B cells and myeloid cells after an allogeneic SCT according to Park et al. and Thiede [35, 36].

2.8.4 Results

Definition of chimerism, as it is described above considers a patient to have CC, when he does not show any evidence or less than 1% of autologous—recipient DNA at any time after allo-hSCT. Patients with both donor and recipient DNA (that increased 5% or more) in any of the samples analysed were defined as having MC. Split chimerism is present if one or more leukocyte lineages are of host and one or more leukocyte lineages are of donor origin [4, 36, 37].

As other studies mentioned above, also our results show there is a relationship between chimerism status and clinical course as well as outcome of allogeneic SCT in non-malignant diseases. From our cohort, 75% (55 patients) reached complete chimerism (CC) monitored by 'FA' and 25% (19 patients) mixed chimerism on different levels. Most of the patients with CC and decreasing or stable MC are alive doing well and are in remission, with a median follow-up time of 4.3 years. All of the patients with high MC (>40% or increasing MC) experienced transplant rejections and almost half of them died. Patients with CC had a higher risk of acute graft-versus host disease GVHD compared with MC patients.

2.8.5 Conclusion

Therefore, mixed chimerism (if there are still low levels of recipient cells) may be welcomed in these patients, as it reflects a decreased allo-response with less acute GVHD. Reduced intensity conditioning (RIC) was more often associated with decreasing or low stable MC compared to myeloablative conditioning, but importantly high MC was not different when using reduced intensity conditioning than with myeloablative conditioning [33, 34].

3. SNP and NP DNA markers in chimerism monitoring by 'RQ PCR'

3.1 Introduction

Chimerism monitoring allows the characterisation of the haematopoietic stem cell origin in the recipient's blood or bone marrow after allo-hSCT. The DNA identification of the person is mainly based on the DNA polymorphisms, which include single-nucleotide polymorphisms (SNPs) due to nucleotide substitutions and insertion or deletion of one or more nucleotides (indels). The late can be multiallelic (STR) and diallelic (biallelic). The extensive bibliographical search for human diallelic indels and its basic properties were determined and selected for chimerism monitoring [13, 38]. The sensitive quantitative real-time PCR analysis using indel polymorphisms can be the useful tool to predict relapse in leukaemia patients after allo-hSCT [39].

3.2 Complete and mixed chimerism monitoring by SYBR green-based real-time PCR method ('RQ PCR')

Tens of biallelic (diallelic) nucleotide polymorphisms specific for the donor and the recipient can be detected by the method of allele-specific real-time PCR.

3.2.1 Cohort

The cohort consisted of 188 patients from University Hospital Bratislava, Slovak Republic and 188 donors (111 from relatives and 77 from national and world registers of the bone marrow).

3.2.2 Methods

The DNA was isolated (NucleoSpin Blood, Macherey-Nagel) from peripheral blood leukocytes (centrifugation 3000 × g/10 min) before allo-hSCT from both donor and recipient and 30, 100, 180 and 365 days after allo-hSCT only from recipient (patient). Concentration of the DNA was measured on NanoPhotometer, Implen and samples were diluted to 10 ng/μl. To get allogenic and autologic informative markers for quantification after allo-hSCT, screening of donor and recipient DNA samples before allo-hSCT was essential. Three 1 μM allele-specific primers (two forward and one reverse or one forward and two reverse) for 11 biallelic nucleotide polymorphic markers were localised on 1st, 5th, 6th, 9th, 11th, 17th, 18th, 20th and X chromosome. Also, two pairs of specific primers (forward and reverse) for monoallelic DNA marker on Y chromosome (amelogenin) and for endogenic control gene GAPDH were used (**Figure 4**) [40]. The amounts for one-well allele-specific PCR reaction on 96-well plate were: 12.5 μl Power SYBR Green (PCR Master mix, Power SYBR green; Applied Biosystems), 1.25 μl 1 μM forward-primer (A or B) and1.25 μl 1 μM reverse primer (C) or vice versa (Sigma Genosys), 5 μl DNA (10 ng/ul), 5 μl DNase, RNase free water to final volume 25 μl. Thermal profile of 7300 Real Time PCR System (Applied Biosystems) for allele-specific PCR: 50°C/2 min, 1×; 95°C/10 min, 1×; (95°C/0.15 min, 60°C/1 min)/50×; and dissociation of amplicons with incorporated SYBR green: 94°C/0.15 min; 60°C/0.30 min; increasing 1°C/min; 95°C/0.15 min. Amplification curves from real-time PCR with following dissociation curves revealed type A, or B of marker (M) allele (MA or MB). For each donor/recipient pair, there are different informative markers for relative quantification and chimerism estimation after allo-hSCT. Relative quantification was calculated and evaluated from amplification plots of the individual PCR reactions on 96-well plate by the gene expression Study software (7300 System SDS Software, Applied Biosystems). Amplification plot of each informative marker before alloTKB was used as the calibrator for relative quantification of measured marker and amplification plot of gene GADPH was used as endogenous control [40].

3.2.3 Results

In most of screened donor/recipient pairs, we have found 2–3 informative autologous and allogeneic markers. An example of donor and recipient (patient) screening for informative NPs DNA markers (M1–M12) by SYBR green-based real-time PCR amplification and following dissociation curves is presented in **Figure 5**. For this donor/recipient pair, recipient's marker 3B (M3B) can be considered as informative autologous marker and can be used for chimerism monitoring after allo-hSCT. Only in three cases, we did not find any of the informative autological DNA markers, which are most convenient (detection <1%) for the measurement of micro chimerism. After allo-hSCT, informative DNA markers found in samples of patient's peripheral blood of patients were quantified. The relative amounts (expressed in %) were evaluated from threshold cycle (cT) values of amplification curves and analysed by Study Software, previously used for a relative quantification of the gene expression. The results of the DNA marker quantification measurements were obtained from (relative quantification) RQ and simultaneously from the charts, which had been constructed automatically [41] and transformed (**Figure 6**). In this figure, chimerism monitoring of AML patient after allo-hSCT is expressed. All patients were regularly monitored, and from the quantification of autologous informative DNA markers, mixed (MC) or

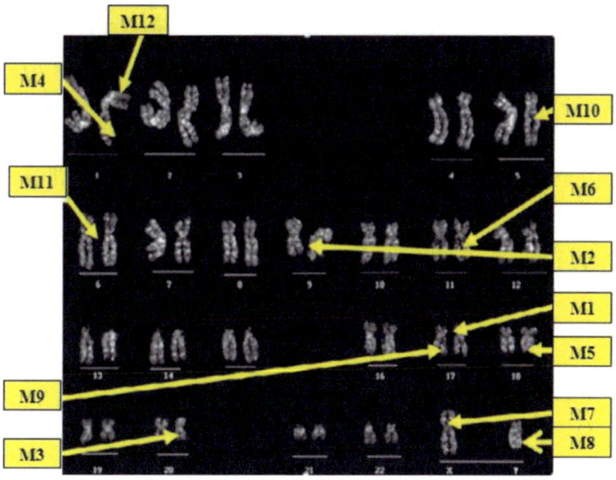

Figure 4.
Localisation of DNA markers (M1-M12) (11NPs).

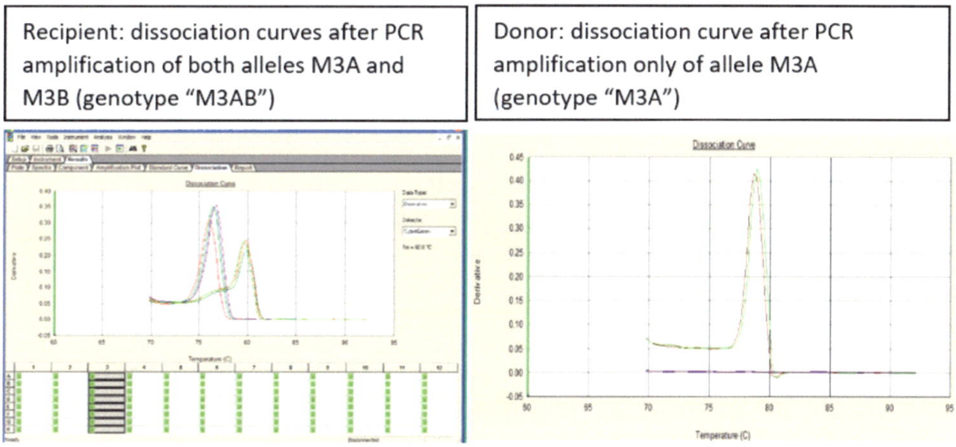

Figure 5.
An example of screening DNA markers M1-M12 by SYBR green based real-time amplification and following dissociation curves. Recipient's marker 3B can be used for chimerism monitoring after allo-hSCT.

complete (CC) chimerism was evaluated. Identification of donor allogenous informative markers have evaluated only semiquantitatively. Cutoff for CC was 0.01% with relative quantification sensitivity RQ = 0.0001. Special time-dependent charts for each patient were archived and sent to doctors in appropriate transplantation units.

3.2.4 Conclusion

We have implemented the method of DNA diagnostics for the detection of micro chimerism (add to cytogenetics and FISH previously used) after allo-hSCT, which is independent from the sex of donor and recipient and reaches sensitivity of <1% (0.01%). The method of relative quantification by real-time PCR is currently routinely used in our clinical practice and can serve clinician as another factor for the patients monitoring after haematopoietic stem cell transplantation and his early intervention if necessary.

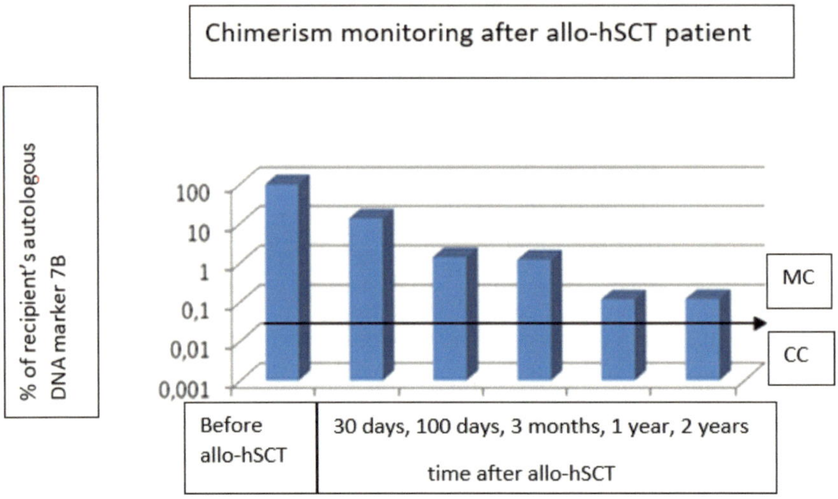

Figure 6.
Chimerism monitoring of AML patient after allo-hSCT by SYBR green based real-time PCR relative quantification method. MC, mixed chimerism; CC, complete chimerism.

3.3 Different malignant and non-malignant diagnosis in our study and their donors provided by 'RQ PCR'

3.3.1 Results

In our diagnostic laboratory, we have analysed samples from patients before and after allo-hSCT with different malignant and non-malignant diagnoses (**Figure** 7).

During the last decades, the number of allo-hSCT among *CML* patients is decreasing due to the drug-targeted treatment and transplantation is mostly indicated in the case of resistance to targeted tyrosine-kinase-inhibitor treatment. In our study, only 9 CML patients were transplanted from the cohort of 188 different malignant and non-malignant diagnosis (patients from University Hospital Bratislava, Slovak Republic), which is only 5%. The majority of allo-hSCT were provided and chimerism was monitored in AML patients (45%); then, ALL patients were 31% and MDS with others non-malignant diagnoses were 19% (11 + 8).

The selection of a donor is a critical element contributing to the success of haematopoietic cell transplantation. Possible donors for allo-hSCT can be HLA identical, haploidentical or mismatched (sibling, relative or unrelated donor). In our study, there were 188 donors (111 from relatives and 77 from Slovak National Bone Marrow Donor Registry and world registers of the bone marrow donors) and 188 recipients (**Table 1**). About 95% haemopoietic stem cells were obtained from peripheral blood by its drug mobilisation. Only 5% stem cells were from the bone marrow.

3.3.2 Conclusion

From our results, it is obvious that assessment of sex-independent donor/recipient method based on SYBR green real-time relative quantification RQ PCR) for chimerism monitoring has been very important due to cohort of different gender donor/recipient pairs. This molecular method has completed cytogenetics and FISH methods used previously for chimerism monitoring. The advantage of 'RQ PCR' compared to methods mentioned above is not only in its higher diagnostic and analytical sensitivity and sex-independent monitoring but also in the fact

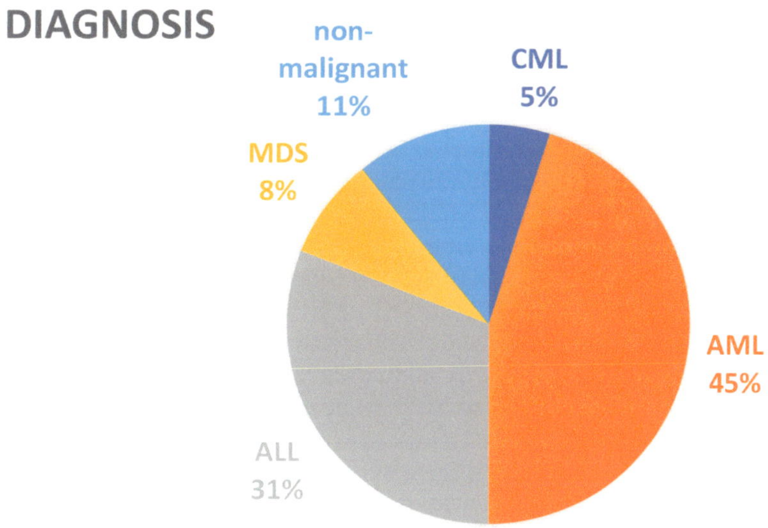

Figure 7.
Different malignant and non-malignant diagnosis in process of allo-hSCT

Types of recipient/donor in allo-hSCT	
Total number of transplant patients-recipients	188
Total number of donors	188
Related donors for allo-hSCT	**111**
Female/female	15
Male/male	42
Sex-mixed	54
Unrelated donors (MUD) for allo-hSCT	77
Female/female	9
Male/male	33
Sex-mixed	35

Table 1.
Types of recipient(patient)/donor variants in the process of allo-hSCT.

that almost 50% of AML patients has not genetic mutation marker to distinguish increasing mix chimerism and no indicator for relapse of primary patient disorder before allo-hSCT.

4. Chimerism evaluation by two different DNA marker sets and molecular methods 'FA' and 'RQ PCR'

4.1 Introduction

The aim of our study was to compare patient's chimerism monitoring by two different DNA marker type sets and molecular methods 'FA' and 'RQ PCR' measured in parallel after allo-hSCT [40, 42]. The subject matter of the first PCR-STR method 'FA' is explained in chapter '2—PCR-STR DNA markers in chimerism monitoring by "FA"'. Informative STR DNA markers were amplified with special fluorescent labelled primers by PCR. Amplicons were separated by the capillary electrophoresis on genetic analyser and then evaluated by fragment analyses GeneMapper software. The basis of the second method 'RQ PCR' (SYBR green-based relative quantification by real-time PCR) to be compared is discussed in the chapter "3—SNP and NPs DNA markers in chimerism monitoring by RQ PCR". Informative SNP and biallelic NP (including DIPs—IN/DEL polymorphic markers) DNA markers were obtained from donor's and recipient's DNA before transplantation by SYBR green-based real-time PCR amplification following dissociation curves analysing screening. Post allo-hSCT chimerism monitoring is provided by relative quantification (RQ-PCR) of SYBR green-based real-time PCR of SNP or NPs informative DNA markers and evaluated by gene expression software. The relative quantity of the donor's and recipient's DNA markers is proportional to total leukocytes and can be expressed as mixed (MC) or complete chimerism (CC) in post-transplant patients.

4.2 Cohort

The cohort consisted of 65 AML, ALL and CML patients from Department of Haematology and Transfusion, Comenius University Medical School Bratislava and 65 donors from national and international bone marrow registers according their HLA compatibility to the individual patient.

4.3 Methods

Whole peripheral blood samples were collected for DNA extraction from both the donor and recipient before transplantation in order to determine an informative marker for two molecular methods mentioned previously. The blood samples of leukaemia patients (AML, ALL and CML) after allo-hSCT (N = 65 pairs) were collected at regular time periods (before allo-hSCT and 30 days, 100 days, 6-month, 1 year, 2 years and 3 years after allo-hSCT) at the Department of Haematology and Transfusion, Comenius University Medical School Bratislava. Isolation of the DNA and chimerism testing was provided in two diagnostic laboratories: Laboratory Diagnostics Medirex, Bratislava and Bone Marrow Transplantation Unit, Bratislava, Slovak republic, EU. RQ-PCR was performed by the real-time PCR system using SYBR green and 12 pairs of specific primers for two allelic variants of DNA polymorphism and GAPDH as endogenous gene control. The cT (threshold cycle) values of informative patient's DNA markers before allo-hSCT were used as calibrator for the relative quantification. The PCR reaction mixtures and DNA were placed on 96-well reaction plates in duplicates separately, not as multiplex amplification set. Relative quantification was evaluated by gene expression software study [40]. The PCR-STR analysis was performed using commercially available STR multiplex amplification kits with fluorescently labelled PCR primers. The quantification of donor and recipient DNA marker's signal was provided by comparing the fluorescence intensity given by the peak area of analysed fragments [20].

4.4 Results

We screened 65 related and unrelated donor/recipient pairs by both molecular methods, and we found at least one informative marker for each laboratory approach mentioned above. The parallel quantifications of DNA (two different informative DNA marker sets used) were provided by both methods, and the estimated chimerism was compared at the same time period after the allogeneic haematopoietic stem cell transplantation. We found that our results were identical only in 2% and the discrepancy was noticed also in 2% between the two methods used. In the case of 1–50% mixed chimerism (MC), similar results were obtained. However, complete chimerism (CC) estimated by the fragment analysis was evaluated as mixed chimerism (MC) by the real-time PCR in 94% patients, mainly in the first half of a year of the post-transplantation monitoring. The example of the parallel monitoring of one patient is shown in **Figure 8**. From this presented results of patient chimerism monitoring, we can see that 30 days after allo-hSCT mixed chimerism was detected by both methods used (FA-MC and RQ PCR-MC). Also 1, 2 and 3 years after allo-hSCT, both methods showed identical complete chimerism results (FA-CC and RQ PCR-CC). But the discrepancy was revealed 100 days after allo-hSCT where complete chimerism was detected by the method FA (FA-CC), but simultaneously mixed chimerism was detected by RQ PCR method (RQ PCR-MC) in the same patient sample.

4.5 Conclusion

The parallel chimerism monitoring of post allo-hSCT leukaemia patients was provided for 3 years. Discrepancy between complete chimerism (CC) detected by the fragment analysis (FA) of PCR-STR DNA markers and mixed chimerism (MC) detected by the real-time PCR of SNP and NP DNA markers was due to the different sensitivity of two methods used. It is also important to note that in different molecular diagnostic approaches also, two different DNA marker sets were used. RQ PCR had the higher sensitivity (<1%) for the detection of the autologous DNA markers than FA (1–5%), so it is better for earlier revealing of eventual relapse. On the other hand, the quantification of donor's DNA markers is more precise estimated by the FA. Both methods compared above are suitable for chimerism assessment after

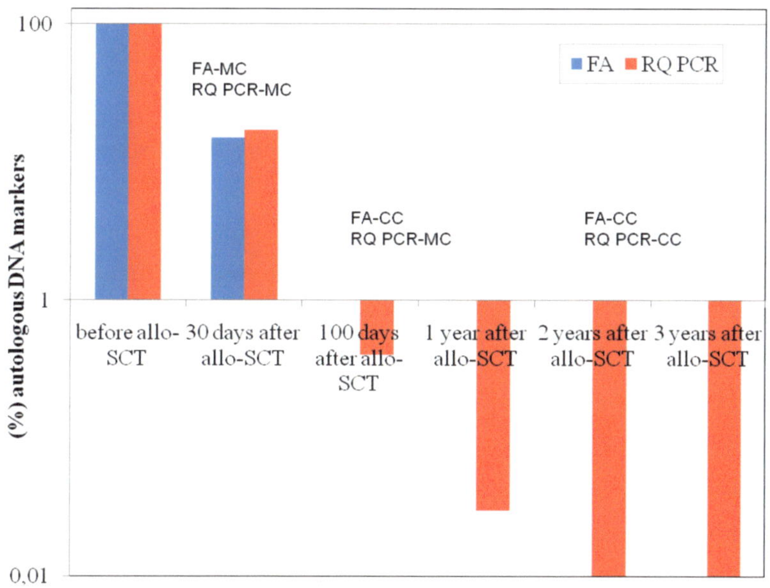

Figure 8.
Parallel monitoring of chimerism of one leukaemia patient after haematopoietic allogeneic stem cell transplantation (allo-hSCT) by two DNA molecular methods in different time periods. FA, analysis of PCR-STR DNA markers by fragment analysis following capillary electrophoresis on Genetic analyser; RQ-PCR, analysis of SNP and NPs DNA markers by relative quantification of SYBR green-based Real-time PCR; CC, complete chimerism (only donor's DNA markers detected in patient); MC, mixed chimerism (recipient's -autologous and donor's DNA markers detected in patient). 100 days after allo-SCT complete chimerism was detected by the method FA (FA-CC), but simultaneously mixed chimerism was detected by RQ PCR method (RQ PCR-MC) due to its different sensitivity.

the allogeneic haematopoietic stem cell transplantation, although nowadays many new kits with different DNA marker sets (STR, SNP, NPs and DIPs) for chimerism monitoring are available.

5. Conclusions

A number of studies have shown that chimerism evaluation based on PCR amplification of polymorphic microsatellite STR markers is a readily applicable technique, informative almost for all patients, but less sensitive then real-time PCR of SNP and NPs DNA method. It is important to notice that complete, mixed chimerism, decreasing chimerism, and increasing chimerism are only the relative terms, because different laboratories have their own criteria to differentiate between complete donor chimerism and mixed decreasing chimerism, based on the method that is used, its sensitivity and local policies [43–45]. However, both provide a powerful tool in post-transplant decision making. They can document engraftment, predict graft failure or rejection, identify those patients who are at the highest risk to develop relapse and clarify the origin of the cells after relapse. According to the changes in chimerism status after transplantation, early implementation of immunotherapeutic measures such as rapid cessation of immunosuppression and donor lymphocyte infusion (DLI) with or without cytokine coadministration can be delivered as prophylaxis and seems to be highly efficacious in restoring CC and decreasing autologous cell contents.

We appreciate the huge Human Genomic Project, because we can use its results also in our small labs and participate on the patient quality of life improvement by chimerism monitoring after allogeneic haematopoietic stem cell transplantation.

Acknowledgements

We thank our parents Milada with Alexander and Valeria with Julius for their example of a life fulfilled with enthusiasm dedicated to the research.

Conflict of interest

The authors declare no conflict of interest.

Abbreviations

ALL	acute lymphoblastic leukaemia
AML	acute myeloid leukaemia
allo-hSCT	allogeneic haematopoietic stem cell transplantation
AA	aplastic anaemia
BFM	bone marrow failure
CC	complete chimerism
CGD	chronic granulomatous disease
CML	chronic myeloid leukaemia
cT	threshold cycle
DIPs	diallelic insertion/deletion polymorphisms
DLI	donor lymphocyte infusion
DNA	deoxyribonucleic acid

FA	fragment analysis
GVHD	graft versus host disease
MC	mixed chimerism
MDS	myelodysplastic syndrome
NPs	nucleotide polymorphisms
OSR	overall survival rate
PCR	polymerase chain reaction
RQ-PCR	relative quantification real-time PCR
SCID	severe combined immunodeficiency
SNPs	single-nucleotide polymorphisms
STR	short tandem repeats
SYBR	Green intercalation dye
WAS	Wiskott–Aldrich syndrome

Author details

Eva Hanusovska[1*] and Sabina Sufliarska[2*]

1 St. Elizabeth University of Health and Social Sciences, Bratislava, Slovak Republic,

2 Children's Medical Practice, Bratislava, Slovak Republic

*Address all correspondence to: eva.hanusovska@gmail.com and sabina.sufliarska@gmail.com

References

[1] Okamoto Y et al. Hematopoietic stem-cell transplantation in children with refractory acute myeloid leukemia. Bone Marrow Transplantation. 2019;**54**(9):1489-1498

[2] Soyer N et al. Allogeneic stem cell transplantation in chronic myeloid leukemia patients: Single center experience. World Journal of Hematology. 2017;**6**(1):1-10

[3] Sullivan KM, Parkman R, Walters MC. Bone marrow transplantation for non-malignant disease. ASH Education Program Book. 2000;**2000**(1):319-338

[4] Khan F, Agarwal A, Agrawal S. Significance of chimerism in hematopoietic stem cell transplantation: New variations on an old theme. Bone Marrow Transplantation. 2004;**34**(1):1

[5] Anderson D et al. The use of skin grafting to distinguish between monozygotic and dizygotic twins in cattle. Heredity. 1951;**5**(3):379

[6] Muller-Berat N, Lion T. Chimerism and Transplant-Related Diagnostics. Leukemia. 2006;**20**:1358-1360

[7] Turkiewicz D et al. Monitoring of hematopoietic chimerism after sex-mismatched allogeneic stem cell transplantation (alloSCT) by dual-color FISH analysis of X and Y chromosomes. Leukemia Research. 2003;**27**(11):993-998

[8] Thiede C et al. Rapid quantification of mixed chimerism using multiplex amplification of short tandem repeat markers and fluorescence detection. Bone Marrow Transplantation. 1999;**23**(10):1055

[9] Ahci M et al. Clinical utility of quantitative PCR for chimerism and engraftment monitoring after allogeneic stem cell transplantation for hematologic malignancies. Biology of Blood and Marrow Transplantation. 2017;**23**(10):1658-1668

[10] Horky O et al. Increasing hematopoietic microchimerism is a reliable indicator of incipient AML relapse. International Journal of Laboratory Hematology. 2011;**33**(1):57-66

[11] Bai L et al. A SYBR green-based real-time PCR method for detection of haemopoietic chimerism in allogeneic haemopoietic stem cell transplant recipients. European Journal of Haematology. 2006;**77**(5):425-431

[12] Bach C et al. Monitoring of hematopoietic chimerism by real-time quantitative PCR of micro insertions/deletions in samples with low DNA quantities. Transfusion Medicine and Hemotherapy. 2015;**42**(1):38-45

[13] Weber JL et al. Human diallelic insertion/deletion polymorphisms. American Journal of Human Genetics. 2002;**71**(4):854-862

[14] Mills RE et al. An initial map of insertion and deletion (INDEL) variation in the human genome. Genome Research. 2006;**16**(9):1182-1190

[15] Kristt D et al. Hematopoietic chimerism monitoring based on STRs: Quantitative platform performance on sequential samples. Journal of Biomolecular Techniques: JBT. 2005;**16**(4):380

[16] Baron F, Sandmaier B. Chimerism and outcomes after allogeneic hematopoietic cell transplantation following nonmyeloablative conditioning. Leukemia. 2006;**20**(10):1690

[17] Bryant E, Martin PJ. Documentation of engraftment and characterization of chimerism following hematopoietic cell transplantation. In: Thomas' hematopoietic cell transplantation. 3rd ed. Wiley Online Library, Blackwell Publishing Ltd.; 2004. pp. 234-243

[18] Bader P et al. Increasing mixed chimerism is an important prognostic factor for unfavorable outcome in children with acute lymphoblastic leukemia after allogeneic stem-cell transplantation: Possible role for pre-emptive immunotherapy? Journal of Clinical Oncology. 2004;**22**(9):1696-1705

[19] Beck JF et al. Relapse of childhood ALL, AML and MDS after allogeneic stem cell transplantation can be prevented by donor lymphocyte infusion in a critical stage of increasing mixed chimerism. Klinische Pädiatrie. 2002;**214**(4):201-205

[20] Dubovsky J et al. Kinetics of chimerism during the early post-transplant period in pediatric patients with malignant and non-malignant hematologic disorders: Implications for timely detection of engraftment, graft failure and rejection. Leukemia. 1999;**13**(12):2060

[21] Ataergin S et al. Donor cell leukemia in a patient developing 11 months after an allogeneic bone marrow transplantation for chronic myeloid leukemia. American Journal of Hematology. 2006;**81**(5):370-373

[22] Bland JM, Altman DG. Statistical methods for assessing agreement between two methods of clinical measurement. International Journal of Nursing Studies. 2010;**47**(8):931-936

[23] Wäsch R et al. Rapid achievement of complete donor chimerism and low regimen-related toxicity after reduced conditioning with fludarabine, carmustine, melphalan and allogeneic transplantation. Bone Marrow Transplantation. 2000;**26**(3):243-250

[24] Chalandon Y et al. Quantitative analysis of chimerism after allogeneic stem cell transplantation by PCR amplification of microsatellite markers and capillary electrophoresis with fluorescence detection: The Geneva experience. Leukemia. 2003;**17**(1):228-231

[25] Koehl U et al. Quantitative analysis of chimerism after allogeneic stem cell transplantation by PCR amplification of microsatellite markers and capillary electrophoresis with flourescence detection: The Frankfurt experience. Leukemia. 2003;**17**(1):232-236

[26] Kreyenberg H et al. Quantitative analysis of chimerism after allogeneic stem cell transplantation by PCR amplification of microsatellite markers and capillary electrophoresis with flourescence detection: The Tuebingen experience. Leukemia. 2003;**17**(1):237-240

[27] Lion T. Summary: Reports on quantitative analysis of chimerism after allogeneic stem cell transplantation by PCR amplification of microsatellite markers and capillary electrophoresis with fluorescence detection. Leukemia. 2003;**17**(1):252-254

[28] Schraml E et al. Quantitative analysis of chimerism after allogeneic stem cell transplantation by PCR amplification of microsatellite markers and capillary electrophoresis with flourescence detection: The Vienna experience. Leukemia. 2003;**17**(1):224-227

[29] Thiede C, Bornhäuser M, Ehninger G. Evaluation of STR informativity for chimerism testing - comparative analysis of 27 STR system

in 203 matched related donor recipient pairs. Leukemia. 2004;**18**(2):248-254

[30] Thiede C, Bornhäuser M, Ehninger G. Strategies and clinical implications of chimerism diagnostics after allogeneic hematopoietic stem cell transplantation. Acta Haematologica. 2004;**112**(1-2):16-23

[31] Barrios M et al. Chimerism status is a useful predictor of relapse after allogeneic stem cell transplantation for acute leukemia. Haematologica. 2003;**88**(7):801-810

[32] Peggs KS et al. Dose-escalated donor lymphocyte infusions following reduced intensity transplantation: Toxicity, chimerism, and disease responses. Blood. 2004;**103**(4):1548-1556

[33] Sufliarska S et al. Establishing the method of chimerism monitoring after allogeneic stem cell transplantation using multiplex polymerase chain reaction amplification of short tandem repeat markers and Amelogenin. Neoplasma. 2007;**54**(5):424-430

[34] Svenberg P et al. Allogeneic hematopoietic SCT in patients with non-malignant diseases, and importance of chimerism. Bone Marrow Transplantation. 2009;**44**(11):757-763

[35] Park M et al. Clinical implications of chimerism after allogeneic hematopoietic stem cell transplantation in children with non-malignant diseases. Korean Journal of Hematology. 2011;**46**(4):258-264

[36] Thiede C. Diagnostic chimerism analysis after allogeneic stem cell transplantation: New methods and markers. American Journal of Pharmacogenomics. 2004;**4**(3):177-187

[37] Willasch A et al. Outcome of allogeneic stem cell transplantation in children with non-malignant diseases. Haematologica. 2006;**91**(6):788-794

[38] Alizadeh M et al. Quantitative assessment of hematopoietic chimerism after bone marrow transplantation by real-time quantitative polymerase chain reaction. Blood. 2002;**99**(12):4618-4625

[39] Jacque N et al. Chimerism analysis in peripheral blood using indel quantitative real-time PCR is a useful tool to predict post-transplant relapse in acute leukemia. Bone Marrow Transplantation. 2015;**50**(2):259-265

[40] Hanušovská E et al. The role of DNA diagnostics in chimerism analysis after allogeneic hematopoietic stem. Cell Transplantation. 2013;**62**:211-217

[41] Hanušovská E. Assessment of chimerism after allogeneic hematopoietic transplantation using SYBR green-based real-time PCR analysis of DNA polymorphism. In: 16thCongress of the European Hematology Association (EHA); 9-12 June 2011; London, United Kingdom. haematologica; 2011

[42] Šufliarska S. Dlhodobé sledovanie pacientov po alogénnej transplantácii krvotvorných buniek. In: Lekárska fakulta. 2. detská klinika. UKOLF2DK, Bratislava Slovakia: Univerzita Komenského; 2010. p. 117

[43] Roug AS, Ommen HB. Clinical use of measurable residual disease in acute myeloid leukemia. Current Treatment Options in Oncology. 2019;**20**(4):28

[44] Tyler J et al. Personalized Chimerism test that uses selection of short tandem repeat or quantitative PCR depending on Patient's Chimerism status. The Journal of Molecular Diagnostics. 2019;**21**(3):483-490

[45] Bader P. Documentation of engraftment and chimerism after HSCT. In: Carreras E et al, editors. The EBMT handbook. Hematopoietic Stem Cell Transplantation and Cellular Therapies. Springer Open; 2019. pp. 143-147

Section 6

Policy Regulation and Data Sharing of Rare Diseases

Chapter 15

International Data Sharing and Rare Disease: The Importance of Ethics and Patient Involvement

Adrian Thorogood

Abstract

Improving our understanding of rare disease and developing new therapies can only succeed through global collaboration. Whole genome sequencing is increasingly being deployed to diagnose rare disease, and can be combined with machine-learning tools that analyze patient photos to identify phenotypes. Clinical interpretation of genomes and phenotypic data in rare disease depends on sharing individual patient data internationally. Data sharing is essential in rare disease contexts, to support the diagnosis of patients, recruitment into trials, the development of precision diagnostics and therapies, and clinical trial transparency. The sharing of rich molecular and phenotypic data presents privacy risks for rare disease patients, though many want to see their data made available to improve their care and advance research. Informed consent, access governance, and access technologies are important to realize the benefits of data sharing while mitigating risks. Rare disease patients should be involved in the design of data sharing governance to ensure it responds to their particular needs and preferences.

Keywords: rare disease, data sharing, law, ethics, consent, privacy, patient involvement

1. Introduction

There is great interest in adopting data-intensive approaches as part of both care pathways and research in rare disease contexts. Indeed, many rare diseases "have no treatments, are incurable, and have a devastating impact on patients and their families" [1]. One of the first areas where whole-genome sequencing is already demonstrating clinical utility is in helping to provide a genetic diagnosis of individuals with rare disease [2]. Whole-genome sequencing can be a powerful tool to resolve diagnoses for patients with rare disease. Receiving a timely and accurate diagnosis can have a number of direct benefits for patients, "enabling a better understanding of their prognosis, more personalized treatment and tailored management and surveillance" [3]. An ethics report from Canada's health technology assessment body, CADTH, recently concluded that genome sequencing could be effective for patients with unexplained developmental disabilities and multiple congenital abnormalities, if responsibly administered [4].

Data-intensive medicine is powered by data sharing. Data sharing practice and policy has long been a hallmark of genomic research. Many health research funders and journals now require researchers to deposit sequence data in repositories or otherwise make data available to the broader research community. "Data sharing enables researchers to rigorously test the validity of research findings, strengthen analyses through combined datasets, reuse hard-to-generate data, and explore new frontiers of discovery" [5]. Data sharing in health care contexts is also growing in importance. The American College of Medical Genetics and Genomics (ACMG), for example, "advocates for extensive sharing of laboratory and clinical data from individuals who have undergone genomic testing" [6]. Data sharing is expected to have a range of benefits, including improving the diagnoses of other patients, informing the development of diagnostic approaches and tools, and powering research. Some have even argued that sharing minimal information about variant interpretations should be the standard of care in genetics [7].

Data sharing is of particular importance in rare disease contexts. Making a diagnosis is often dependent on many forms of data sharing. Databases of population genetic variation are needed as a reference to help filter out benign variants from test results. Comparison of family trios can help filter candidate disease-causing variants even further. Making a genetic diagnosis available through publications or public genetic variant databases can offer confirmation and can inform and accelerate the diagnosis of future patients. Data-intensive approaches are not limited to genomic data. Facial recognition technologies such as Face2Gene can inform diagnosis based on images of facial morphology [8]. Because the meaning of all this data is not fully understood, data-intensive medicine for rare disease depends on adoption of a learning health system approach. In learning health systems, rich data are generated as part of routine clinical care and are subsequently made available for quality improvement and research. Data sharing between rare disease clinicians, laboratories and scientists can help to refine interpretive techniques and analysis pipelines. Images and videos of facial morphology can be used to train machine-learning algorithms and improve diagnostic tools [9].

The impetus to make genomic and health-related data collected as part of routine clinical care available for research is stronger in the rare disease context, where there are numerous barriers and limited incentives. These data could also serve as a rich resource for natural history studies to better understand the progression of rare diseases, for biomarker discovery, as registries to recruit patients into precision clinical trials, and as a resource for ongoing surveillance of the clinical and cost effectiveness of rare disease therapies.

Biobanking and biobank networks are essential infrastructure for genomic research, which require collection and analysis of biospecimens [10]. Biobanks are organized collections of samples and associated data. Samples have to be collected, stored, and shared following scientific and technical standards in order to be comparable. Biobanks must meet standards of quality and size to be scientifically valuable. Biobank networks are established to enable aggregation of samples and data from geographically disperse patients. This is essential in the rare disease context. Fostering standardization is a complicated challenge for biobank networks. In the era of Big Data, the value of biobanks increasingly lies in their datafication. Datafication includes: (1) the collection of rich associated demographic, health and clinical information about patients, and (2) the analysis of samples to generate molecular, imaging or other forms of biological data. Of course, the quality and compatibility of data collected or generated is also essential to aggregation of data across biobank networks. In order to attract researchers and additional resources to understudied areas like rare disease, biobank networks and datafication are key. This article will focus primarily on data sharing, but the reader should keep in mind that the generation of data from biological samples is an essential step, one that is organizationally and scientifically non-trivial.

Little will be achieved for rare disease patients without collaboration and international data sharing. No single institution, laboratory, or even country is likely to encounter a sufficient number and diversity of patients with a given rare disease to be able to advance research alone. In the next section, I review some major data-driven initiatives to improve rare disease care and research. These learning health system approaches, powered by international data sharing, are essential to deliver data-intensive medicine for rare disease. International data sharing does raise concerns about the privacy of patients with rare disease. I discuss issues of privacy and consent in data-intensive rare disease medicine and research. However, it is important to note that many rare disease patients want to make their data available to improve their care and to support research. It is therefore important that patients are involved in the development and implementation of data sharing governance to ensure the benefits of data sharing are achieved while managing risks to patient privacy.

2. Rare disease data sharing initiatives

This section discusses the importance of data sharing for rare disease, across the research lifecycle, from diagnosis and basic research, to clinical trial transparency, to health technology assessment.

2.1 Diagnosis and drug discovery

A number of national and international initiatives have emerged to demonstrate the potential of data to improve rare disease patient care and to accelerate research. All of these initiatives seek to adopt data-intensive approaches to accelerate rare disease diagnosis. They adopt learning health system strategies, which involve collecting rich data as part of routine clinical care and making these data available for research to improve diagnostics and therapies. Finally, the initiatives all recognize the importance of international data sharing in the rare disease context.

The Genomics England 100,000 Genomes Project has "committed to sequencing 100,000 whole human genomes, from 70,000 patients, by the end of 2018" [11], with a focus on rare and infectious diseases [12]. This project will facilitate the introduction of genomic medicine in NHS care while contributing to the personalization of its medicine [11]. Clinicians are hoping to achieve earlier diagnoses and develop more effective treatments with this data [13]. Researchers also hope to gain a better understanding of cancer.

Genome Canada has proposed a national, clinical genomics project, which aims to advance precision medicine for all Canadians, with an initial pilot focused on rare disease [14]. The proposal is to introduce genomic testing as part of clinical care. The data will then be made available as a research platform. The vision is to establish a national cohort, perhaps through a federation of provincial datasets.

The European Joint Program on Rare Diseases (EJP RD) brings 130 institutions together across 27 EU Member States as well as Canada, Armenia, Georgia, Israel, Norway, Serbia, Switzerland and Turkey, to accomplish its two main goals: [15].

1. "To ***improve*** the integration, the efficacy, the production and the social impact of research on [rare disease] through the development, demonstration and promotion of Europe/world-wide sharing of research and clinical data, materials, processes, knowledge and know-how

2. To ***implement*** and further *develop* an efficient model of financial support for all types of research on [rare disease] (fundamental, clinical, epidemiological,

social, economic, health service) coupled with accelerated exploitation of research results for benefit of patients" [15].

To achieve its objectives, the EJP-RD has developed a five pillars structure subdivided in various themes and activities such as Joint Transnational Calls for collaborative research projects; a common virtual platform for discoverable data and resources for rare disease research; capacity building and training of patients and researchers in rare disease research and processes, all to accelerate the validation, use and development of innovative methodologies tailored for clinical trials in rare diseases [15].

Through the Breaking Barriers to Health Data Project, the World Economic Forum is "partnering with genomics institutes in the United Kingdom, the United States, Canada and Australia" [16] to pilot a governance framework "to support the effective and responsible use of federated data systems to advance rare disease diagnostic and treatment-related research" [16]. Federated data systems enable researchers to query a distributed network of secure databases. The individual-patient data remains hidden in each of the secure nodes. This pilot project aims to demonstrate a proof-of-concept for federated data systems, accompanied with an economic analysis and a scalable governance framework [16].

An example of a commercial initiative to overcome the geographic barriers to rare disease research is the start-up RDMD [17]. This company aims to generate a rich, regulatory-grade biobank, database, and registry of patients with rare disease from across the United States (US) and internationally. The start-up leverages the rights of patients in the US and in other countries to request access to their health records and biospecimens for onward transfer to RDMD. RDMD then looks to enter into partnerships with pharmaceutical companies to accelerate their research into rare disease therapies. Patients are provided with access to their aggregated and structured medical record through an app.

2.2 Clinical trial transparency

Improving the transparency of clinical trials has been an important public health priority for regulators and policy-makers in recent years. Clinical trial transparency encompasses the registration of clinical trials before recruitment, the timely dissemination of results—whether positive or negative, and the sharing of individual patient data supporting those results [18]. Sharing of individual patient data enables reproducibility studies to confirm the validity of results, and facilitates meta-analyses. Transparency can also accelerate research and reduce duplicative trials that waste resources and expose participants to unnecessary risks. Regulators increasingly publish the clinical data submitted by pharmaceutical companies seeking market approval [19]. Some sponsors also proactively make individual patient data available. There are now several data sharing platforms that facilitate clinical trial data sharing, including Yale Open Data Access project (YODA) [20], ClinicalStudyDataRequest [21], and Vivli [22].

Ensuring that the results of clinical trials as well as the underlying data are made available is perhaps more important for rare disease clinical trials. Regulators sometimes allow more flexibility and accept greater clinical uncertainty to accelerate approvals of drugs for rare diseases with high unmet need. This is because of the "unique challenges that hinder efficient and effective traditional clinical trials, including low patient numbers, limited understanding of disease pathology and progression, variability in disease presentation, and a lack of established endpoints" [1]. Where there is greater uncertainty over the meaning of research data, there is a greater need for transparency to support regulators, prescribing physicians, and patients. Sharing individual patient data does raise concerns about patient privacy, discussed below. The tension between transparency and privacy, however, tends to be overstated, as benefits can be promoted and risks can be reduced through governance mechanisms. Moreover, rare disease patients are generally supportive of greater transparency, as long as their privacy is protected, appropriate steps are taken to seek their consent, and patient groups are involved in the design of data sharing governance.

2.3 Access to medicines

Even where approved medicines are available for rare disease, an additional hurdle is convincing health technology assessment bodies that these medicines—which are often very expensive per patient—are cost-effective [23]. There is often significant uncertainty over the clinical and economic value offered by rare disease therapies, in part because of the limits to generating clinical evidence in small patient populations. One potential solution to accelerate patient access is through managed access programs. Where countries offer these programs, drugs may be given early approval despite some uncertainty over value, under the condition of ongoing collection of data to fill in evidentiary gaps. Real world evidence is collected through post-market surveillance to confirm the drug delivers value. Post-market surveillance, however, is challenging and requires effective data sharing strategies and infrastructure. Moreover, it is important to involve patients in decisions to approve drugs where there is greater uncertainty over benefits and risks. Patient can also be engaged in establishing the conditions under which a drug would meet or fail to meet the conditions of a managed access agreement. Indeed, patients are increasingly involved in health technology assessment to ensure that the drugs are delivering the clinical, economic, and personal value that matters to them [24]. Given the diverse burdens of disease on rare disease patients and their caregivers, they have important perspectives on the true value that can be delivered by new therapies.

3. Privacy

Data-intensive medicine, and the research, biobanking, and data sharing that necessarily accompany it, all raise privacy concerns for patients. In the Big Data era, increasingly rich data are being generated as part of clinical care and research protocols. Traditionally, privacy in research was primarily protected by removing or separating identifiers from research data. Rich, multi-dimensional health data can no longer be definitively de-identified. Genomic data for example is rich, unique to the individual, stable over time, and shared across families. It also contains potentially sensitive information about the health predispositions of individuals and their families. Genomic data therefore raise particular concerns about the limits of de-identification [25]. But the problem is broader than just genomic data. A recent study also showed that 99.98% of American can be reidentified from a database with less than 15 demographic attributes [26]. Re-identification is increasingly seen as an inherent risk in research. This risk increases as the dimensionality of data increases, as more publicly available data becomes available, and as new statistical re-identification tools emerge. If patients are re-identified, sensitive information about their health may be disclosed to unauthorized third parties, including employers, insurers, and family members, and may be used to discriminate against or stigmatize the individual or their family. Sharing patient data with clinicians and researchers around the world may heighten concerns over privacy. Where data are copied and distributed to many different parties, there is a greater potential for a breach of confidentiality or security, and lower confidence that the breach will be identified and rectified.

Rare disease patients may face a greater risk of re-identification or subsequent harm. Rare disease patients may be easier to single-out in a dataset, given their unique genotypes and phenotypes, and the small number of participants in a study. Rich data is often collected or generated about rare disease patients, such as whole genome sequences and pictures and videos of their phenotypes. In order to match similar patients to inform a diagnosis, or to conduct a study with an acceptable sample size, information about rare disease patients must often necessarily be shared beyond institutions and national borders. Moreover, in part because of institutional and geographical barriers to care and participation in research, many rare disease patients share rich health information about themselves online with patient support groups or researchers. In fact, there are numerous academic and commercial research efforts that enable remote participation of rare disease patients to overcome geographic barriers [27]. The public availability of patient information could potentially increase the risk of re-identification in research datasets.

At the same time, many patients with rare disease see the important clinical and scientific value of data sharing and are willing to participate if research involves appropriate consent processes, safeguards, and patient involvement. A number of solutions have evolved to reduce the tension between privacy and openness. The first solution is to develop more transparent consents about how data are shared. This is recommended by the Global Alliance for Genomics and Health (GA4GH) Consent Policy [28]. Consent is discussed in greater detail in the next section. The second solution is through safeguards and governance, including robust de-identification, security protections, and access controls. Responsible data governance aims to maximize uses of data that benefit science and society, minimize risks to data subjects, and strike a proportionate balance where these interests come into conflict [29]. Risks of data breaches or misuse when sharing data can be significantly reduced through governance mechanisms including due diligence review of access requests by an expert committee, data access agreements that protect participant privacy, and ongoing monitoring of data use. Sharing data within secure cloud environments can enhance security and accountability by limiting the distribution of copies of datasets. Federated network technologies now allow researchers to submit search queries or run research analyses across multiple secure patient databases, without ever having to access the patient results. The World Economic Forum is exploring such an approach specifically for international rare disease research (see above). A third solution, also discussed below, is greater patient involvement in the design or research and data sharing governance, to ensure their input on priorities and the balancing of risks and benefits under uncertainty.

There is also a risk of too much privacy protection in the rare disease context. Data privacy laws are tightening globally in response to concerns over commercial and law enforcement surveillance practices. Europe's *General Data Protection Regulation* (GDPR) is now in force, and California will soon be introducing its own comprehensive consumer data privacy regime [30]. The GDPR imposes stricter, more formal procedural and security safeguards for the protection of personal data, particularly for special categories of data, for example, health and genetic. It also imposes higher consent standards with regards to the purposes of processing, and transfers between organizations and across borders. Different national and institutional interpretations of the GDPR have hampered international health research collaborations [31]. Formal legal safeguards and strict transparency requirements leave organizations with less flexibility to share samples and data about rare disease patients, especially internationally, even where researchers seek explicit patient consent and/or patient involvement in data sharing governance.

4. Consent

This section considers three issues concerning consent in data-intensive medicine for rare disease. The first concern is that it is impossible to fully specify all the potential users and uses of patient data at the time of collection. A common solution when seeking consent to research and sharing of samples and data is seeking broad consent to future not-fully-specified uses accompanied with ongoing governance. A second issue is re-use or sharing of legacy collections of samples and data that have significant scientific and societal value but where the original consent is absent or is silent about key matters. A third issue is consent in the pediatric context, which raises special concerns about capacity, protection from harm and exploitation, inclusion, and shared decision-making. Arguably, the tension between promoting science and respecting individual autonomy is greater in the rare disease context.

4.1 Broad consent

The International Rare Diseases Research Consortium (IRDiRC) in collaboration with the GA4GH has shared template consent clauses for rare disease research [32]. These clauses emphasize some of the special characteristics of rare disease research, such as the collection of photos and videos of patient phenotypes, the participation of and feedback of health findings to family members, as well as the imperative of international data sharing to support both research as well as to match patients to inform diagnoses. This initiative also demonstrates the importance of engaging patients in the development of research governance and consents.

Biobanking and data sharing aim to make samples and data available for research that cannot be fully specified at the time of recruitment and collection. This present risks to patient autonomy: how much information can and should be provided at the time of consent? What kinds of meaningful choices can and should be offered to patients about who can access their samples and data? As samples and data are typically stored for long periods of time, can and should patients be able to withdraw consent or change their preferences over time? Broad consent—consent to not-fully-specified research uses coupled with ongoing governance—has been adopted in many research contexts internationally, is now expressly permitted under the US Common Rule and recognized under the EU GDPR (rec 33) [33].

Especially where samples and data are collected in clinical care contexts, there is concern that sharing those samples and data for research may be done coercively, or that patients may have limited knowledge or comprehension. Moreover, rare disease patients may see data sharing as a necessity for receiving a diagnosis, or to advance research on a cure, and thus may feel compelled to forgo their privacy. Where consents cover a broad set of purposes, this can be seen as coercively tying purposes together, unless patients are given granular choices. But these kinds of arguments can result in inefficient sharing and use of data that precludes effective care and research, and that contradicts the wishes of many rare disease patients. Broad consent may be especially important in rare disease, given the scarcity of data and the risk of losing that data if every subsequent use is subject to re-consent. There is also an argument that rare disease data, again considering its scarcity, should be made available for a wide range of purposes, including diagnostic matchmaking, research to discover new biomarkers, natural history studies to better understand the nature of a rare disease, and the recruitment of individuals into precision medicine clinical trials. Generating multiple siloed resources for multiple different purposes is simply not feasible.

4.2 Legacy collections

Legacy collections of samples and data are those collected without consent or without consent covering core consent elements required to conduct research or data sharing. These collections present an ethical dilemma: they often continue to have great scientific and societal value if shared and used for research, but the consent to do so is missing or insufficient. This is particularly a problem in biobanking, where samples are often collected many years before they are able to be distributed, aggregated, or analyzed. As the years pass, scientific and data sharing practices can change, and regulatory and ethical frameworks can evolve. As a result, the existing consents may become insufficient. One could argue the ethical dilemma is even more pressing in rare disease contexts, because of the high unmet need for research into novel diagnostics and therapies, as well as the associated practical difficulties of recruiting geographically disperse patients and collecting samples.

Solutions have been developed for legacy collections that aim to strike an appropriate balance between making them available for research, while also making best efforts to communicate with and respect the expectations of patients. When seeking to study or share legacy collections, an important starting point is to assess the existing consent materials (if applicable) [34]. If core elements of consent are met, then the research may be able to proceed. If the consent is silent on the desired research or data sharing, then patients should be recontacted to renew their consent. If permitted by applicable norms, it may also be sufficient to notify the patients and provide them with an opportunity to opt-out. In many cases, however, re-consent or re-contact will be impossible if patients can no longer be found. In such cases, some jurisdictions allow research ethics committees (RECs) to alter or waive consent requirements, as long as certain conditions are met. In Canada for example, a consent alteration/waiver is available where research is minimal risk, consent is impracticable, the alteration/waiver will not adversely harm individuals, there are appropriate safeguards in place, and there has been no clear refusal by the individual (art 3.7B (samples); art 5.5A (identifiable information)) [35].

Where consent is silent, an ethics waiver may be more easily justified. Where consent makes a specific commitment (e.g., guarantees data will be kept confidential, or will only be used for a specific research project), it may be harder to justify a waiver. Because consent is often take-it-or-leave-it, however, it is not necessarily clear if the commitment was determinant to the patient's decision, or what the patient would have preferred. An active refusal by the patient to participate in research or data sharing is a more clear-cut case [36]. For example, the patient may have been offered the option to participate in research or to share their data and may have refused. Indeed, the revised US Common Rule for research on human subjects in the US prohibits use of an ethics waiver when a patient has rejected a broad consent (§46.116) [37]. Practically, however, given the limits of tracking systems, it is unclear how these refusals can be tracked and respected over time.

Typically, ethics waivers are used to approve a specific research project using legacy collections, but in some cases, they have also been used to approve the deposit of data into international databases for onward sharing. The GA4GH recommends ethics waivers under certain conditions for international sharing of genomic and health-related data [34].

A final consideration offering some additional flexibility in rare disease contexts is patient involvement. Patient groups or representatives may lend moral support to a particular interpretation of an existing consent, or to a particular decision to re-use or share legacy collections with an ethics waiver. This can help to alleviate uncertainty over what patients would have wanted in cases of uncertainty. If core consent elements are legally required, however, such modifications will not be possible.

4.3 Consent and capacity: pediatrics

An additional challenge that tends to be overlooked in data sharing discussions is that many patients with rare disease are minors, who are generally legally presumed to lack the capacity to consent to genetic testing, research participation, or release of personal data on their own [38]. Moreover, a number of rare diseases involve intellectual disability, which may diminish the decision making capacity of rare disease patients. Regulatory frameworks developed in the context of experimental research are traditionally protectionist, aiming to ensure vulnerable individuals are protected from harm and exploitation. These frameworks place several limitations on research involving minors. Where research is allowed, additional safeguards must be in place for minors. The guiding legal and ethical principle is the best interests of the child, though this principle is somewhat modified in the research context. A modified best interests limitation is only allowing research if it offers direct benefit to the individual or to individuals with a similar age or condition, and that the benefit is favorable vis-a-vis the individual risks, as determined by a REC. Where research is permitted, the minor is protected by parental (or legal guardian) representation, who must provide informed consent. The parent would be provided with detailed information about the research and would be asked to consent on behalf of the child.

This protectionist approach has been somewhat modified both by public health and human rights concerns. From a public health perspective, the inclusion of children in research is imperative to ensuring that the standard of care improves for conditions that predominantly affect children. Given the physiological differences between children and adults, drugs demonstrated to be safe and effective for adults may not be so for children. Human rights instruments and discussions have also highlighted the principle of non-discrimination, which argues that some attempts to protect children ultimately result in their exclusion from participation in society.

Another important human rights and ethical principle is respect for the developing autonomy of the child. Mature-minor exceptions address the developing capacity of minors to make decisions. These regimes allow exceptions for children below the age of majority to make certain their own decisions (e.g., for health care) if they demonstrate their capacity to understand information and appreciate the consequences of decisions. Regardless of who has ultimate legal capacity to consent, children should generally be given appropriate opportunities to be involved in decisions concerning them. Many health research ethics guidelines recommend that children should be involved in decisions through assent, where the child is provided with age appropriate information and asked if they would like to participate, and dissent, where a clear objection to participation must also generally be respected by researchers. Dissent is more clearly applicable in experimental research, such as distress caused by a needle, than in data-intensive research.

Based on the principle of inclusion, as well as practical implications, the GA4GH Pediatric Task Team has argued that those who generate pediatric data as part of research or clinical care have an obligation to offer minors and their parents an opportunity to share their data, so as to benefit the care of children in the future [39]. The best interests of the child are ensured in this context through the benefit–risk assessment, ongoing data governance (to maximize scientific and societal benefits while minimizing risk), parental representation and informed consent, and the child's involvement through assent processes.

5. Patient involvement

This section discusses patient involvement (also referred to as patient engagement) in the governance of research, challenges to involving patients effectively and responsibly, and how rare disease patients may be involved specifically in the governance of biobanking and data sharing.

Respect for communities is an important ethical principle in health research. According to Charles Weijer *et al.* researchers have "an obligation to respect the values and interests of the community in research and, wherever possible, to protect the community from harm" [40]. This principle is also prominently featured in the international health research ethics guidelines of the Council for International Organizations of Medical Sciences and World Health Organization: "[r]esearchers, sponsors, health authorities and relevant institutions should engage potential participants and communities in a meaningful participatory process that involves them in an early and sustained manner in the design, development, implementation, design of the informed consent process and monitoring of research, and in the dissemination of its results" (Guideline 7) [41]. Communities are not only defined geographically, but include subpopulations affected by or able to influence research. Patients affected by a particular condition are clearly a key stakeholder in related research.

The involvement of patients and patient advocacy organizations across the research, drug-development, and delivery of care life cycle is increasingly practiced and is the subject of numerous national and international research ethics guidelines. Patient involvement is when patients "meaningfully and actively collaborate in the governance, priority setting, or design and conduct of research" [42]. The term patient is understood broadly to include "those having or a risk of having a medical condition, their families, and their caregivers" [43]. Patients have intimate, lived experience with and understanding of their medical condition, and how symptoms affect their everyday lives. These perspectives can inform the priorities, goals, and conduct of research and the ultimate value new diagnostic tools and therapies can deliver to patients.

The CIOMS/WHO guidelines also reflect the importance of engaging patient communities in the governance of research. Patients have valuable perspectives on both the potential value of research and the acceptability of associated physical and privacy risks. Patients also have perspectives on how consent documentation can meaningfully communicate the nature of research, its benefits and risks, and the safeguards in place to limit risks. Patient involvement in the governance of research can supplement the efforts of RECs to ensure the ethical conduct of research. There is a spectrum of patient involvement approaches, from feedback through surveys or workshops, to advisory boards, to formal leadership roles within research, to patient-led initiatives where patient groups decide when and how to engage experts [44].

Patient involvement can involve important costs and potential delays for research. There is a risk that involvement initiatives successful in specific research and community contexts are extrapolated by policy-makers or oversight bodies into generic ethical requirements [45]. Researchers alone cannot be expected to bear the financial and administrative burden of patient involvement without appropriate support from funding agencies and institutions. Imposing specific forms of involvement as an ethical requirement may also encourage a compliance mentality where researchers want to get it out of the way rather than developing meaningful community and partnership with patients. Systemic barriers and negative perceptions can discourage patients from meaningfully engaging with researchers. Patients are already dealing with the burden of living with a disease and potentially also the burden of participating in research. It may therefore be difficult for them to visit research sites in order to participate in unpaid involvement activities. Patients may also have negative perceptions that they will not actually be listened to [42]. Some critics have highlighted that patient involvement is usually designed to advance an institutional agenda rather than truly give a voice to all patients [45]. Involvement activities do not necessarily mean that patients have significant decision-making power. Researchers may preferentially seek to engage with patients who have considerable experience as research participants, as well as experience with research involvement activities, which may reduce opportunities to hear other voices.

The organizational governance of patient advocacy groups is often informal, which raises concerns about democratic representation and managing conflicts of interest. There can often be major differences of opinion within a patient community. Some patient advocacy groups receive significant financial support from pharmaceutical companies and may not have formal processes in place for declaring and managing these conflicts [46]. Patient involvement challenges may be exacerbated in rare disease contexts. Patient involvement for rare disease may be difficult for the same reasons that doing research on rare disease is difficult. Patients may be small in number, geographically dispersed, and may have very heterogeneous experiences with the disease. This makes it hard to survey patients about their views on research. Many patients with rare disease struggle to even receive an accurate diagnosis, which may affect their ability to identify with and organize a specific community in the first place.

Patients are also increasingly engaged in the governance of biobanking and data sharing. YOURDNAYOURSAY is an interactive, international, online survey exploring public perspectives about the international sharing of genomic and health-related data. The results of the survey address public fears over potential harms, public willingness to release their data, and how trust differs between organizations [47, 48]. A European survey specific to rare disease patients found they were supportive of data sharing to improve research and health care, as long as steps were taken to provide individual patients with meaningful choices, to protect patient privacy, and to provide patients with transparent information about how their data are shared and used [49]. Patients can also be engaged in the design of governance documents for biobanks and databases, such as access policies, privacy safeguards, and consent forms (see previous sections). This involvement can provide assurances that governance strikes an appropriate balance between openness and promotion of science with protection of participant privacy. In many cases, patients may be highly supportive of greater openness in research and their perspectives may serve as a counterweight to overly protective stances by oversight bodies like RECs. Patients may also participate directly on biobank access committees, influencing decisions about which researchers receive samples and data, for which research projects.

Patient involvement in the governance of biobanking and data sharing can raise tensions between community control and scientific openness. In particular, the value of biobanks and data sharing is often dependent on their integration into networks allowing integration of multiple resources to increase statistical power. This is particularly true for rare disease. There is a recognized need for harmonized ethical and legal governance of biobanks and databases to enable such integration. One potential solution is for involvement activities to address the importance of harmonization with patient groups, to make sure this value is taken into account in the co-development of governance [50]. Another potential solution is to develop more concerted public involvement efforts in the development of international standards for biobank and data sharing governance.

6. Conclusion

Rare disease research continues to be hampered by lack of academic and commercial incentives and practical barriers to conducting research involving small, geographically dispersed populations. This results in limited understanding of rare diseases, delayed diagnoses and a lack of therapeutic options for patients. There is hope that international biobank networks and data sharing can improve care and advance research into rare disease. Research ethics concerns about protecting patient privacy, enabling individuals to make informed decisions, and involving patients in governance deserve concerted and nuanced attention in these contexts. Standard governance approaches may need to be re-calibrated for rare disease contexts, given the necessity of openness, high unmet need, and the willingness of many rare disease patients to contribute to biobanks and databases, despite minor privacy risks. This is not to say that rare patients do not care about privacy or about being offered meaningful choices. Involving patients in the governance of biobanks and data sharing, while appropriately highlighting the importance of international collaboration, can help to ensure these activities ultimately improve the prospects of those with rare disease.

Acknowledgements

The author would like to thank Genome Canada, Genome Quebec, and the Canadian Institutes of Health Research for funding support, the hosts of the International Symposium on Rare Diseases held in Santiago, Chile in September 2019, and Kristina Kékesi-Lafrance for helping with the preparation of the chapter.

Author details

Adrian Thorogood
Centre of Genomics and Policy, McGill University, Canada

*Address all correspondence to: Adrian.thorogood@mcgill.ca

References

[1] Mulberg AE, Bucci-Rechtweg C, Giuliano J, Jacoby D, Johnson FK, Liu Q, et al. Regulatory strategies for rare diseases under current global regulatory statutes: A discussion with stakeholders. Orphanet Journal of Rare Diseases. 2019;**14**(1):36

[2] Might M, Wilsey M. The shifting model in clinical diagnostics: How next-generation sequencing and families are altering the way rare diseases are discovered, studied, and treated. Genetics in Medicine. 2014;**16**(10):736-737

[3] Wright CF, FitzPatrick DR, Firth HV. Paediatric genomics: Diagnosing rare disease in children. Nature Reviews Genetics. 2018;**19**(5):253-268

[4] CADTH. Genome-wide sequencing: ethical considerations [Internet]. 12 November 2019. 37 p. Available from: https://www.cadth.ca/sites/default/files/hta-he/he0020-genome-wide-sequencing-ethical-considerations.pdf [cited: 17 December 2019]

[5] National Institutes of Health. DRAFT NIH Policy for data management and sharing [Internet]. November 2019. 4 p. Available from: https://osp.od.nih.gov/wp-content/uploads/Draft_NIH_Policy_Data_Management_and_Sharing.pdf [cited: 17 December 2019]

[6] ACMG Board of Directors. Laboratory and clinical genomic data sharing is crucial to improving genetic health care: A position statement of the American College of Medical Genetics and Genomics. Genetics in Medicine. 2017;**19**(7):721-722

[7] Wright CF, Ware JS, Lucassen AM, Hall A, Middleton A, Rahman N, et al. Genomic variant sharing: A position statement [version 2; peer review: 2 approved]. Wellcome Open Research. 2019;**4**(1):22

[8] Gurovich Y, Hanani Y, Bar O, Nadav G, Fleischer N, Gelbman D, et al. Identifying facial phenotypes of genetic disorders using deep learning. Nature Medicine. 2019;**25**(1):60

[9] Hallowell N, Parker M, Nellåker C. Big data phenotyping in rare diseases: Some ethical issues. Genetics in Medicine. 2019;**21**(2):272-274

[10] Dove ES. Biobanks, data sharing, and the drive for a global privacy governance framework. The Journal of Law, Medicine & Ethics. 2015;**43**(4):675-689

[11] NHS England [Internet]. 100,000 genomes project; [about 2 screens]. Available from: https://www.england.nhs.uk/genomics/100000-genomes-project/ [cited: 10 December 2019]

[12] Department of Health and Social Care [Internet]. DNA mapping to better understand cancer, rare diseases and infectious diseases. 5 July 2013 [about 3 screens]. Available from: https://www.gov.uk/government/news/dna-mapping-to-better-understand-cancer-rare-diseases-and-infectious-diseases [cited: 10 December 2019]

[13] NHS England [Internet]. 100,000 genomes project; [about 2 screens]. Available from: https://www.gov.uk/government/news/dna-mapping-to-better-understand-cancer-rare-diseases-and-infectious-diseases [cited: 10 December 2019]

[14] Genome Canada, Canadian genomics partnership for rare diseases (CGP4-RD): Mission statement. Available from: https://www.genomecanada.ca/en/programs/precision-health-strategy/canadian-genomics-partnership-rare-diseases-cgp4-rd-mission

[15] EJP RD [Internet]. About EJP RD [about 2 screens]. Available from:

http://www.ejprarediseases.org/index.php/about/ [cited: 10 December 2019]

[16] World Economic Forum [Internet]. Breaking barriers to health data project; [about 3 screens]. Available from: https://www.weforum.org/projects/breaking-barriers-to-health-data-project/ [cited: 10 December 2019]

[17] Constine J. RDMD attacks rare diseases with data mined from health records [online]. TechCrunch; 2018. Available from: http://social.techcrunch.com/2018/08/20/rdmd/

[18] Bruckner T. (TranspariMED) [written in close consultation with Cochrane, CRIT and Transparency International's Pharmaceuticals and Healthcare Programme]. Clinical trial transparency: Aa guide for policy makers [Internet]. UK. 2017. p. 40. Available from: https://docs.wixstatic.com/ugd/01f35d_def0082121a648529220e1d56df4b50a.pdf [Transparency International Report] [cited: 17 December 2019]

[19] European Medicines Agency [Internet]. Transparency; [about 9 screens]. Available from: https://www.ema.europa.eu/en/about-us/how-we-work/transparency [cited: 17 December 2019]

[20] Krumholz HM, Waldstreicher J. The Yale open data access (YODA) project—A mechanism for data sharing. New England Journal of Medicine. 2016;**375**(5):403-405

[21] ClinicalStudyDataRequest [Internet]. Our mission; [about 1 screen]. Available from: https://clinicalstudydatarequest.com/Default.aspx [cited: 17 December 2019]

[22] Vivli: Center for Global Clinical Research Data [Internet]. About Vivli: Overview; [about 2 screens]. Available from: http://vivli.org/about/overview/ [cited: 17 December 2019]

[23] Menon D, Clark D, Stafinski T. Reimbursement of drugs for rare diseases through the public healthcare system in Canada: Where are we now? Healthc Policy. 2015;**11**(1):15-32

[24] Perfetto EM, Oehrlein EM, Boutin M, Reid S, Gascho E. Value to whom? The patient voice in the value discussion. Value in Health. 2017;**20**(2):286-291

[25] Gymrek M, McGuire AL, Golan D, Halperin E, Erlich Y. Identifying personal genomes by surname inference. Science. 2013;**339**(6117):321-324

[26] Rocher L, Hendrickx JM, De Montjoye YA. Estimating the success of re-identifications in incomplete datasets using generative models. Nature Communications. 2019;**10**(1):1-9

[27] Rothstein MA, Zawati MN, Knoppers BM. Regulatory landscape of international irect-to-participant (DTP) genomic research: Time to untie the Gordian knot? The Journal of Law, Medicine & Ethics. 2019;**47**(2):1-14

[28] Global Alliance for Genomics and Health (GA4GH) in their Consent Policy. 2019. Available from: https://www.ga4gh.org/work_stream/regulatory-ethics/

[29] Council of Canadian Academies. Accessing health and health-related data in Canada [Internet]. 2015. 260 p. Available from: https://cca-reports.ca/wp-content/uploads/2018/10/healthdatafullreporten.pdf [cited: 17 December 2019]

[30] General Data Protection Regulation (GDPR), Regulation (EU) 2016/679 [Internet]. 2016. Available from: https://eur-lex.europa.eu/legal-content/EN/TXT/PDF/?uri=CELEX:32016R0679 [cited: 17 December 2019]; California Consumer Privacy Act of 2018, A.B. 375 [cited: 28 June 2018]

[31] Rabesandratana T. Researchers sound alarm on European data law. Science. 2019;**366**(6468):936

[32] Nguyen MT, Goldblatt J, Isasi R, Jagut M, Jonker AH, Kaufmann P, et al. Model consent clauses for rare disease research. BMC Medical Ethics. 2019;**20**(1):55

[33] Contreras JL, Knoppers BM. The genomic commons. Annual Review of Genomics and Human Genetics. 2018;**19**:429-453

[34] Global Alliance for Genomics and Health. Consent policy [Internet]. 2019. 6 p. Available from: https://www.ga4gh.org/wp-content/uploads/GA4GH-Final-Revised-Consent-Policy_16Sept2019.pdf [cited: 17 December 2019]

[35] Canadian Institutes of Health Research, Natural Sciences and Engineering Research Council of Canada, Social Sciences and Humanities Research Council. Tri-council policy statement: Ethical conduct for research involving humans—TCPS 2018 [Internet]. 2018. 211 p. Available from: https://ethics.gc.ca/eng/documents/tcps2-2018-en-interactive-final.pdf [cited: 17 December 2019]

[36] Gainotti S, Turner C, Woods S, Kole A, McCormack P, Lochmüller H, et al. Improving the informed consent process in international collaborative rare disease research: Effective consent for effective research. European Journal of Human Genetics. 2016;**24**(9):1248-1254

[37] Revised common rule, Electronic Code of Federal Regulations, 45 CFR 46 [Internet]. 2018. Available from: https://www.ecfr.gov/cgi-bin/retrieveECFR?gp=&SID=83cd09e1c0f5c6937cd9d7513160fc3f&pitd=20180719&n=pt45.1.46&r=PART&ty=HTML [cited: 17 December 2019]

[38] Dalpé G, Thorogood A, Knoppers BM. A tale of two capacities: Including children and decisionally vulnerable adults in biomedical research. Frontiers in Genetics [Internet]. 2019;**10**:289. Available from: https://www.frontiersin.org/articles/10.3389/fgene.2019.00289/full [cited: 2 May 2019]

[39] Rahimzadeh V, Schickhardt C, Knoppers BM, Sénécal K, Vears DF, Fernandez CV, et al. Key implications of data sharing in pediatric genomics. JAMA Pediatrics. 2018;**172**(5):476-481

[40] Weijer C, Goldsand G, Emanuel EJ. Protecting communities in research: Current guidelines and limits of extrapolation. Nature Genetics. 1999;**23**(3):27-80

[41] Council for International Organizations of Medical Sciences (CIOMS) [in collaboration with the World Health Organization (WHO)]. International ethical guidelines for health-related research involving humans [Internet]. 2016. 119 p. Available from: https://cioms.ch/wp-content/uploads/2017/01/WEB-CIOMS-EthicalGuidelines.pdf [cited: 17 December 2019]

[42] CIHR. Draft CIHR ethics guidance for developing research partnerships with patients [Internet]. 2019. 42 p. Available from: https://ktcanada.org/wp-content/uploads/2019/04/ethics_guidance_developing_research-en.pdf [cited: 17 December 2019]

[43] Hoos A, Anderson J, Boutin M, Dewulf L, Geissler J, Johnston G, et al. Partnering with patients in the development and lifecycle of medicines: A call for action. Therapeutic Innovation & Regulatory Science. 2015;**49**(6):929-939

[44] Deverka PA, Gilmore D, Richmond J, Smith Z, Mangrum R, Koenig BA, et al. Hopeful and concerned: Public input on building a trustworthy medical information

commons. The Journal of Law, Medicine & Ethics. 2019;**47**(1):70-87

[45] Johannesen J. The trouble with Patient and Public Involvement (PPI) [Internet]. Session presented at: 2018 Cochrane Colloquium. Edinburg, UK; 2018. Available from: https://johannesen.ca/2018/09/the-trouble-with-patient-and-public-involvement-ppi-keynote-at-cochrane-colloquium-2018/ [cited: 10 December 2019]

[46] von Tigerstrom B. The patient's voice: Patient involvement in medical product regulation. Medical Law International. 2016;**16**(1-2):27-57

[47] Milne R, Morley KI, Howard H, Niemiec E, Nicol D, Critchley C, et al. Trust in genomic data sharing among members of the general public in the UK, USA, Canada and Australia. Human Genetics. 2019;**138**:1237-1246

[48] Middleton A, Milne R, Thorogood A, Kleiderman E, Niemiec E, Prainsack B, et al. Attitudes of publics who are unwilling to donate DNA data for research. European Journal of Medical Genetics. 2019;**62**(5):316-323

[49] Courbier S, Dimond R, Bros-Facer V. Share and protect our health data: An evidence based approach to rare disease patients' perspectives on data sharing and data protection-quantitative survey and recommendations. Orphanet Journal of Rare Diseases. 2019;**14**(1):175

[50] Thorogood A. Towards Legal Interoperability in International Health Research. University of Toronto (School of Graduate Studies—Theses). 2019. 203 p. Available from: http://hdl.handle.net/1807/98411 [cited: 17 December 2019]